Medicine Transformed

Medicine Transformed

HEALTH, DISEASE AND SOCIETY IN EUROPE

1800–1930

———— Edited by Deborah Brunton ————

Manchester University Press

Manchester and New York

distributed exclusively in the USA by Palgrave

Published in association with

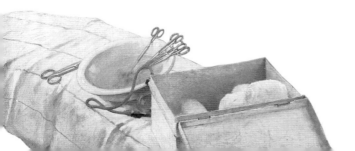

This publication forms part of an Open University course: A218 *Medicine and Society in Europe, 1500–1930*. The complete list of texts that make up this course can be found in the Preface. Details of this and other Open University courses can be obtained from the Course Information and Advice Centre, PO Box 724, The Open University, Milton Keynes MK7 6ZS, United Kingdom: tel. +44 (0)1908 653231; e-mail general-enquiries@open.ac.uk

Alternatively, you may visit the Open University website at http://www.open.ac.uk where you can learn more about the wide range of courses and packs offered at all levels by The Open University.

To purchase a selection of Open University course materials, visit the webshop at www.ouw.co.uk, or contact Open University Worldwide, Michael Young Building, Walton Hall, Milton Keynes MK7 6AA, United Kingdom for a brochure: tel. +44 (0)1908 858785; fax +44 (0)1908 858787; email ouwenq@open.ac.uk

Published by Manchester University Press; written and produced by The Open University

Manchester University Press
Oxford Road, Manchester
M13 9NR
www.manchesteruniversitypress.co.uk

The Open University
Walton Hall, Milton Keynes
MK7 6AA

Distributed exclusively in the USA by Palgrave, 175 Fifth Avenue, New York, NY 10010, USA

Distributed exclusively in Canada by UBC Press, University of British Columbia, 2029 West Mall, Vancouver, BC, Canada V6T 1Z2

First published 2004. Reprinted 2004

Edited, designed and typeset by The Open University

Printed and bound in the United Kingdom by The Bath Press, Bath

Colour plates printed in the United Kingdom by Nicholson & Bass Ltd

British Library Cataloguing in Publication Data: data available

Library of Congress Cataloging in Publication Data: data available

ISBN 0 7190 6735 9 paperback

1.3

Contents

Preface

This is the second of two books of specially commissioned essays that form the main teaching texts of a Level 2 Open University course: A218 *Medicine and Society in Europe, 1500–1930*. The course aims to demonstrate how social, political and cultural contexts shaped medical thought and practice between 1500 and 1930. This way of approaching the history of medicine differs from traditional accounts, which in the main have focused on the achievements of individuals. In both books, the contributors engage with this approach, and guide readers through some debates provoked by it. The books are intended to appeal to as wide an audience as possible, including students of history and of medicine, as well as the interested general reader.

A feature of the main teaching texts is the inclusion of exercises designed to allow readers to explore a selection of primary and secondary source materials, which are published in companion volumes. For convenience, these companion volumes are referred to in the text as 'Source Book 1' and 'Source Book 2'. For readers who do not have access to the companion volumes, a full bibliographic list of the extracts reproduced in them is supplied at the end of each chapter.

The four books that make up the series are:

The Healing Arts: Health, Disease and Society in Europe, 1500–1800, edited by Peter Elmer (Book 1)

Health, Disease and Society in Europe, 1500–1800: A Source Book, edited by Peter Elmer and Ole Peter Grell (Source Book 1)

Medicine Transformed: Health, Disease and Society in Europe, 1800–1930, edited by Deborah Brunton (Book 2)

Health, Disease and Society in Europe, 1800–1930: A Source Book, edited by Deborah Brunton (Source Book 2)

Readers are not expected to have undertaken any previous historical or medical study; all concepts are explained in the text and a glossary at the end of the book provides a guide to terminology. Entries in the glossary are emboldened in the text, usually at their first occurrence.

Many people have been involved in the production of this book. I would like to thank my colleagues at The Open University: Silvia De Renzi, Peter Elmer, Ole Peter Grell and James Moore for their help and support. Special thanks are due to the huge team of consultant authors – Jonathan Andrews, Roger Cooter, Stephen Jacyna, Hilary Marland, Maxine Rhodes, Thomas Schlich, Paul Weindling and Michael Worboys – for their enthusiasm for the project, prompt responses to queries, and their patience and good humour during the Open University's rigorous editorial processes. This book would never have appeared without help behind the scenes from Robert Doubleday and Adrian Roberts (course managers), Jane Lea and Audrey Linkman (visual resources), Liliana Torero de Clements, Janet Fennell and Kerry Lawrence (course unit assistants), Ray Munns (cartographer), Pam Higgins (graphic designer) and Charles Harris (compositor). Above all, I would like to thank the editors, Hazel Coleman, Christine Considine and Rachel Crease, for their tireless editing under huge pressure and unfailing kindness to authors and myself. Their contribution is evident on every page of this book.

Deborah Brunton

Contributors

Jonathan Andrews is Senior Lecturer in the History of Medicine at Oxford Brookes University

Deborah Brunton is Lecturer in the History of Medicine at The Open University

Roger Cooter is Professorial Fellow at the Wellcome Trust Centre for the History of Medicine at University College London

L.S. Jacyna is Senior Lecturer at the Wellcome Trust Centre for the History of Medicine at University College London

Hilary Marland is Reader in the Department of History at the University of Warwick

James Moore is Reader in the Department of the History of Science, Technology and Medicine at The Open University

Maxine Rhodes is an Associate Lecturer with The Open University and Community Liaison Manager in the Centre of Community and Lifelong Learning at the University of Wales, Newport

Thomas Schlich holds the Canada Research Chair in the History of Medicine at the Department of Social Studies of Medicine, McGill University, Montreal

Paul Weindling is Professor of the History of Medicine at Oxford Brookes University

Michael Worboys is Professor at the Centre for the History of Science, Technology and Medicine at the University of Manchester

Acknowledgements

Grateful acknowledgement is made to the following sources for permission to reproduce material in this book:

Tables

Table 2.2: Marland, H. (1987) *Medicine and Society in Wakefield and Huddersfield 1780–1870*, Cambridge University Press;

Table 7.1: La Berge, A.E.F. (1992) Table 1: 'Correlation of wealth and mortality rates in 12 districts of Paris', in *Mission and Method*, Cambridge University Press;

Table 12.1: Garrison, F.H. (1970) *Notes on the History of Military Medicine*, George Olms Verlag AG.

Every effort has been made to trace all the copyright owners, but if any have been inadvertently overlooked, the publishers will be pleased to make the necessary arrangements at the first opportunity.

Introduction

Deborah Brunton

The nineteenth and early twentieth centuries saw a radical and comprehensive transformation in medicine. Until the nineteenth century, medical ideas and practices had remained fundamentally the same for hundreds of years. In 1800, the first signs of change were just becoming apparent. Practitioners began to abandon the idea that ill health originated in an imbalance of fluids or energies – the so-called 'humoral theory', which had dominated western medicine since classical times – and to think of disease as a localized phenomenon, based on organic changes in the solid organs and tissues of the body. Hospitals and other health-care institutions, which had been on the margins of medical care, offering shelter to the poorest, began to expand in numbers and size. In particular, the hospital began to acquire its modern, multifaceted role as a place of research and teaching as well as care. The old order of practitioners, with its division into physicians, surgeons and apothecaries, was also beginning to break down; however, practitioners who had received a formal medical education remained poorly distinguished from a host of 'irregular' practitioners (see my note on terminology below), who competed with them for business. By 1800, a new type of medical man – the general practitioner – had appeared. Trained in both surgery and medicine, he quickly became the dominant provider of medical services.

In other respects, medicine in 1800 had changed little since 1700 or even 1600. The way in which disease was understood was beginning to change, but these new ideas did not immediately result in a new system of therapeutics. Practitioners continued to use traditional remedies to cure their patients' disorders, prescribing drugs to promote the body's evacuation of noxious material and specifying an appropriate diet and nursing care, to support the body's own healing resources. Although institutional care was expanding, it remained the exception, not the rule. Most illnesses were still dealt with within a domestic setting, and the vast majority of the population paid directly for the services of nurses and practitioners. The state played a minor role in medicine. Governments took short-term action to deal with serious epidemics and in some countries they provided medical care for the very poorest classes.

By 1930, a recognizably modern medicine had emerged. Medicine was now thought of as 'scientific'. Knowledge of disease no longer relied on subjective judgements made by practitioners' unaided senses and clinical skills. Instead, the study of the body's processes was the subject of laboratory research, whereby physiological phenomena were explored through experiment and objectively measured. Practitioners now understood disease in terms of processes that occurred at the cellular level: infectious diseases resulted from the action of microscopic pathogens, while other complaints resulted from malfunctions within the complex physiological processes of the body. This new understanding of disease paved the way for new and improved therapeutic strategies. Surgery acquired enormous prestige, as new techniques allowed the repair of injuries that had previously been fatal and the cure of hitherto untreatable conditions. Practitioners had at their disposal more potent forms of old drugs, such as aspirin and morphine, and a handful of brand-new chemical drugs, such as Salvarsan, used to treat syphilis. Physiological research made possible the treatment of deficiency diseases, and metabolic disorders such as diabetes, with vitamins and hormones. Infectious diseases could be treated or prevented using sera and vaccines. One of the most significant developments in medicine since 1800 was the rise of preventive medicine. At the beginning of the nineteenth century, sporadic action was taken against only a handful of diseases. By 1930, populations were subjected to constant surveillance to monitor disease patterns, and were the targets for educational programmes, sanitary reform, isolation and immunization, all of which had combined to markedly reduce deaths from a number of infectious diseases, including smallpox and cholera. Although infectious diseases would continue to claim large numbers of victims (in 1918–19, an influenza epidemic swept the globe, killing millions), nevertheless, medicine had begun to affect epidemiological patterns. ('Epidemiology' is the science of epidemics.)

By 1930, much of the institutional structure of modern medicine was in place. The medical profession had acquired a recognizably modern form: unified, self-regulating, it held high authority and power in society, not only dictating how the sick should be treated but also prescribing 'healthy' diets, behaviours and lifestyles for everyone. Practitioners who lacked a recognized training or qualification were marginalized as purveyors of 'irregular' or 'unorthodox' medicine. Institutions had become centres for the treatment of the acutely ill. Hospitals continued to expand in number and acquired their modern place at the centre of medical care, offering high-tech, high-quality care to the whole population. The asylum was accepted as the best place to treat mental illness and clinics offered a wide range of services to outpatients. Much of this dramatic growth in institutions was due to states taking on an increased responsibility for health. By 1930, governments had become significant providers of care to a wide section of society through state-funded hospitals, clinics and welfare centres. From the turn of the century, inspired by fears of national and racial degeneration, governments sponsored campaigns designed to educate the population about the benefits of maintaining a healthy lifestyle and avoiding infection. Despite medicine's undoubted increased ability to cure and to prevent disease, people continued to worry about their health – then, as now, they were 'getting better and feeling worse'.

While historians have always seen the nineteenth and early twentieth centuries as a period of profound change, their understanding of the history of that period has itself changed radically over time, reflecting developments within the discipline. Early historians of medicine focused on intellectual developments: they looked back into the historical record to find the origins of modern medical theories, therapies and institutions. Many focused their research on the rise of scientific medicine. Not surprisingly, at a time when medicine seemed to offer ever more effective treatment, these historians chose to portray medicine as a story of progress and sought to describe change, not to explain why medicine changed. Thus medicine appeared to develop under its own momentum: new ideas about the body and disease were portrayed as having driven improvements in therapeutics and the expansion of institutional medicine, unaffected by the wider social, intellectual, political and cultural contexts. For example, the history of surgery consisted of lists of 'first' operations made possible by two 'great leaps forward' – anaesthesia and antisepsis.

However, since the 1980s, the history of medicine has been dominated by another approach – that of the social history of medicine. Researchers now see medicine as a social phenomenon, whose ideas and practices do not develop through their own inexorable logic, but are shaped by wider forces. Thus, for example, understandings of the body and of disease were influenced by a wider intellectual context and the institutions in which knowledge was generated and disseminated. Social historians of medicine have also shown how medicine affects society: how it can serve as a resource for claims of authority and expertise. Reflecting a wider trend to study 'history from below', they have sought to understand medicine from the viewpoint of contemporary patients and practitioners. Rather than ridiculing past therapies as useless and positively dangerous, they have pointed to the need to understand the ideas and beliefs underpinning practice, and to recognize in them a rational response to ill health.

The emphasis on the social aspects of medicine has inspired research into previously unexplored topics. Historians have studied the role of women in medicine – as practitioners, nurses, healers and patients. A reassessment of Europe's colonial past has prompted new studies of medicine in the colonial enterprise. Other fruitful areas for research include medicine in war, the understanding and treatment of mental illness, health education and welfare programmes, and the medical care offered to children and the elderly. This approach has also prompted a critical re-evaluation of earlier work. For example, new studies suggested that the rise of the laboratory in mid-nineteenth-century Germany owed much to wider changes in German culture, in particular to an enthusiasm for *Wissenschaft* – the pursuit of knowledge for its own sake – rather than, as previously thought, to the discovery of new cures.

Medicine Transformed aims to provide an introduction to the major developments in medicine in Europe between 1800 and 1930. Change did not, of course, end in 1930, but given the need to limit the length of this book, we have chosen not to tackle the complex impact of the Second World War or the arrival of the National Health Service. This volume does not attempt to give a comprehensive description of the changing face of medicine. Instead, the thirteen essays explore a selection of topics that have been the focus of research since the 1980s. Most of the chapters examine a particular set of developments within a particular aspect of medicine, but two chapters explore medicine in specific contexts – in European colonies and in wartime. All the essays are written by scholars active in the field. Reflecting current historiography, they aim not only to describe important developments, but also to explore why and how change was accomplished, and to set medicine in its social and political contexts. Most of the essays aim simply to introduce readers to a selection of historical studies within their specific topic, examining how our understanding has changed over time. However, Chapters 11 and 12 take an explicitly historiographical approach, and these discussions of asylums and of military medicine are structured around the changing accounts of these topics. All the chapters stand as separate essays, and maintain the distinctive voice of each author. Brief cross-references within the text and marginal notes help to knit the material together. Each chapter is accompanied by a selection of images. These are not intended simply to make the pages more interesting. Rather, they are used as historical sources, and each image has a caption which explores the meanings (intended and unintended) conveyed by it. Colour plates 5 to 14 are designed to function as a 'visual essay', exploring the power of the medical profession. These portraits of practitioners reflect the social status enjoyed by medical men and women, and reveal the many ways in which medical practitioners acquired power: through the possession of specialist knowledge and skills (which granted them power over patients and respect from their peers), and through service to the community, state and nation.

Rather than being organized chronologically, the essays are grouped according to their common themes. Chapters 1 to 4 deal with some of the most important innovations in medical ideas and institutions. They show that the adoption of new ideas is a complex process, which affects medical practice, the function of institutions, the status of different groups of practitioners, and the relationships between patients and practitioners. Chapter 1 uses the sociologist Nicholas Jewson's classic paper 'The disappearance of the sick-man' as a springboard to explore the major developments within medical thinking in the nineteenth century. Stephen Jacyna introduces a historiographical dimension to the discussion by examining how Jewson's conclusions have been modified by the work of other historians. Chapter 2 explores the rise of hospitals to their central place in modern medicine. Hilary Marland shows how the roots of the modern hospital lie in the eighteenth century, and how changes in the size, organization and architecture of the institution are related to its medical and social functions. A crucial part of hospital development was the increasing use of surgery to treat disease as well as to repair injuries to the body. In Chapter 3, Thomas Schlich shows us that to understand the history of surgery we need to look beyond technical developments, and to appreciate how professional, theoretical and technical changes are interlinked. Similarly, in Chapter 4, I examine the rise of laboratory medicine by going beyond the lists of fundamental discoveries made in nineteenth-century laboratories. Instead, I look at the varied functions of labs, and contrast the rapid acceptance of biomedical ideas with the more hesitant adoption of new diagnostic techniques and the very slow fulfilment of the promise of new cures.

Chapters 5 and 6 explore developments within the medical profession in the nineteenth century. Both chapters analyse the processes of professionalization, setting them in their social context, and examine how professional boundaries are established so as to include and exclude certain groups of practitioners. In Chapter 5, I look in detail at the ways in which the occupation of medicine changed during the nineteenth century. I then discuss whether we should interpret these changes as a coherent process of professionalization, consciously driven by practitioners with the aim of acquiring a new status, or as a series of undirected and sometimes unrelated reforms which owed much to economic considerations. In Chapter 6, Maxine Rhodes examines the effect of professionalization on women practitioners and nurses. Rhodes explores how a social context that emphasized the particular caring qualities of women meant that many male practitioners were reluctant to readmit women to the medical profession and helped to shape the nursing profession.

Chapters 7 to 10 explore the developing role of the state in preventive medicine. They discuss the strategies used against a range of diseases, from mid-nineteenth-century sanitary reform to twentieth-century social medicine, and show how political considerations shaped public health policies. The chapters fall into two pairs. In Chapter 7, I look at nineteenth-century public health measures, and challenge the assumption that reform in this area was a great triumph for medicine. Rather, the understanding of disease patterns and public health practices were rooted in political, as well as medical, concerns. I also analyse the historiographical debates on the effect of sanitary reforms. In Chapter 8, Michael Worboys looks at how these public health strategies were used in European colonies, and discusses the development of tropical medicine, with its distinctive body of practices. By comparing health policies in a number of colonies, Worboys shows how colonial medicine was not simply informed by a desire to spread medical enlightenment to 'dark' continents, but was used as a political tool to advance trade and to control unrest among indigenous peoples. Chapters 9 and 10 examine twentieth-century health policies aimed at halting a perceived 'degeneration' in the health of populations. In Chapter 9, which follows on from the developments described in Chapter 7, Paul Weindling explores the impact of the germ theory on public health practice and the rise of social medicine – schemes to improve the overall health of the population through improved diet, birth control, and the prevention and treatment of specific diseases. Weindling shows how these new policies overlapped with older public health programmes, making it difficult to assess their effect on health and disease. In Chapter 10, James Moore explores one particular aspect of social medicine – eugenics – which sought to control ill health by welfare programmes to ensure the health of babies and children, and by preventing the birth of unhealthy infants. Moore reveals the role of wider political and cultural norms in the adoption of these policies through a detailed analysis of eugenic medicine in different European countries.

Chapters 11 and 12 take a distinctively historiographical approach to the discussion of the rise of the asylum and of war medicine. Rather than chronologically tracing developments within these fields, the chapters review how historians have explored these problems. As this approach poses greater challenges to the student, we have placed these chapters near the end of the book. In Chapter 11, Jonathan Andrews focuses on one central problem: why did the asylum become accepted as the best place for the treatment of the mentally ill in the nineteenth century? He discusses a number of the explanations put forward by historians, both social and medical. This chapter gives a flavour of the historical process, showing how ideas put forward by historians are challenged and modified by later researchers, often as a result of using different sources. In Chapter 12, on the relationship between war and medicine, Roger Cooter examines how historians have moved from the view that war fostered the development of medicine to the idea that, although war provides a climate favourable to the development of military medicine, it has a limited effect on civilian medicine. He ends the chapter by questioning whether historians should draw a clear distinction between military medicine and civilian medicine.

Chapter 13 provides a conclusion to the whole book by surveying the availability of medical services in the early twentieth century – from health promotion to domestic and institutional care. In this chapter, I challenge the assumption that greater provision of medical services through the state meant better care for all, arguing that fundamental inequalities remained: the poorer classes had more limited access to care and received care of a poorer quality than their wealthy counterparts. I also explore the issue of 'medicalization' – that is, the expansion of the power of practitioners to dictate not only the behaviour of the sick, but also that of healthy people. I conclude that, although practitioners did exert considerable power and influence, even in the 1930s patients continued to control their own treatment through self-diagnosis and therapy, and by selecting where and when to apply for help from medical professionals.

What picture of medicine emerges from these essays? Certainly, it is clear that the history of medicine in the nineteenth and early twentieth centuries is not a simple story of progress; of new theories and knowledge leading to more effective and ever more widely available therapies. If one conclusion stands out it is the extraordinarily complex links between ideas, practices, institutions, disease, society, culture, politics and the medical profession. New medical theories were adopted because they were supported by influential medical practitioners; practitioners acquired power as a result of holding institutional posts; institutions fulfilled social as well as medical roles; public health policies were adopted and new institutions built because they fitted with wider political objectives.

In addition, a number of important themes recur throughout the book. The authors show that the relationship between medical theory and medical practice is highly complex. It has often been assumed – by practitioners and historians – that better understandings of the body and of disease led to more effective therapy. A number of case studies presented in this book show that this was not an inevitable step. 'Hospital medicine' inspired no novel therapeutic strategies. New drugs and therapies emerged from laboratory-based research only very slowly. The adoption of new ideas and practices was also complex, their success depending in part on the status of the innovator and whether influential practitioners believed that new ideas would add to or detract from their established status and authority.

The material also demonstrates that institutions were shaped by their multiple functions. Hospitals, clinics and asylums fulfilled the (sometimes conflicting) demands of patient care, teaching and research. They were also crucial to professional advancement, supplying a ladder of more and more senior and prestigious posts by which an individual practitioner could rise in his or her profession. But, as in the case of the nineteenth-century asylum, institutions also provided a means by which groups of practitioners could garner credibility and prestige for their particular areas of medical practice. These institutions had functions outside the medical sphere. Charitable institutions fulfilled important social objectives: they were a vehicle to heal divisions between social classes and political cliques. For governments of all political colours – from enlightenment Sweden to Fascist Italy – funding for hospitals and clinics demonstrated the benevolent concern of states and monarchs for their peoples and helped to secure a healthy and productive workforce and army.

This brings us to another major theme: the idea that medicine was deeply influenced by politics. This is perhaps most obvious in the field of preventive medicine, which was mainly funded by governments. The public health strategies of states were guided by wider political objectives and economics – to quell social unrest and, in the colonies, to promote trade. Medicine was also a means to express national pride, through the funding of new research institutes for distinguished researchers.

The final theme is the growing power of the medical profession. At the level of the individual encounter between patient and practitioner, practitioners gradually acquired more and more power, mediated by specialist knowledge, an esoteric language with which to describe disease and technologies with which to interrogate the patient's body. However, not all patients were equally powerless: while poor patients in hospitals had little say over their treatment, wealthy patients used their financial clout to maintain some control. The profession also collectively gained power and authority as experts on all sorts of medical issues. By the twentieth century, practitioners had considerable influence on government health policies and the work of institutions.

A picture of European medicine also emerges from the pages of *Medicine Transformed* – one in which the broad continuities in the development of medicine are more striking than the differences. In some ways, this seems counter-intuitive. Social conditions varied hugely across Europe: from countries experiencing rapid industrialization and urbanization, such as Britain, to rural Sweden. Patterns of disease were markedly different across the Continent. More importantly, the rise of individual nation-states, and the emergence of government as a provider of medical services, would seem to militate against common medical developments. Often, governments responded in quite different ways to the same problem. For example, when faced with epidemic cholera, they adopted strategies that placed varying emphasis on quarantine, isolation and sanitary improvement. And yet, despite this divergence, in the medical sphere nineteenth-century Europe was a continent held together by similarities, rather than riven by difference. Medical practitioners across Europe shared the same ideas about the body and disease, and used the same medical treatments. Students travelled across Europe to pick up new skills and new knowledge from hotbeds of research. The rise of medical publishing facilitated the exchange of information across national boundaries. From the 1880s, practitioners and health administrators met in international congresses to discuss ideas and policies and to examine health-care strategies adopted in other countries. It is easy to see how, from the late nineteenth century, such exchanges could have resulted in common public health strategies being adopted across the Continent: around the beginning of the twentieth century, welfare programmes were copied and adapted by different European governments. However, it is more difficult to see what exchanges informed the earlier, parallel developments in medical institutions and of the medical profession from Britain to Russia and France to Norway.

Finally, a word on terminology. As the occupation of medicine changed in the nineteenth century, the titles used to describe those people who practised medicine also changed. Practitioners themselves used these terms rather loosely. In the late nineteenth century, a British practitioner graduating from medical school with a degree might describe himself as a physician, a surgeon, a general practitioner or a medical practitioner. (Although many held the title of doctor, practitioners rarely described themselves as 'a doctor' in official records until the twentieth century.) Our strategy is to adopt a consistent form of terminology, based on contemporary usage. 'Practitioner' is used as a general term to describe physicians, surgeons, consultants and GPs, all of whom had received a formal medical education. We use 'medical men' as a convenient synonym for practitioners until the 1870s, since there were almost no women practitioners at this time. We use the term 'elite' to describe the well-educated, well-connected and well-paid practitioners who formed the *crème de la crème* of the profession in the nineteenth century. The term 'consultant' refers to specialist consulting practitioners, who performed little or no general practice – a group that appeared in substantial numbers only in the twentieth century. Practitioners without a formal medical education, who offered orthodox forms of therapy, are called 'irregular' practitioners or 'healers'. Those who practised unorthodox forms of medicine, such as herbalism or homeopathy, are referred to as 'unorthodox practitioners' even if they had been trained in orthodox medicine.

1

The Localization of Disease

L.S. Jacyna

Objectives

When you have completed this chapter you should be able to:

- distinguish the major stages in the development of modern medicine;

- understand how the locus of medical knowledge and research has since 1800 shifted to different sites;

- appreciate how such changes have impinged on the social relations of medical practice.

1.1   Introduction

The nineteenth century witnessed fundamental changes in western medicine. These were evident in medical theory: the ways in which the workings of the body in health and disease were understood. They were also apparent in medical technology: the techniques and instruments that doctors used to investigate the bodies of their patients. The spaces in which medical knowledge was developed and applied also underwent transformation. These reorientations had a major impact on the social relations of medicine, and in particular on the patient–doctor relationship. The final product of these trends was the creation of modern medicine as we recognize it today.

The changes that occurred were complex and interrelated. They proceeded at various rates in different parts of the western world, and the effect of local circumstances makes generalization difficult. Nonetheless, certain common patterns can be discerned. A framework to address these issues was provided during the 1970s by the sociologist N.D. Jewson. He described a shift from 'bedside medicine' to 'hospital medicine' and then to 'laboratory medicine' and charted changes not only in the locations in which medical knowledge was generated but also in how medicine was practised, and in the power relations between patients and practitioners. This chapter uses Jewson's thesis as a springboard to explore the major developments in medicine in the course of the nineteenth century. It also explores a number of case studies in which historians have sought to apply the general notions advanced by Jewson to particular institutions, individuals and locations, to see if the bold generalizations contained in Jewson's model stand up to close historical scrutiny. Do his essential elements remain intact? Do we need to qualify some of his claims?

1.2   The disappearance of the sick man

You will read some of Waddington's work as part of Chapter 5.

Nicholas Jewson worked in the sociology department of the University of Leicester. His colleagues there included Ivan Waddington, who himself made a notable contribution to the emerging field of the social history of medicine. Whereas Waddington's work is characterized by fine-grained empirical studies, Jewson, in two influential articles published during the 1970s, attempted to provide an over-arching view of the essential features of the history of modern western medicine.

Jewson is especially concerned with what he calls 'the disappearance of the sick-man' from **medical cosmology** in the period 1770–1870 (by 'medical cosmology' Jewson means knowledge, practice, practitioners and patients). He first discussed these issues in a 1974 paper entitled 'Medical knowledge and the patronage system in eighteenth-century England' (Jewson, 1974), in which he tried to show how the form of the medical systems during this period was influenced by the power exercised by the patient (this is described below as 'bedside medicine'). He later broadened the scope of his analysis. In his 1976 article 'The disappearance of the sick-man from medical cosmology, 1770–1870' (Jewson, 1976) he tried to show how the social relations that had underpinned eighteenth-century medicine were supplanted by novel arrangements, which also had consequences for the prevalent forms of medical knowledge. (Jewson always refers to the 'sick-man'; however, he means all patients, male and female.)

Jewson maintains that at the beginning of this period a system known as 'bedside medicine' prevailed in the western world. Diseases were thought to result from imbalances in the body's fluids or energies, and health reflected a state of balance. Therapeutic practices, such as bloodletting and the use of medicines to stimulate or evacuate fluids from the body, restored the disrupted equilibrium. Under this cosmology, the patient was conceived as a 'conscious human totality'. In other words, no sharp dichotomies were set between mind and body. The sick man, or sick woman, was, moreover, not seen as an isolated individual; his or her social circumstances and life history were deemed relevant to the diagnosis and treatment of the current complaint.

Within the system of bedside medicine – which Jewson sees as characteristic of the eighteenth-century medical world – the patient exercised a significant amount of autonomy and power. This was based, ultimately, on economic considerations. The doctor relied on the patient's fees for his livelihood; conversely, the paying patient could choose a practitioner who met his or her needs and tastes. But the degree to which patients and practitioners had a shared knowledge of medicine (Jewson calls this 'epistemological parity') also had important implications for the clinical encounter. The educated lay person was sufficiently well versed in medical theory to be able to converse almost as an equal with the practitioner on the nature of his or her condition. The sick man's account of his illness (or 'narrative', as it is often called) was at the centre of the encounter between patient and practitioner, and formed the basis of diagnosis.

Around 1800 a significant shift occurred. A new medical cosmology – 'hospital medicine' – began to displace the older regime. This shift was first evident in post-revolutionary France, but its effects were eventually felt throughout the western world. As the name suggests, hospital medicine was characterized by a change in the space in which medical knowledge was elaborated and applied. While the typical setting for bedside medicine was domestic, a location in which the patient exercised most power, under the new regime the hospital came to assume a dominant position. The hospital was, in the words of Erwin Ackerknecht, the doctor's 'bailiwick' (Ackerknecht, 1967).

The balance of power between patient and doctor was further altered by economic and epistemological considerations. First, the patient was no longer the doctor's 'patron'. Hospital patients all came from the poorest classes and were treated free of charge. The practitioner looked for recognition and remuneration not to those he treated but to his professional peers. Second, the understanding of disease that emerged under hospital medicine was increasingly couched in terms and concepts that were alien to lay understandings of health and disease. A marker of this change in medical theory, for example, was the increasingly esoteric language in which medical men expressed themselves, using technical terms unfamiliar to most patients.

Under bedside medicine, the conceptualization of illness tended to be holistic, seeking to place the patient's condition in the wider context of his or her lifestyle and biography. Hospital medicine, on the other hand, was oriented towards abstracting the most salient features of the illness and correlating these with the pathological changes taking place within the organs of the body. Its impulse was, in other words, towards the localization of disease – from the whole body (Jewson's 'sick-man') to a diseased organ or tissue.

The realization of this programme depended on three principal techniques. In the first place, the patient was subjected to rigorous physical examination. The clinician's unaided senses were increasingly supplemented in these enquiries by a variety of instrumental aids, of which the stethoscope was perhaps the most significant. Second, should the illness prove fatal, the patient's body was as a matter of routine subjected to **autopsy**. The main aim of these post-mortem examinations was to correlate symptoms evident during life with morbid alterations, or 'lesions', evident in the body after death. These dual procedures are referred to as the **clinico-pathological** method. Finally, the results of large numbers of such enquiries were subjected to statistical analysis in order to reveal significant patterns.

The hospital was for a number of reasons well suited to investigations of this kind. It was only in such an environment that sufficient numbers of similar cases were gathered for clinical and pathological scrutiny. The hospital patient's dependent, and relatively powerless, position made it possible to pursue practices that would have been impossible under an earlier medical regime. Physical examination came to involve an ever-greater degree of intrusion on the patient's body. Some degree of nudity was often involved, and the doctor would touch the patient with his hands and sometimes with instruments. Often these examinations extended to the parts of the body that were traditionally viewed as 'private'. Conventional codes of decorum and decency were thus routinely violated in the name of medical necessity. The transgressive nature of medical practice was especially obvious when the patient was female. (Medical practitioners during this period were almost invariably men. Very few women qualified as doctors until the 1870s.) Autopsy, moreover, involved the flagrant flouting of lay attitudes towards the proper treatment of the body after death.

Another aspect of the shift in the power relations between patient and doctor lay, according to Jewson, in the contrasting priorities embedded in bedside and hospital medicine. The former system laid most emphasis on prognosis (predicting the course of illness) and therapy. These were the patient's main concerns. Hospital medicine, in contrast, prioritized the diagnosis and classification of morbid conditions. The fate of the individual sufferer was of less consequence than what this 'case' might contribute to the wider pool of medical knowledge. In other words, the patient ceased to be a person – Jewson's 'sick-man' with his or her own agenda and understanding – and became instead a diseased body to be probed and ultimately dissected by the practitioner.

Around the middle of the nineteenth century, a new medical cosmology, which Jewson calls 'laboratory medicine', supervened on these structures and practices. Laboratory medicine originated in the German-speaking states. It was character-ized by an insistence on studying vital processes with the tools and concepts of chemistry and physics. It thus espoused a **reductionist** view of the organism. 'Reductionism' refers to the view that no fundamental difference exists between the processes that occur in living bodies and those that are found in the inorganic world. Laboratory medicine regarded the clinico-pathological method as inadequate. Instead, it sought the seat of disease at the cellular level, or in the biochemical processes at work in the body.

Pathogenic changes at these levels could not be discerned by the clinician at the patient's bedside; their analysis required a new set of skills and a new locus. The principal space for the advancement and application of medical knowledge now became the laboratory. The use of these facilities was entrusted to highly trained scientific researchers. In the later part of the nineteenth century, and still more in the twentieth century, it became increasingly common for specimens taken from patients to be sent to such laboratories for purposes of diagnosis.

Laboratory medicine reinforced certain tendencies already inherent in the preceding regime. In particular, the marginalization of the patient's perspective inherent under hospital medicine became still more marked. The laboratory scientist was in no way economically dependent on the patient: his patron was the academic system within which he pursued his career. In most cases, indeed, the laboratory scientist would have no direct contact with the patient; all he would see would be the particular sample of body fluid or tissue specimen that had been forwarded for analysis. Conversely, the terms in which the eventual diagnosis of the condition was conceived would have been still more alien to the patient: a vast gulf had opened up between what might be called the personal phenomenology of disease and the technical terms with which the medical profession worked.

Exercise

Read 'Hospital and laboratory medicine' (Source Book 2, Reading 1.1). This extract is taken from Jewson's 'The disappearance of the sick-man'. Even though you have read an overview of Jewson's ideas, you may find this piece quite hard to follow. (The diagrams of bedside, hospital and laboratory medicine provide a handy summary.) Jewson uses the language of sociology, rather than history. Notice that the article is entirely taken up with the discussion of ideas, and with concepts concerning the relationships between knowledge and practice, patients and practitioners. Jewson provides no detailed historical evidence to back up his arguments.

Jewson's argument is open to criticism of various kinds. It is highly schematic and somewhat simplistic. Nonetheless, provided its limitations are acknowledged, it provides a useful framework for understanding the major transformations that have occurred in western medicine since 1800. These may be summarized as the shift away from a 'person-oriented' to an 'object-oriented' medical cosmology. The patient, conceived as a concrete individual, was increasingly analysed by the medical gaze into ever smaller parts, first organs and then cells. The patient's individuality became ever more irrelevant as he or she became a 'case' or a 'specimen' exemplifying certain general medical principles. This object-oriented world-view is sometimes referred to as 'scientific medicine' or 'techno-medicine'.

This way of viewing the history of medicine is also valuable because it draws attention to the intimate connections between forms of medical theory and the social relations within which these principles and practices are implemented. Jewson is aware of the importance of economic considerations – the 'medical marketplace' – in determining what medical systems flourish in any particular epoch. He also draws attention to the different power relations between doctor and patient that underlie each medical cosmology.

The relationship between Jewson's and Foucault's writing is discussed in more detail later in the chapter.

The originality of Jewson's account lies in its long trajectory. Other authors had previously noted the major shift in medical thinking at the end of the eighteenth century that was associated especially with the Paris hospitals. The most influential account of this shift in thinking was Michel Foucault's *The Birth of the Clinic* (first published in 1964, translated into English 1973).

1.3 Medicalization of the hospital

The hospital in modern western society is regarded as the pre-eminent medical institution. In terms of function, it is devoted entirely to the accommodation, diagnosis and treatment of the sick. In some cases, the hospital may also perform the ancillary function of serving as a centre for medical education. Medical considerations govern the admission, management and discharge of patients.

The development of the hospital is discussed more fully in Chapter 2.

It is important to grasp, however, that medical domination of the hospital is a relatively recent development. For much of their history, hospitals performed a much more diverse role than that with which they are associated today. In medieval and early modern Europe, they acted as repositories for various classes of inmate, only some of whom would be classed as medical cases. While doctors might have a role within these establishments, hospital management was usually in the hands of other groups. In Catholic countries, hospitals were often religious institutions run by monks or nuns. In eighteenth-century Britain, hospitals were charitable institutions funded by voluntary contributions; the running of the hospital was entrusted to the most prominent subscribers, most of whom were not medically qualified.

Is Jewson right to point to the rise of the hospital as a site for the production of new forms of medical knowledge and practice in the late eighteenth century? Many historians have described a process of 'medicalization' of the hospital beginning in the later eighteenth century and becoming more pronounced in the course of the nineteenth century. While Jewson sees important changes occurring in the hospitals of post-revolutionary Paris, later research has shown that similar developments took place in Britain. Mary E. Fissell has provided a detailed study of the unfolding of this process in an English provincial hospital, the Bristol Infirmary. The infirmary was founded in 1737 as a charitable institution run by lay governors with the power to admit patients whom they regarded as deserving. In the course of the century, however, the governors progressively abdicated their authority, while the medical staff of the hospital claimed more power for themselves. Fissell is, moreover, concerned to show how these developments impinged on lay understandings of health and disease.

Read 'Surgeons and the medicalisation of the hospital' (Source Book 2, Reading 1.2), in which Fissell discusses changes in the governance and functions of the Bristol Infirmary in the course of the eighteenth century. What lay behind these changes? Does Fissell's work back up Jewson's ideas? What were the implications of the fact that a significant proportion of practitioners trained in the infirmary went on to serve in a variety of institutional capacities?

Fissell provides support for Jewson's thesis and shows how the Bristol hospital was geared increasingly to the needs of teaching and research, as well as to patient care. She describes how the surgeons attached to the hospital came to play an increasingly prominent role in the running of the hospital. They did this chiefly because of changes in the way in which surgeons were trained. Previously, young surgeons had learned their trade as apprentices to established practitioners. In the course of the century, however, this was replaced by a system where pupils learned by walking the wards of the hospital and attending lectures given by prominent surgeons. As the infirmary became a more important site for medical education, from which the surgeons derived significant income and status, so they had a greater interest in regulating such matters as admissions in a way that would best suit the needs of teachers and students. One consequence of these developments was the emergence of a new sense of identity among medical men: they came to see themselves as being less akin to other tradesmen, who learned their business by apprenticeship, and more as professional gentlemen. It was their shared experience of training in the hospital that was the basis of this new identity (Figure 1.1). The fact that many of these students spent at least part of

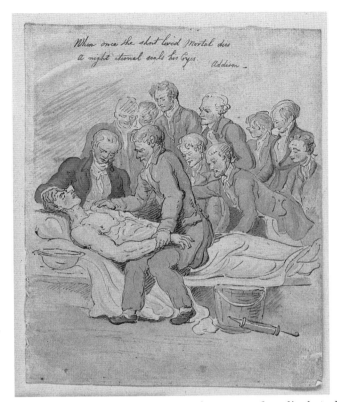

Figure 1.1   In this watercolour, two doctors and a group of medical students gather round the bedside of a dying patient – a vomit bowl, enema and bucket testify to their efforts to treat him. The caption – 'When once the short lived mortal dies/A night eternal seals his eyes' (Addison) – is a reminder of the finality of death. The presence of so many people observing the final moments of the patient's life shows how the demands of teaching override the normal rituals of death. Here, the large group of students, unknown to the patient, replaces the handful of close relatives or friends who would normally sit with a patient in his last hours. At least the students are shown to be quiet and orderly, and struck by the solemnity of the moment: there are accounts of students in the Paris hospitals (discussed later in the chapter) climbing on to the patient's bed to get a better view of their teachers lecturing on a case. Wellcome Library, London

their subsequent careers in various civilian and military institutions meant that they were introduced to forms of practice that differed from the classic clinical encounter between a practitioner and a fee-paying private patient that Jewson regards as characteristic of the eighteenth century.

These issues can be explored further through the surviving letters of medical students of the period. Hampton Weekes was a student at St Thomas's Hospital in London in the early years of the nineteenth century. His friend Owen Evans studied at St Bartholomew's. An extract from their correspondence is shown below. Both of these hospitals had been among the first to develop medical schools.

The extract gives substance to Jewson's claims about the objectification of the patient under hospital medicine. It also amplifies Fissell's suggestion that hospital training helped foster a sense of professional identity that distanced medical men from their patients and from the community at large.

OE to HW, St Bartholomew's Hospital, 2 January 1797

We have of late been froze out of the Dissecting Rooms so that till now again that part of my business has been at a stand ... I am sorry to say Subjects [bodies] are very scarce in proportion to what they formerly were & they charge a most exorbitant price for blood Vessel subjects & Extremitys; they charge 4 Guineas for a Muscular Subject. – I have during the season spent a great deal of time in the Dissecting Room assisting one or another & sometimes help Mr. Abernethy's Man get the Subject ready for Lecture; I assure you the more I know of Anatomy the fonder I am of it which I hope will be of some encouragement to you ... I am of opinion for a Man to make himself a good Anatomist sh[oul]d. attend only to that subject; I would the next Course if I could, attend only to this, but in the situation in which I am in I cannot; as I must attend to the Patients in the Hospital & go round with the Physicians as well as the Surgeon which takes up a great deal of time.

(Ford, 1987, p.35)

This passage raises a number of points. Evans refers to the bodies he dissects as 'subjects'. He draws no distinction between whole bodies and body parts. What does this tell us about his attitude to these cadavers? He complains about the cost of obtaining the bodies; for him, they are *commodities*. It is likely that a majority of the 'subjects' dissected by medical students in this period were obtained illegally. The practice of grave-robbing was commonplace and engendered deep hostility and suspicion in the community towards the medical profession.

Next, here are extracts from two letters written within the space of a month by Hampton Weekes to his father (who was a surgeon). In them, Weekes describes his first and subsequent reactions to witnessing surgical operations.

St Thomas's, 24 September 1801

Now for fainting ... dont suppose I was carried off as a dead man Dr, but I felt a something indescribable as I have heard you say & took myself off just as they had taken hold of the Artery with the Tenaculum [a surgical instrument] & immediately recovered, I wont do so again I think for I will persue the means you recommend, I can dissect I know, & could have performed the operation myself.

(Ford, 1987, p.44)

St Thomas's, 8 October 1801

[A]t both Hospitalls I have seen several operations since I wrote last & mind nothing about it, the more the poor devills cry ye.[the] more I laugh with ye. rest of them.

(Ford, 1987, p.49)

Within a remarkably short time, Weekes's initial squeamishness about attending operations has been replaced by an emphatic show of nonchalance. Indeed, he stresses his own and his fellow surgeons' callousness: they laugh at the screams of the patient. Note that he sees dissection as preparing him technically for operative surgery. It may also have helped the trainee surgeon to view the body as an object and so foster the insensitivity necessary to performing operations (Richardson, 1988).

Fissell's account is significant because it describes events in a provincial English hospital – a location that might be thought peripheral to the mainstream of change in the medical world. At this time, Paris was the centre of new developments in medical knowledge. Yet many of the features usually associated with Paris medicine of the late eighteenth and early nineteenth centuries – large-scale clinical training, hands-on dissection, and the clinico-pathological method – can already be seen in Bristol, at least in outline. Other historians have shown that similar developments can be discerned in places like London and Vienna during the same era. I shall now turn to developments in the Parisian hospitals in the period following the French Revolution of 1789.

1.4   Paris medicine and its dissemination

Jewson claims that events in France following the Revolution provided conditions for major transformations in medical thought and practice. The forms of medicine that emerged from these local circumstances were to have a global impact. Jewson does not, however, go into detail about how the political upheavals of the period came to impinge on the medical sphere. Although one of his medical epochs is called 'hospital medicine', he has remarkably little to say about the nature of hospitals in France during this period.

The Revolution impinged on most aspects of French society, including medicine. Established medical institutions, such as the faculty of medicine in Paris, were viewed with suspicion by the revolutionaries because of their connections with the *ancien régime*. Consequently, in the early stages of the Revolution there was a widespread dismantling of the existing mechanisms of medical education and licensing. For a period, something akin to a free market in the provision of medical services was encouraged. The revolutionaries were ill disposed to the huge urban hospitals they inherited and at one stage there were proposals that these be shut and replaced by care for the sick in the community. It was thought that at most a few small hospices might be needed to care for those who had no family to tend to them.

These somewhat utopian proposals were soon overtaken by events. Successive French governments were forced to reconsider their attitudes to medical provision and education, in part because of pressing practical demands. Between 1793 and 1814, France was almost continually at war. There was a constant demand for competent doctors to serve in the armed services, and institutions to train these practitioners were urgently required. There was, moreover, a sense in which successive regimes recognized that among the rights of the citizen in the new French republic was a right to health and to adequate medical treatment.

Instead of seeking to abolish hospitals, therefore, the authorities began to strive to place them on a better footing in order to meet these obligations (Figure 1.2).

The process of reconstruction began in 1794 with a proposal to create three new *écoles de santé* (schools of health) in Paris, Strasbourg and Montpellier. These schools were to be democratic, in that they were to admit students of all backgrounds. Posts within them were to be filled by a system of open competition known as the *concours*. The new system of medical training was to be strictly practical and empirical in its orientation, eschewing what was seen as the sterile scholasticism of the *ancien régime* when students were taught medicine only through lectures and books, in favour of observation at the bedside and dissection – strategies that were also adopted at the Bristol Infirmary. In this regard, the medical reformers of the 1790s showed a clear debt to the ideology of the

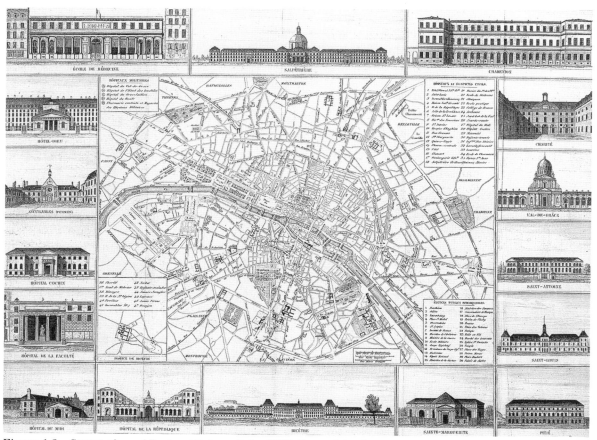

Figure 1.2   Street plan of Paris with hospitals, 1855. From this plan you can get a sense of the number of hospitals in Paris, and their size and grand appearance. After the French Revolution, when Paris was at its height as a centre for teaching and learning, around 5,000 students a year flocked to the hospitals, with their 20,000 inpatients (a total greater than the number of hospital inpatients in the whole of England at this time). Clinical teaching was centred on the Hôtel-Dieu, Charité, Salpêtrière, St Louis, Maternité and Children's hospitals. Wellcome Library, London

Enlightenment. Their viewpoint was best summed up by Antoine Fourcroy, one of their number, when he declared, 'reading little, seeing and doing much: this will be the basis of the new teaching' (Ackerknecht, 1967; La Berge and Hannaway, 1998).

Another important feature of the new system was the abolition of the traditional distinction between the teaching of surgery and the teaching of medicine. This had a number of significant consequences. Surgical **pathology** had tended to deal with local disturbances of the solid parts of the body. Physicians' pathology, on the other hand, was more humoral and systemic in its orientation. As surgical modes of thinking came to pervade all medical thinking, localist notions that had previously been applied to the surface of the body were now used to explicate changes taking place in its deeper recesses (Maulitz, 1988).

There was widespread agreement that the best place for medical students to gain the practical knowledge they needed was the hospital. Here, they would be exposed to a critical mass of patients that would enable them to gain vital diagnostic and therapeutic skills. The hospital was, moreover, increasingly seen as a site where new medical knowledge could be developed. It was, in short, the premier site for medical *research* as well as teaching. Foucault designated these changes as the 'birth of the clinic' (Foucault, 1973). In his book of that name, Foucault described the emergence of new medical ideas in the post-revolutionary Paris hospitals. Diseases were no longer seen as phenomena that were unique to each patient, changing over time and affecting different parts of the body. Diseases were now seated in a particular organ or tissue, and the slight differences in the pattern of symptoms observed in each patient were unimportant. However, Foucault was interested not simply in the discovery of new 'facts': in this, as in much of his writing, he was interested in the emergence of a new discourse (the process he called 'discursive formation'). Discourses provide a language, concepts and ideas and thus shape the way we think about phenomena. The Paris hospitals saw the emergence of the 'clinician's gaze' – a way of looking at the patient and 'seeing' disease which no longer dealt with environment or lifestyle, but focused on the organic changes occurring in the spaces within the body. For Foucault, this new way of seeing and thinking turned the body into an object that could be understood by scientific knowledge, and the foundation for the emergence of the human sciences. For Foucault, knowledge and power are intimately linked: as practitioners developed a new discourse of disease, they acquired a new power within the clinical relationship. Within the 'clinic' the patient occupied an entirely subservient position. He or she became teaching material to be probed and examined during life and, as you have seen in the extract from the Evans letter, a 'commodity' to be dissected after death. Foucault has written of a tacit 'contract' that legitimated this exploitation of the hospital patient. In return for free medical assistance, the poor made their bodies available to the medical gaze. (For a vivid depiction of the power relationships between patient and practitioner, see Plate 5.) Jewson acknowledges Foucault's work in his 1976 article. He remarks, for instance, on the similarity of his own concept of medical cosmology to Foucault's notion of 'discursive formation'. Both Jewson and Foucault are in some sense seeking to expose the role of power in the creation of systems of medical knowledge. Despite these similarities, however, it is important to note that between the two authors there are profound differences in approach. Jewson employs a notion of power as an essentially repressive, manipulative agency located in determinate social loci. For Foucault, power pervades society and plays a positive, creative function.

Since the publication of *The Birth of the Clinic* and Jewson's article, a number of historians have produced detailed studies of the Paris hospitals. The next reading, by Dora B. Weiner, is an account of the patient's experience in one such hospital.

Exercise

Read 'The inpatient' (Source Book 2, Reading 1.3). To what extent does Weiner's account of the experience of the inpatient accord with Foucault's notion of 'the clinic'? How does the image of the Paris hospitals compare with Fissell's account of the Bristol Infirmary?

Discussion

Weiner provides evidence to support Foucault's and Jewson's picture of the hospital as a centre for research. She stresses that the whole post-revolutionary hospital system was geared to teaching and research. Medical criteria now came to predominate in admissions. Despite the presence of nuns on the wards, the hospital was an increasingly secular institution where doctors were the dominant figures. One way in which medical research into particular disorders was fostered was the creation of specialist institutions, a trend followed in many late eighteenth-century hospitals. The bodies of deceased patients were subjected to routine autopsy to elicit further information. All these features correspond to Foucault's account of the most salient features of the clinic. While both Weiner and Fissell suggest that doctors had considerable power over what went on in hospital, Weiner provides a picture of a vast system of institutions stretching across the city and sharing a common purpose. Fissell describes one quite small institution in which a handful of practitioners taught a small number of students. She provides an important corrective to the view – implicit in Jewson's article – that medical authority increased inexorably in the period after 1800 by showing that the poor could and did offer resistance to encroachments upon their bodies. She suggests that in the Bristol Infirmary, patients did have some power – relatives would refuse permission for post-mortem examinations. In contrast, Weiner's patients seem to lack any power or control over their treatment or destiny.

In the Paris hospitals, the clinician's gaze was not limited to the external signs and symptoms of illness: techniques of physical examination were developed that allowed practitioners to visualize pathological changes deep within the body. The most famous is the use of the stethoscope. Among the first students trained at the new Paris School of Medicine was a young Breton called René Théophile Hyacinthe Laennec (1781–1826). After a period as a surgeon in the military hospitals of Nantes, Laennec came to Paris as a student in 1801. He attended the course of Xavier Bichat (1771–1802), one of the founders of pathological anatomy, and became a friend of Gaspard-Laurent Bayle (1774–1816), another important figure in the establishment of the discipline. Laennec also attended the lessons of Jean-Nicholas Corvisart (1755–1821), who was, among other things, Napoleon's personal physician.

Corvisart is noted for reviving interest in thoracic percussion, a technique first discussed in 1761 by the Austrian physician Leopold Auenbrugger (1722–1809). Inspired by the observation that wine casks emitted different sounds when they were struck, depending on how full they were, Auenbrugger had speculated that percussion might supply information about the state of the body cavities. It was only in the nineteenth century, however, that this suggestion was extensively adopted. Corvisart, in particular, promoted percussion as a clinical technique, and translated Auenbrugger's work into French in 1808. The method consisted of the doctor tapping the patient's body with his hand to elicit a sound. Percussion

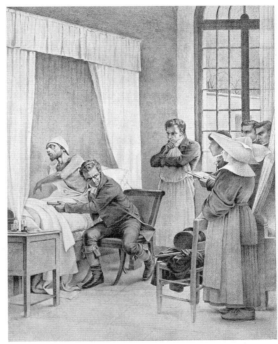

Figure 1.3   René Laennec auscultating a patient at the Necker Hospital, 1816. This is a rather romanticized image. The thin and obviously sick patient (compare with the patient in Gervex's painting, shown in Plate 5) is the centre of attention for Laennec and his fellow doctors, who look on in concern. A medical student (holding a notepad and pen, in the group on the right) acts as clinical clerk, recording the patient's symptoms. The image demonstrates how rapidly Laennec's name was linked to the use of the stethoscope – although in fact in this painting Laennec is shown performing immediate auscultation, applying an ear directly to the patient's chest in order to hear sounds from the lungs. In his hand, he holds an early stethoscope – a simple wooden tube – which was used in mediate auscultation. Wellcome Library, London

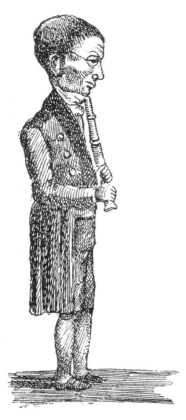

Figure 1.4   René Laennec, self-portrait, 1824.
Compare the image in Figure 1.3 with this rather
self-deprecating cartoon in which Laennec shows
himself holding a long stethoscope. Reproduced
courtesy of Académie Nationale de Médecine,
Paris

became one of the principal techniques of physical examination by which doctors
achieved insights into morbid changes occurring in the patient's body.

After graduating, Laennec gained a reputation as an expert in pathological
anatomy. He also developed a fashionable practice among the elite of Parisian
society. In 1816, he was appointed physician to the Necker Hospital in Paris, a
position that gave him access to a wide range of patients and the opportunity to
make numerous post-mortem examinations. It was during this period that
Laennec introduced the innovation for which he is chiefly remembered: mediate
auscultation. This was a development of immediate auscultation, where the
doctor applied his ear directly to the patient's body. While some information might
be derived by this means, immediate auscultation entailed a number of difficulties.
It involved a degree of direct contact between patient and doctor that both might
find embarrassing or distasteful.

Apparently by accident, Laennec discovered that some medium between the
patient and the doctor's ear actually enhanced the audibility of sounds emanating
from the body. At first, he used a rolled-up paper for this purpose; later, he
substituted a solid wooden cylinder (Figures 1.3 and 1.4). Laennec called this
instrument a stethoscope. The name was derived from the Greek words for 'chest'
(*stēthos*) and 'to examine' (*skopein*) (Duffin, 1998).

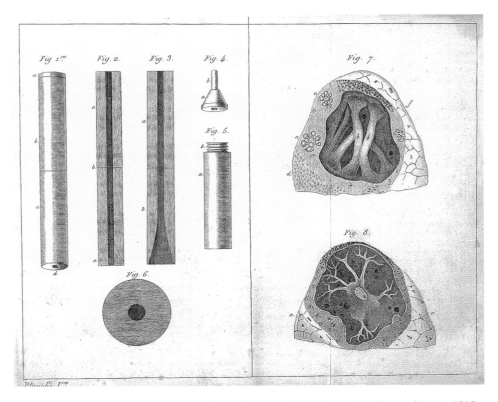

Figure 1.5 Stethoscope and lungs, from Laennec's *De l'auscultation médiate*, 1819, plate 1. The page on the left shows the design of Laennec's stethoscope. The page on the right shows the type of condition that can be detected using the instrument – the lung of a patient who died from severe tuberculosis. This plate can be read as a summary of the Paris school – the investigation of disease by physical examination during life, and the correlation of those symptoms after death through dissection. It also graphically shows how the patient has ceased to be the 'sick man' described by bedside medicine, suffering from a disease whose form and progress reflect his constitution and lifestyle. Instead, the patient has been reduced to a diseased organ (or rather, part of a lung) which is used to demonstrate the typical lesions caused by tuberculosis – the large cavities containing bands of tissue or obliterated blood vessels, and smaller tubercles (on the left-hand side of the top diagram). Wellcome Library, London

In 1819, Laennec published his *Traité de l'auscultation médiate* in which he outlined the advantages of the technique. The book provided an exposition of the clinico-pathological method. Laennec described the clinical signs associated with many diseases of the lungs and heart. He distinguished the sounds made by different conditions that might otherwise be confused with one another. He also developed an elaborate vocabulary to describe the various sounds investigators would hear when they applied the stethoscope to the body of the patient. For instance, he gave the name 'pectoriloquy' to the unusual audibility of the patient's voice through the chest that was sometimes detectable by the stethoscope. He associated this sign with a localized cavity in the lung caused by tuberculosis (Figure 1.5).

Laennec's work thus typifies the growing emphasis on physical signs as the basis of diagnosis. The patient's own account of his or her symptoms was, at most, of secondary importance in establishing the character of the condition. This emphasis on the lesions underlying the sounds and other signs discernible at the patient's bedside reinforced the tendency for doctors to turn their attention away from external appearances to deep pathology. At the same time, the development of an esoteric descriptive language further widened the gulf between lay and professional understandings of disease. The stethoscope can also be seen as the forerunner of other diagnostic instruments, such as the laryngoscope and the ophthalmoscope, that came into use later in the nineteenth century (Reiser, 1978).

Although the stethoscope was greeted with scorn by some conservative practitioners, it was widely recognized as representing a major medical advance. Thus, John Forbes (1787–1861), the British physician, author and editor, who translated Laennec's work into English, declared in 1821 that '(if his [Laennec's] new diagnostics are as certain as he affirms) he may be said to have realized the wish of the antient [*sic*] philosopher, and to have placed a window in the breast through which we can see the precise state of things within'.

Here is Forbes's translation of one of Laennec's case histories.

> 392. CASE. (No. xxxvii. of the Author...) PHTHISIS PULMONALIS. – *Tuberculous excavation producing the metallick tinkling.* A woman, aged 40, came into the Hospital 29th January, having been affected with cough for five months, and which had increased since her confinement, three months ago. At this time the respiration was short and quick, and difficult; the chest resounded pretty well in the back and left side before, – but better on the right side; there was distinct pectoriloquism near the junction of the sternum and left clavicle, and the same phenomenon, but less distinct, on the same side where the arm joined the chest; the sound of the ventricles was dull, and the heart gave hardly any impulse. Two days after, by means of the cylinder [the stethoscope], we distinguished a sound resembling fluctuation, in the left side, when the patient coughed, and the *metallick tinkling* when she spoke. Succussion [shaking] of the trunk did not produce the sound of fluctuation. From these results the following diagnostic was given: *very large tuberculous excavation in the middle of the left lung, containing a small quantity of very liquid tuberculous matter.* The patient dies five days after this.
>
> (Laennec, 1821, p.392)

What means does Laennec employ to determine the nature of the patient's complaint? How does this differ from the means by which a physician from a previous era might have arrived at a diagnosis?

Laennec seems to have employed percussion and immediate auscultation in his initial examination of the patient. He also resorted to 'succussion', or shaking the patient, to see what sounds were emitted from the chest. This was an ancient technique referred to in the Hippocratic corpus. These methods were later supplemented by use of the stethoscope – the 'cylinder'. By these means, Laennec felt able to visualize the lesion in the lung underlying the patient's symptoms. In an earlier era, physicians relied on the patient's own account of their illness – its history, progress and possible cause – and on information about their lifestyle, when formulating a diagnosis. There is remarkably little in this case history about the patient's life history or social circumstances.

In the original text, the case history is followed by a report on the autopsy carried out twenty-four hours after the patient's death, which confirms this diagnosis. Laennec was sometimes criticized for being preoccupied with diagnosis and indifferent to therapeutics. This imputation is consistent with the more general stereotype of Paris medicine. Ironically, teachers in Paris are often portrayed as urging a more active, 'hands-on' approach to teaching and diagnosis but at the same time shunning contemporary 'heroic' therapeutics, with its active blood-letting and large doses of medicine. Instead, they preferred to give full rein to the healing powers of nature, a position known as therapeutic scepticism. Laennec was sensitive to such claims and maintained that auscultation could, at least in some cases, assist treatment. Surgeons had since ancient times sought to remedy cases of empyema (accumulation of pus in the chest) through the operation of thoracentesis (making an incision into the body cavity). However, the difficulty of identifying the correct spot for the incision was widely acknowledged by surgeons. Laennec maintained that the stethoscope could solve this problem by localizing the effusion with much greater precision than had previously been possible.

Laennec's anxiety to show the therapeutic potentials of his new technique indicates that leading members of the Parisian school were not as indifferent to improving methods of treatment as is sometimes suggested. Laennec's contemporary and rival François-Joseph-Victor Broussais (1772–1838) combined a strong interest in pathological anatomy with an optimistic therapeutic outlook, advocating an active treatment regime, including bloodletting. In fact, the view of Parisian therapeutic scepticism – that treatment was of little use, and most diseases were cured by natural processes – was to a large extent manufactured by British and American doctors who had studied in France but who wished to underline their own commitment to treating and curing patients.

Nonetheless, it is true that hospital medicine of the first half of the nineteenth century was more notable for its contributions to understanding the organic seat of disease and illuminating the physical signs by which these conditions were manifested than in devising significant new treatments. It may, however, be argued that therapeutic scepticism served a valuable, if negative, purpose by demonstrating that many of the therapies previously deployed by practitioners were ineffective.

Because of the work of Laennec and his colleagues, Paris became recognized in the first third of the nineteenth century as the world centre for medical theory and technique. As a result, students from throughout Europe and from North America flocked there to learn the clinico-pathological method in the Parisian hospitals. These included such notable British practitioners as Thomas Hodgkin (1798–1860).

Hodgkin travelled to Paris in 1821, where he studied with Laennec. He returned to England with a stethoscope and delivered a lecture on the instrument to his fellow students at a meeting of the Guy's Hospital Physical Society. In 1825, he was appointed lecturer in morbid anatomy and curator of the Pathology Museum at Guy's Hospital Medical School. There, he combined his clinical investigations with extensive work in pathological anatomy. He was instrumental in building up an impressive museum illustrating the action of disease on different parts of the body. In 1832, he described the form of cancer that bears his name.

Among Hodgkin's colleagues at Guy's Hospital was Richard Bright (1789–1858), another notable exponent of the clinico-pathological method. Bright is especially linked with the identification of structural changes in the kidney associated with particular conditions. He also made extensive use of chemical analysis in his researches, and his work may therefore also be seen as an early example of laboratory medicine. The fact that a great deal of laboratory work was undertaken by clinicians within hospitals demonstrates that Jewson's sharp distinction between hospital and laboratory medicine is difficult to sustain. Jewson may also be faulted for glossing over the great variety of establishments gathered under the umbrella term 'laboratory'. (This point is discussed in greater depth in Chapter 4.)

1.5   The patient's perspective

Medical history has, for the most part, been written from the doctor's point of view – in a way mirroring the demotion or even erasure of the patient's viewpoint that Jewson sees as characteristic of the shift from bedside to hospital medicine. More recently, however, historians have attempted to recover the patient's perspective. These efforts can be seen as part of a more general endeavour to write 'history from below' – that is, to seek to give due weight to the stories and experiences of marginalized groups such as women and workers.

Thus, Fissell has tried to show how the developments she describes in late eighteenth- and early nineteenth-century Bristol would have impinged on the poor who attended the Bristol Infirmary. In line with Jewson's ideas, she argues that one immediate consequence of the shift towards a more 'object-oriented' medical cosmology was a downgrading of the importance of the patients' own words and perspectives in the clinical encounter. Whereas in an earlier era patients' own accounts of how they became ill and of the symptoms they experienced were at the heart of diagnosis, these became increasingly devalued as doctors came to rely more on physical signs. Biographical details embodied in patients' own understandings of disease were mostly irrelevant to the professional discourse they encountered on entering the hospital. Case histories accordingly contained scant detail about patients' lives and circumstances before they turned to an account of physical signs.

Because the needs of the medical student rather than of the patient were now paramount, infirmary surgeons felt no need to adapt their practice to match the patient's expectations. The hospital patient became a mere 'case' exemplifying certain pathological principles. Should the patient die, their body was appropriated for autopsy in order to complete their instructive purpose: while 'vernacular medicine looked backward to the cause of illness, hospital medicine looked forward to dissection' (Fissell, 1991, p.163).

A comparable dissociation of lay and professional culture was evident in therapeutics. The extensive range of botanical remedies employed outside the hospital was replaced within by an almost exclusive reliance on bleeding. This was well suited to an institutional regime where routine and economy was of greater importance than individualized treatment. But general bleeding was also appropriate to the new regime: 'this style of therapy bypassed the patient's account of him or herself because it relied on the body's own response; the patient's body served as its own monitor of therapeutic efficacy' (Fissell, 1991, p.161). In other words, the clinician was able to disregard the patient's own account of his or her feelings and perceptions. 'Objective' physical signs dictated when bleeding was required, and the pulse was used to judge when sufficient blood had been drawn.

The turn of the nineteenth century thus saw a 'fragmentation of a common understanding held by practitioner and patient' (Fissell, 1991, p.170). It is difficult to gauge patients' responses to these changes: most of the records of medical practice were produced by doctors and, as you have seen, the patient's point of view does not figure prominently in these documents. One indication of popular feeling, however, is fierce resistance to the appropriation of dead bodies for dissection and autopsy, as Fissell suggests.

A few records embodying a patient's viewpoint do survive, and these can prove particularly instructive in testing some of the claims made by Fissell about the changing nature of the clinical encounters that have been outlined. In cases of chronic disease, well-off patients would often consult several practitioners over an extended period of time. In order to keep a record of the advice they received, the patient might compile a dossier, both for his or her own benefit and for the guidance of doctors consulted for the first time. These documents may be considered as forerunners of the case notes that accompany patients through various clinical encounters in modern practice. One significant difference, however, is that it was the patient who played the dominant role in compiling these dossiers, and consequently they can shed light on his or her perspective. One such dossier was created by James Scott, an Edinburgh accountant in the 1820s.

Scott was a man of means. Edinburgh was itself a major medical centre. He could afford, however, to travel to London in order to consult the most distinguished practitioners there. He also appears to have gone to Paris to seek further advice. His case provides a rare insight into elite private practice which complements the work of historians such as Fissell on the experience of the hospital patient.

Exercise

Read 'Mr Scott's case' (Source Book 2, Reading 1.4).

1   In what sense is this case 'typical', and in what sense is it exceptional?

2   To what extent does it differ from the discussion of the experience of hospital patients provided by Weiner in Source Book 2, Reading 1.3?

3   Who is the author of the record of this case?

Discussion

1   Scott's case is more typical of Jewson's eighteenth-century bedside medicine than of nineteenth-century hospital medicine. Because he was wealthy, Scott enjoyed the position of 'patron' in the doctor–patient relationship: he paid fees to the practitioners he saw, and could choose whom to consult. There is evidence that he possessed a certain amount of medical knowledge and could converse with these doctors about his case. They, in turn, in most instances made an attempt to explain their opinions to him. In other respects, however, his case diverges from what might be expected. For instance, he seems to have *expected* physical examination as part of these consultations rather than seeing it as a form of impropriety. (One wonders if a female patient may have felt differently.)

2   Scott was very different from the patients in the Paris hospitals, who had no control over which practitioner took charge of their case. While manners and deportment were a consideration in the choice of some of the doctors consulted, it is evident that other criteria were also relevant; in particular, a reputation for specialist expertise might also incline a paying patient to seek out an individual practitioner.

3   Because the history of Mr Scott's case is a composite document, the question of authorship is complex. The dossier reveals an elaborate process of negotiation between the patient and the various doctors he encountered that belies any simple notion of who was dominant in the clinical encounter.

As you have seen in the first part of this section, Jewson's thesis is in many respects supported by more detailed historical studies. In particular, his claims about a growing rift between lay and medical perceptions of disease, about the growth of an 'object-oriented' medicine, and a corresponding diminution in the power of the patient in the clinical encounter, are all borne out by the work of Fissell and Weiner. The account of Mr Scott's case shows, however, that 'bedside medicine' was, in some social settings, still practised in the nineteenth century.

Certain patients were still able to function as 'patrons' who exerted considerable influence on the form of the clinical interaction. The question is thus which of these types of practice was the more typical or definitive of the medicine of the period? You should not think in terms of different systems of medicine supplanting one another, but of degrees of coexistence of two systems.

1.6   The rise of laboratory medicine

The reform of medical teaching throughout Europe is described in greater detail in Chapters 3 and 5.

You will recall that Jewson claims that around 1850 a further major change occurred in western medicine, when the locus of medical authority shifted from the clinic to the laboratory. This term covers establishments involved in the pursuit of such basic medical sciences as physiology and biochemistry as well as laboratories that provided services that were of more immediate use in the diagnosis of disease. The latter were, for obvious reasons of convenience, usually situated within the premises of the hospital – indeed, simple chemical and microscopic tests were often performed in side-rooms attached to hospital wards. You have seen that Richard Bright was one notable example of a medical man who succeeded in bridging the gap between laboratory and hospital ward.

For most of the first half of the nineteenth century, France was acknowledged as the world centre for medical innovation and training. After 1850, however, the focus of activity began to shift eastwards, towards German-speaking central Europe. While France was particularly associated with the pursuit of hospital medicine, the German universities became the centres for the application of laboratory science to medical theory and practice.

There are a number of reasons for Germany's pre-eminence in this field. German universities were among the first to develop a research culture: that is, to insist that academic staff should seek to add to the fund of knowledge through original enquiry rather than merely disseminating established truths. Because of the political fragmentation of the German states before 1871 (Plate 3), various governments had vied to establish prestigious universities within their borders and had competed to attract the best staff. As a result, it became possible for talented scientists to pursue full-time academic careers. Prominent scientists were also able to demand resources to maintain the laboratory facilities their research demanded.

Within these university laboratories, novel patterns of scientific work began to emerge. Previously, individuals had tended to pursue investigations alone or in loose association with others who had similar interests. In the nineteenth-century German universities, however, collaborative work by teams of researchers came to be the norm. Typically, an eminent professor would create a 'school' around himself by training talented pupils and assigning them related research projects. Later in the nineteenth century, this system became systematized, as the PhD (doctor of philosophy degree) emerged as the formal token of such research training. A PhD is usually gained by submitting a dissertation displaying evidence of original research.

As a result of these favourable circumstances, Germany was acknowledged by the last quarter of the nineteenth century as the pre-eminent centre for scientific research. Scientists in other nations, notably Britain, could only envy the facilities that were available to their German colleagues. While German superiority was evident in most departments of science, it was especially marked in physiology, pathology and other branches of medical investigation. Germany differed from both France and Britain in that throughout the nineteenth century medical education remained centred in universities.

The rise of laboratory medicine involved a major shift in the locus of medical authority. No longer was knowledge about health and disease to be sought merely through clinical enquiry coupled with post-mortem examination – the essential elements of 'hospital' or 'Paris' medicine. Instead, the laboratory came to be seen as the site at which the most fundamental and reliable information about the workings of the body, and the causes of disease and its possible cures were to be found. The term laboratory needs to be widely construed in this regard to connote not only a set of physical spaces but also certain characteristic attitudes and methodologies. These included a drive to measure and to subject phenomena to experiment rather than simply to observe, and new technologies to carry out these operations (Cunningham and Williams, 1992).

The prototype for the application of laboratory science to medicine was the rise of medical microscopy. Microscopes had been in use since the seventeenth century. Influential physicians such as Thomas Sydenham (1624–89) had, however, denied that the instrument had any application to medicine. Prominent nineteenth-century doctors, including Bichat and Laennec, shared this scepticism. Doubts about the value of the microscope were based in part on the optical defects of the instrument, but there was also a feeling that such gadgets were a mere distraction from the true source of medical knowledge – clinical observation.

After 1830, some of the optical problems that had dogged earlier microscopic investigations were overcome. Around the same time, a number of German scientists began to make systematic use of the new, improved compound microscopes that were becoming available to elucidate the minute structure of the living body. The outstanding result of these enquiries was the promulgation in 1838 by Theodor Schwann (1810–82) of the cell theory. This maintained that all living tissues were composed of the same elementary component – the cell (Figure 1.6). Research schools emerged in academic centres such as Berlin and Breslau, where students learned to use the microscope and where coherent programmes of investigation were pursued.

The new role of the laboratory was made possible, then, by improvements to the design of microscopes, which eradicated the spherical aberration associated with older designs and gave the viewer a much clearer picture of minute structures. The development of new dyes made it possible selectively to stain certain cells and structures to make them show up more clearly. Researchers also had to invent new ways of teaching, in order to show cellular structures to students. Figure 1.7 shows one solution – a microscope which accommodated three observers. The design did not catch on, however, and instead, teachers prepared sets of similar slides that students could view using their own apparatus.

In 1858, Rudolf Virchow (1821–1902), a product of the Berlin school, produced a major work entitled *Cellular Pathology*. He argued that the cell theory was the

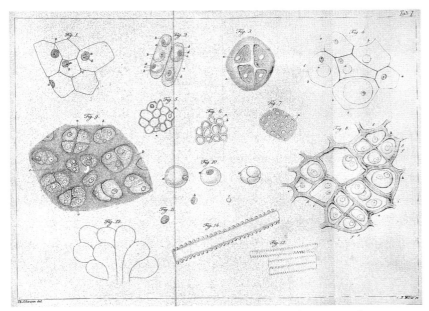

Figure 1.6   Theodor Schwann, cell structures under a microscope, from *Mikroskopische Untersuchungen*, 1839. Cells had been described in plant material from the seventeenth century, but Schwann was one of the first researchers to show that all animal tissues were also composed of cells. Cells were the fundamental units of life, and all possessed a nucleus and an outer membrane. This drawing from Schwann's textbook clearly shows these cellular structures. Wellcome Library, London

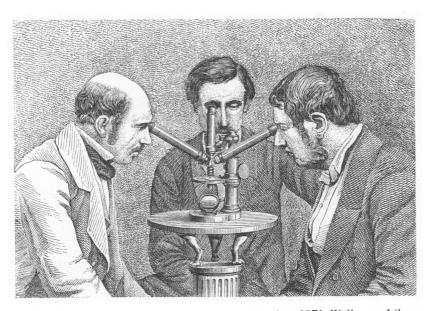

Figure 1.7   Microscope with three eyepieces, engraving, 1871. Wellcome Library, London

necessary foundation for scientific medicine. All disease, he maintained, was the result of disruption to normal cellular function. Microscopic disease processes produced characteristic changes at the cellular level. Virchow saw his work as the culmination of the movement towards the anatomical localization of disease that had begun with Giovanni Battista Morgagni (1682–1771) – professor of anatomy at Padua University and author of one of the first books on pathological anatomy – and then been developed by the Paris school of the early nineteenth century. Thanks to the insights yielded by the microscope, it was now possible to discern the most primitive seat of disease at the level of the cell. As you have seen, Jewson views these developments as the prelude to the atomization of the patient into his or her constituent cellular components.

The initial impact of the microscope was therefore in the area of basic biomedical science. But there were soon attempts to apply the instrument to the more immediate ends of medical practice. As early as 1843, Guy's Hospital in London set up a microscopy department. Advocates of the microscope argued that an examination of specimens taken from patients might yield fresh insights into disease.

It might even place diagnosis on a more certain and scientific footing. Doctors sometimes disagreed about whether suspicious growths were cancerous and therefore potentially life-threatening. The clinical signs were often ambiguous, yet important therapeutic decisions hinged on the determination of such issues, such as whether or not to amputate a breast when a lump was detected. From the 1840s onwards, there were claims that the microscopic examination of tissue samples could provide reliable answers to these questions. If this assertion were allowed, important implications would follow. The clinician would be obliged to delegate the adjudication of crucial issues to the pathologist armed with the microscope. There would, in other words, be a key shift in medical authority.

Not all clinicians were prepared to concede the claims of the proponents of the microscope. Some stoutly defended the continued validity of a medical epistemology based on attention to the symptoms of disease visible to the naked eye. In varying degrees, they cast doubt on the contribution that novel laboratory technologies could make to medical reasoning and practice. The introduction of the microscope into medicine in the mid-nineteenth century thus initiated important debates about the true foundations of medical knowledge and practice. It also gave rise to competing notions of the path medicine should take if it was to progress.

Some of these issues can be illustrated by the career of John Hughes Bennett (1812–75), a leading British proponent of laboratory science in general and of the microscope in particular. After studying medicine in Edinburgh, Bennett spent two years in Paris. There he absorbed the main tenets of the Parisian method: careful clinical investigation coupled with routine autopsy. While on the Continent, however, Bennett was also introduced to the use of the microscope. He became convinced of both its utility to clinical practice and its importance to the advancement of medical knowledge.

When he returned to Edinburgh in 1841, Bennett was the first British teacher to offer a course in practical microscopy for medical students. He also gave clinical instruction in which he sought to propagate the Paris method. He insisted, however, that the naked-eye examination of post-mortem appearances, with which Bichat and Laennec had been content, must be supplemented by an investigation of morbid changes apparent only through microscopic investigation. As pathologist to the Royal Infirmary of Edinburgh, Bennett had access to extensive post-mortem material. He published accounts of many cases where lesions invisible to the unaided eye had been revealed through the use of the microscope. In his view, the microscope additionally possessed an important role in the diagnosis of certain conditions.

Bennett was a passionate advocate of what he called 'rational medicine'. He argued that medical progress depended on better understanding of the normal processes at work in the body. Disease was no more than a perversion of the physiological norm. Medical education should therefore be geared towards inculcating physiological knowledge before conducting the student towards scientific pathology. In 1848, Bennett was appointed professor of the Institutes of Medicine at Edinburgh University. In this capacity, he promoted the introduction of laboratory training to the medical curriculum. This consisted at first of medical microscopy – or **histology**, as it became known – but was later extended to include practical physiology more generally, including physiological chemistry.

Bennett's claims struck a chord with some of his contemporaries. Many, especially among the student body, saw him as the advocate of all that was progressive in current medical thinking. But he also provoked more hostile reactions. In particular, some of his peers strenuously resisted the suggestion that the clinician should defer in matters of diagnosis to the histologist. Thus James Syme, one of Bennett's Edinburgh colleagues, warned in 1865:

> against paying undue attention to the system of minute investigation at present so much in fashion. I am no enemy to the microscope, and, on the contrary, believe that much useful as well as curious information may be obtained through its assistance; but I beg to remind you that the utmost amount of knowledge derived from this source can never supply the want of acquaintance with the form, structure, and relations of the parts, which are obvious to the unaided senses of sight and touch.
>
> (Syme, 1865, p.526)

Syme was a surgeon and thus especially sensitive to the suggestion that microscopic examination should supersede traditional methods of diagnosing such conditions as cancer. In a review of one of Bennett's publications, William Tennant Gairdner averred that:

> the practical surgeon – who calls that tumour *cancerous* which stretches out on every side ... its straggling limbs – who calls that tumour *malignant* which, wherever situated is accompanied by diseased glands and sallow complexion ... – will not readily surrender these practical and important ideas to any considerations derived from minute structure.
>
> (Gairdner, 1848–9, pp.543–4)

The microscope was to impinge on the practice of medicine in a way that Bennett could scarcely have imagined. In the final decades of the nineteenth century, the germ theory of disease gained increasing credence. This maintained that many diseases were caused by micro-organisms invisible to the naked eye. These germs could, however, be seen through the microscope in properly prepared specimens. The technique was considered to give novel certainty to the diagnosis of conditions that presented ambivalent clinical signs. By the end of the nineteenth century, most major hospitals were equipped with laboratories where specimens taken from patients could be tested for the presence of **bacteria**. These were often also the same places where histological examinations occurred. New medical specialists trained in the techniques applied in these laboratories came to prominence during this period.

Exercise

Read the following case history from an 1883 article by J. Dreschfeld, professor of pathology at the Royal Infirmary, Manchester. How does it resemble and how does it differ from Laennec's case, quoted earlier (p.16)? Does the fact that the patient was a 'gentleman' have any effect on the record?

> A.S., aged 31, a gentleman whom I had known for years, and treated for various ailments, but who, though from a phthisical family history, had himself never suffered from cough, and was in the enjoyment of very good health, consulted me on December 27th for haemoptysis [blood in the spittle], which had attacked him on the morning of that day. He could not in any way account for it, except for a very slight fall he had on December 25th, which, however, did not hurt him in any way. The physical examination showed absolutely normal relations; neither was there loss of flesh, loss of appetite, or pyrexia. Examination of the sputa on December 29th showed abundance of tubercle bacilli.

(Dreschfeld, 1883, p.305)

Discussion

Like Laennec, Dreschfeld used the techniques of physical examination to try to account for the blood in the patient's sputum. These would have included an examination of the chest by means of the stethoscope. The investigations failed, however, to detect any abnormality. Dreschfeld then turned to microscopic examination of a sample, which revealed the presence of the micro-organism that caused tuberculosis, making a diagnosis possible. The fact that A.S. was a 'gentleman', a personal acquaintance and a private (not hospital) patient, may explain why the patient's narrative of the onset of his complaint is reproduced in greater detail than in most hospital case histories. Like Mr Scott, A.S. is able to discuss his complaint with his practitioner.

It is difficult to gauge patients' responses to the rise of laboratory medicine. Most would have been unaware of the procedures now being employed to diagnose their conditions and to indicate appropriate treatments. The terms in which these diagnoses were framed, involving esoteric language drawn from histology, pathology and **bacteriology**, would have been unintelligible to all but a few. This was itself an indication of the growing gulf between lay and medical culture.

One aspect of laboratory medicine did, however, provoke a popular response. Experimental physiology was predicated on the assumption that certain truths about the workings of the body could not be gleaned by an analysis of cadavers or specimens derived from dead animals. These processes could be studied only in the living organism through experimental techniques known generically as 'vivisection'. Because in most cases such procedures induced pain and ultimately death to the animal involved in the experiment, vivisection caused considerable moral revulsion.

The last quarter of the nineteenth century saw the rise of a vocal anti-vivisection movement, especially in Britain. Protests at untrammelled experimentation on animals achieved a measure of success with the passage in 1876 of the Cruelty to Animals Act. This placed certain restrictions on physiologists wishing to employ vivisection; they were obliged to meet certain conditions and to obtain a licence from the Home Office for their proposed research.

Women were prominent in the anti-vivisection movement. There was a marked overlap between anti-vivisection and the movement for female suffrage. Analogies were often drawn between the suffering inflicted on experimental subjects and the intrusive, painful and demeaning procedures performed on women during gynaecological examinations. There was also a wider sense among the poor that the same spirit that motivated vivisection might encourage medical men to experiment on charity patients in public hospitals.

It should be noted, however, that the medical profession was itself divided on the subject. The anti-vivisection movement counted many doctors among its members. These either rejected the claim that vivisection was a necessary means to improved medical knowledge or maintained that the ethical objections to these practices outweighed any benefits that might accrue.

1.7   Conclusion

A number of general themes emerge from this discussion of trends in medical theory and practice after 1800. In the first place, it is clear that changes in medical theory cannot be viewed in isolation. They impinged on medical practice, and this in turn had major implications for the relations between doctor and patient. In other words, there were close correlations between knowledge and power.

The tendency, identified by Jewson and others, has been towards an ever greater separation of medical understandings of the body in health and disease from those entertained by lay persons. Thus, while an educated eighteenth-century patient might hope to converse on near equal terms with his or her physician about their condition, by the end of the nineteenth century doctors were basing their diagnoses and planning their therapies on theories that would have meant little if anything to those they treated. This led to a form of disenfranchisement: the patient was obliged either to accept the doctor's judgement on trust or to seek advice elsewhere. It should be noted that the nineteenth century was also the period in which a legion of alternative medical systems, such as **homeopathy**, first came to the fore. These sects provided a resort for those unwilling to submit to the dictates of the ruling medical discourse. The fact that they were characterized as *alternative* medicines does, however, emphasize the growing dominance of conventional **allopathic** medicine.

Conversely, the rise of hospital and laboratory medicine facilitated the consolidation of the medical profession. Medical training was now underpinned by a shared educational experience in which indoctrination in scientific principles played a key role. There were differences of emphasis between western nations, and even within the same country. For instance, in Britain a significant group of elite practitioners continued to emphasize humanistic attainments, rather than scientific accomplishment, as the foundation of their practice. By the beginning of the twentieth century, however, the notion of the doctor as applied scientist was largely unchallenged.

When it came to validating this commitment in terms of therapeutically important advances, for most of the nineteenth century there was little to show. The work of pathological anatomists such as Laennec may have revealed the organic seat of many diseases, but these developments did little to benefit the patient; indeed, the Paris school became associated with therapeutic scepticism. Similarly, while the microscope yielded major insights into the functioning of the body at the cellular level and revealed how the disruption of cell life led to disease, these revelations offered little if anything in way of new treatments. It was only with the emergence of bacteriology in the last quarter of the nineteenth century that the case for the potential of scientific research to promote human welfare became more plausible.

Where does this leave Jewson's thesis about the changing medical cosmology? The detailed historical studies explored in this chapter suggest that the essential features of his thesis are correct – not least that there is a strong connection between medical knowledge and the power relations between patient and practitioner. In the late eighteenth and early nineteenth centuries in both Britain and Paris, as hospitals became medicalized, the patient became an object. While alive (on the ward and during operations), they were observed by staff and students. When dead, their corpses became 'subjects' to be stolen, dismembered and dissected.

However, the historical studies also suggest that we have to qualify Jewson's ideas. They show that the shifts from bedside to hospital medicine, and from hospital to laboratory medicine, were not inevitable – they occurred at specific times and in particular places, where circumstances supported new forms of medical practice. While hospital patients might be rendered powerless, their relatives did not accept that bodies should be routinely subjected to autopsy or dissection – and in Bristol, they were furious at the removal of body parts for teaching or autopsy. Mr Scott's case shows us that while hospital patients had little power over their diagnosis and treatment, for wealthy patients the power relations typical of bedside medicine

Chapter 4 deals with the development of laboratory medicine in much greater detail.

continued to function. Patients consulted the practitioner(s) of their choice, and had expectations about how medical men would approach their cases. If their expectations were not met, they would take their custom elsewhere. While patients continued to patronize doctors, at the same time those practitioners were making use of the new knowledge and new techniques associated with hospital medicine.

References

Ackerknecht, E.H. (1967) *Medicine at the Paris Hospital*, Baltimore: Johns Hopkins University Press.

Cunningham, A. and Williams, P. (eds) (1992) *The Laboratory Revolution in Medicine*, Cambridge: Cambridge University Press.

Dreschfeld, J. (1883) 'On the diagnostic value of the tubercle bacillus', *British Medical Journal*, vol.1, pp.304–6.

Duffin, J. (1998) *To See with a Better Eye: A Life of R.T.H. Laennec*, Princeton: Princeton University Press.

Fissell, M.E. (1991) *Patients, Power and the Poor in Eighteenth-Century Bristol*, Cambridge: Cambridge University Press.

Ford, J.M.T. (ed.) (1987) *A Medical Student at St Thomas's Hospital, 1801–1802: The Weekes Family Letters*, London: Wellcome Institute for the History of Medicine.

Foucault, M. (1973) *The Birth of the Clinic*, New York: Pantheon.

Gairdner, W.T. (1848–9) review of *On Cancerous and Cancroid Growths* by J. Hughes Bennett, *Monthly Journal of Medical Science*, vol.9, pp.543–4.

Jewson, N.D. (1974) 'Medical knowledge and the patronage system in eighteenth-century England', *Sociology*, vol.8, pp.369–85.

Jewson, N.D. (1976) 'The disappearance of the sick-man from medical cosmology, 1770–1870', *Sociology*, vol.10, pp.225–44.

La Berge, A. and Hannaway, C. (1998) *Constructing Paris Medicine*, Amsterdam: Rodopi.

Laennec, R.T.H. (1821) *A Treatise on Diseases of the Chest*, London: T. & G. Underwood.

Maulitz, R. (1988) *Morbid Appearances: The Anatomy of Pathology in the Nineteenth Century*, Cambridge: Cambridge University Press.

Reiser, S.J. (1978) *Medicine and the Reign of Technology*, Cambridge: Cambridge University Press.

Richardson, R. (1988) *Death, Dissection and the Destitute*, Harmondsworth: Penguin.

Syme, J. (1865) 'Introductory lecture to a course of clinical surgery', *Lancet*, vol.2, p.526.

Source Book readings

N.D. Jewson, 'The disappearance of the sick-man from medical cosmology, 1770–1870', *Sociology*, 1976, vol.10, pp.228, 235–8 (Reading 1.1).

M.E. Fissell, *Patients, Power and the Poor in Eighteenth-Century Bristol*, Cambridge: Cambridge University Press, 1991, pp.136–7, 140, 144, 146–7 (Reading 1.2).

D.B. Weiner, *The Citizen-Patient in Revolutionary and Imperial Paris*, Baltimore: Johns Hopkins University Press, 1993, pp.177–83 (Reading 1.3).

S. Jacyna, 'Mr Scott's case: a view of London medicine in 1825' in R. Porter (ed.) *The Popularization of Medicine 1650–1850*, London: Routledge, 1992, pp.254–65 (Reading 1.4).

2

The Changing Role of the Hospital, 1800–1900

Hilary Marland

Objectives

When you have completed this chapter you should be able to:

- describe the evolution of hospitals from small-scale enterprises to major institutions;

- understand how hospitals were influenced by broader social and economic forces as well as by developments in medicine;

- show how the aims and interests of subscribers and medical staff were reflected in the work of hospitals;

- understand some of more negative interpretations of the quality of hospital care.

2.1 Introduction

From the mid-eighteenth century, right across Europe, hospitals began to take on a 'modern' form and to become the sites of healing we know today. In earlier centuries, they had been primarily places of shelter for the poor and indigent, small-scale enterprises often run on a shoestring of charitable donations and small-scale funding – bit-part actors in the supply of medical care. By the twentieth century, they had become large, numerous, highly 'medicalized' institutions with a leading role in curative medicine. How did hospitals evolve in this way? What drove these changes – was it to do solely with medical care and medical practitioners, or were wider cultural factors involved? How successful were nineteenth-century hospitals in curing their patients? This chapter attempts to answer these questions. Much of the available literature centres on hospitals in Britain, where hospitals developed in a broadly similar way to their European counterparts, although with much less government involvement. At present there are few studies comparing nineteenth- and twentieth-century hospitals in different countries, and so I focus in this chapter mainly on the British experience.

The chapter starts with a brief introduction to the hospital in 1800, showing that the roots of modern hospitals had been put down by the eighteenth century, and that they were already undergoing slow but incremental change. I then move on to explore the growth of hospitals, and the rise of specialization and specialist institutions. The shift from multi-functional organizations to institutions with a clear focus on medical and surgical care and teaching was a complex process, and was slightly different in each institution. Rather than try to give a detailed chronology of this development, therefore, I explore three of the most important aspects of hospital development – design, medical and social functions. The purposes of hospitals were concerned not simply with patient care but with the interests of their founders and funders and their medical staff. Finally, I end the chapter by looking at two 'negative' interpretations of modern hospital development: first, the 'birth of the clinic', which, it has been argued, promoted the power of scientific medicine and resulted in a downgrading of patients' engagement in the healing process; and second, the notion that hospitals did more harm than good, or at least had little impact on overall death rates and general well-being. It has been suggested that rather than curing their patients, hospitals in the eighteenth and nineteenth centuries were 'gateways to death', with high mortality rates resulting from poor standards of care and hygiene and exposure to infection.

2.2   Hospitals in 1800

By 1800, hospitals already had a long history. In Europe, they had been founded from the time of the Middle Ages, and many were still functioning in the eighteenth century. (A handful even survived in their original buildings well into the twentieth century.) Medieval hospitals were founded by the church as part of its remit to succour the sick and needy. They were paid for by endowments from rich donors. The Great Hospital at Norwich, for example, was founded in 1249 by the bishop of Norwich, Walter de Suffield. The development of hospitals throughout Europe closely followed town expansion and the growth of trade. Florence, for example, with its wealthy merchant community, had no fewer than thirty recorded institutions in 1338, geared to alleviating the condition of the poor and maintaining authority in the city. In Turin, too, the city government became involved in the administration of hospitals as part of its effort to maintain welfare provision and order. Most of these hospitals were small, 'multi-functional' institutions accommodating pilgrims and travellers, sheltering the poor, and treating the residents of monasteries and the sick of the district. Most provided minimal medical care, but patients benefited from nursing, rest and good food. There were also plague and leper hospitals, used to isolate people suffering from infectious diseases.

The seventeenth and eighteenth centuries saw a rapid expansion in the number of hospitals in Europe. This growth was made possible by new sources of funding. In continental Europe, governments became involved in hospital provision. They were inspired partly by Enlightenment thinking, which believed in the power of knowledge and reason to enhance social progress and prosperity, including the conquest of disease. At a time when a large and productive population was seen as the key to national prosperity and strength – a political theory called **mercantilism** or cameralism – European states invested in new medical services to ensure that their people were healthy and productive. Franz Xavier Fauken (1740–94), physician and chief designer of the vast new hospital in Vienna, the Allgemeines Krankenhaus, put the mercantilist argument for such a massive institution:

> The state loses nothing through the expenditure [for the hospital]; the products of the land will be used for it, and the small amount of money which will go out of the land every year for medicines which must be

imported will be generously recompensed, through the preservation of so many citizens who would otherwise perhaps have been lost or made permanently ill, and of whom one can never have too many ... since it is customary to draw conclusions concerning the health of the state from the number of useful inhabitants.

(quoted in Thompson and Goldin, 1975, pp.109–13)

New government-funded hospitals were opened across Europe. The Allgemeines Krankenhaus (Figure 2.1) was rebuilt and reopened in 1784 by Emperor Joseph II (1765–90) (Risse, 1999, pp.262–9). In Germany, the Juliusspital opened in Würzburg, and the Krankenspital in Bamberg. In Denmark, the grand Frederiks Hospital was built in Copenhagen in 1758 (Thompson and Goldin, 1975, p.115). In Sweden, too, the government began to fund hospitals. The Serafimer Hospital opened in Stockholm in 1752, and between 1765 and 1800, thirty county hospitals were built (Brandstrom and Tedebrand, 1993, pp.27–8). In France, hospitals flourished, though they had a chequered history. Research based on a source from the 1790s suggests that there were almost 2,000 hospitals by the late eighteenth century. Before the revolution, Paris hospitals were taken over by the state, but in the early nineteenth century they began once again to welcome private charity (Jones, 1989).

In contrast to the Continent, there were few hospitals in Britain. Most medieval hospitals had been abolished by Henry VIII (1509–47) in 1545. Only five hospitals

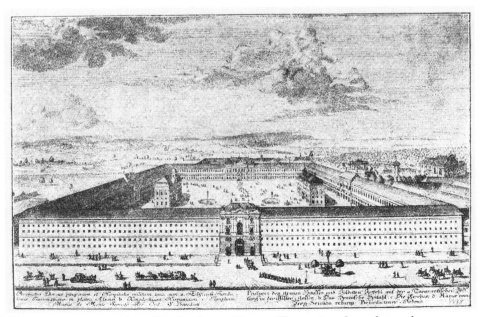

Figure 2.1   Allgemeines Krankenhaus, Vienna. The vast scale and grand appearance of the hospital was a statement about the power of the state and the concern of its leader, the emperor, for his people. The 2,000 beds were divided between the sick, the insane, pregnant women and foundlings. It was staffed by 15 physicians, 15 surgeons and 140 nurses. Wellcome Library, London

were functioning by the early eighteenth century, all in London – St Bartholomew's, St Thomas's, Christ's, Bridewell and Bethlem. They were run by the city authorities, and financed by private, lay donations, housing the old and infirm as well as the sick. A wave of new hospital-building in the eighteenth century was made possible by charitable giving, with local, private funding (hence these are often called **voluntary hospitals**) and very little state involvement. The movement to build new hospitals began with the founding of the Westminster Hospital in 1720, followed by Guy's (1724), St George's (1733), the London (1740) and the Middlesex (1745). Hospital development also took place in prosperous county towns and cathedral cities such as Winchester, Bristol, York and Bath. Large urban centres such as Liverpool, Newcastle and Manchester acquired hospitals in the late eighteenth century. Funds were collected through annual **subscriptions** – ranging from a few shillings to a few guineas – from the wealthier classes living nearby. While most of these new hospitals had some aristocratic patronage, the 'middling sort' – local gentlemen, businessmen, tradesmen, clergymen, solicitors and a small number of wealthy female subscribers – were the backbone of financial support. These subscribers took a role in the running of the hospital, providing letters of admission which testified to the character of potential patients and serving on the boards of governors, which were in overall charge of the institution. Local doctors supported hospitals by giving their services free of charge, and many also paid into the hospitals' coffers (Porter, 1989).

Whether funded by the state or by charity, eighteenth-century hospitals had a rather different function from their medieval counterparts. Increasingly, they were exclusively for the sick poor, while other institutions took over their old welfare role. Mixed institutions housing the sick, infirm, mentally ill, old and injured were reformed and their patients segregated into different classes. In France, two main types of hospital emerged: the *hôpitaux-généraux* housed all manner of problem people – the sick, foundlings, beggars, vagabonds and prostitutes – and the *hôtels-dieu* were infirmaries and refuges for the indigent poor. As hospitals gradually became places of care for the sick, they became more 'medicalized', employing doctors and nurses. In Catholic countries, nurses were drawn from religious sisterhoods such as the Daughters of Charity, who had a range of nursing skills, knew about the use of drugs and could carry out simple surgical procedures. In the British voluntary hospitals, practitioners would visit inpatients several times a week, and an apothecary or house surgeon oversaw the day-to-day care of patients. The apothecary was often joined by a matron, who devoted her time to household concerns, and by a small number of nurses. However, not all sick people would be admitted to hospitals, which were intended to serve the 'deserving poor' and 'objects deserving of charity' – primarily respectable labouring men temporarily prevented from working because of sickness and too poor to pay doctors' bills. The infirmaries excluded numerous categories from admission: children, 'incurables', domestic servants, the mentally ill, epileptics, pregnant women, consumptives, those suffering from venereal diseases or other infectious conditions, 'the chronic, terminal, or infectious' (Borsay, 1999; Risse, 1986).

The eighteenth century also saw the creation of some specialist hospitals for particular groups of patients or those suffering from specific conditions. This facilitated the treatment of large numbers of patients and, as you have read in

Chapter 1, fitted with the demands of teaching and research. Navy and army hospitals were created to preserve the health of the armed forces and to raise their morale. The Haslar Hospital, near Portsmouth (founded in 1761), had 1,884 beds, making it the largest hospital in Britain, with some wards set aside for specific disorders such as smallpox, consumption, dysentery and scurvy, as well as cells for lunatics. Lying-in hospitals, where pregnant women could have their babies under medical supervision, offered care and sanctuary. They dealt with large numbers of women, including single mothers, many of whom were domestic servants. They also provided facilities for midwives and medical students to observe women in labour. Such hospitals were set up throughout Europe, including several in London, such as the British Lying-in Hospital, the City of London, Queen Charlotte and Royal Maternity hospitals. A few fever hospitals, dealing particularly with typhus, were set up in the late eighteenth century, usually in response to severe epidemics.

In Britain, private lay philanthropy also provided for the setting up of dispensaries, which offered care to outpatients (though some did have a handful of beds for inpatients). Dispensaries treated cases of disease normally excluded from hospitals, including smallpox, measles, typhus, influenza, diarrhoea, dysentery, cholera and syphilis, as well as a wide variety of medical and surgical cases, including injuries resulting from accidents. The first General Dispensary was established in 1770 in Aldersgate Street, London, by the Quaker physician John Coakley Lettsom, and similar institutions soon followed in Stroud (1774), Bristol (1775) and Newcastle (1777) (Lane, 2001, p.90). By 1800, Britain had 38 general dispensaries with around 100,000 annual admissions (Loudon, 1981, p.324). In the late eighteenth and nineteenth centuries, many dispensaries were established in the increasingly populous and prosperous manufacturing towns of the north of England. From 1792 onwards, for example, the Doncaster Dispensary was the major provider of medical assistance in the town; Doncaster did not acquire an infirmary until 1867 (Figure 2.2). Dispensaries were organized and funded in a similar way to hospitals, but required less capital expenditure. Outpatients were much cheaper to treat than inpatients, and often only a small building was used as a base from which to run the institution.

The eighteenth-century emphasis on a medical-care function was reflected in European hospital design. Among the most influential writers on the subject was the French surgeon-anatomist and health activist Jacques Tenon (1724–1816). He pointed out that healing or medical principles had little part to play in the planning of hospitals in the past, and argued that the hospital should now become literally a medical machine, an instrument to cure, '*un instrument qui facilite la curation*'. His hugely influential *Mémoires sur les hôpitaux de Paris* (1788) presented a shocking account of conditions in French hospitals (like many reformers, he may have exaggerated in his eagerness to advocate change), and formulated new goals for these institutions. He put forward new ideas on hospital design, paying great attention to the wards, beds, windows, air volume, water supply, sewage disposal, privies, heat, light, ventilation, hygiene, food, length of stay, cost, and the role of the doctors, nurses and other personnel. Based on science and reason, Tenon's ideas informed the design of hospitals across Europe and moulded the modern, curative hospital (Thompson and Goldin, 1975, pp.135–9). The Allgemeines Krankenhaus,

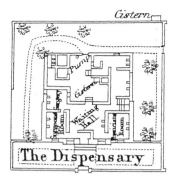

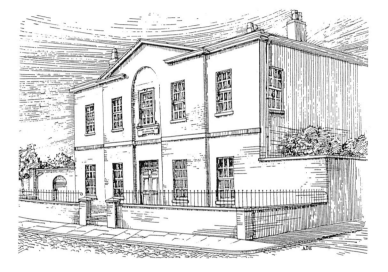

Figure 2.2   Doncaster Dispensary, 1792–1867. These images show the small and simple premises that housed the institution in the mid-nineteenth century. The building looks like a large dwelling-house. Inside, the largest space is given over to a waiting room, with smaller rooms allotted to the surgeon, physician and a surgery. Larger dispensaries might have several consulting rooms, and a separate dispensing room where the poor could collect medicines. Reproduced from Marland (1990), p.26

for example, was purpose-built with an eye to cleanliness, ventilation and the segregation of patients. It employed large numbers of physicians and surgeons, and epitomizes the transformation of the hospital into a place of healing dominated by medical aims. It became a model for hospital-building across the German-speaking countries. Major hospitals built on the same principles were opened in Prague (1789), Berlin (1768) and St Petersburg (1762–96).

2.3   The growth of hospitals

These shifts towards more intensive medical care, more specialized design and an increase in the number of hospitals continued into the nineteenth century. In Britain by the early part of the nineteenth century, no respectable town of any size would be without a hospital, while larger centres might boast several dispensaries and specialist hospitals. The number of voluntary hospitals grew dramatically. In 1861 in England and Wales, there were 230 voluntary hospitals with 14,800 beds, one-third of these in London. The number of beds tripled between 1861 and 1911. A similar pattern occurred in Holland, where the number of hospitals grew from around 80 in 1890 to 250 in 1920 (Van der Velden, 1996, p.63). Norway had just 18 hospitals in 1853, but this number had doubled by 1900.

There was also a huge expansion in the number of different types of hospital. In Britain, the old general hospitals were complemented by an increasing number and range of specialized hospitals. This was an extension of the earlier trend to set up separate wards for particular complaints, and reflected the new understanding of disease as a localized phenomenon centred on specific organs or tissues. By the 1860s, there were at least 66 specialist institutions in London, including the Royal Hospital for Diseases of the Chest (1814), St Mark's Hospital for Diseases of the Colon and Rectum (1835), the Royal Orthopaedic Hospital (1841), Great Ormond Street Hospital for Sick Children (1852) and the National Hospital for Nervous Diseases (1860). This pattern was replicated across Europe: children's hospitals were set up in Paris (1802), Berlin (1830), St Petersburg (1834) and Vienna (1837); and ophthalmology became an established area of practice, with specialist clinics and hospitals established in London, Glasgow, Paris, Utrecht and Berlin. The nineteenth century also saw the creation of small 'cottage' hospitals serving towns or villages. The first was founded in 1859. By 1875, there were 148 cottage hospitals in England and Wales, and by 1900 they provided one-tenth of the voluntary hospital beds. They offered little in the way of specialized care, only basic facilities and nursing, but they provided an important service, particularly in rural areas where they gave doctors access to hospital beds (Cherry, 1996). All these new hospitals were funded through charity. They treated the 'deserving poor', mostly working men and women. The middle and upper classes who funded them were never admitted as patients. They would not have wished to mix with poor people, or to be seen to ask for charity; instead, they received all their medical care at home.

In the late nineteenth century in Britain, the state became a major provider of hospital care for the poorest classes through **Poor Law hospitals**. From Elizabethan times, local parish authorities had collected rates to pay for the support of people unable to work – the aged, orphans, the sick and the infirm. The sick had received care and treatment in their own homes. In 1834, the ancient right to welfare was fundamentally reformed by the Poor Law Amendment Act. The New Poor Law, as it is often called, gathered the old church parishes into large unions, and established elected boards of guardians to administer all forms of welfare. The Act was passed in an effort to bring down expenditure on welfare. It sought to deter people from applying for relief. Those who could not work were housed in workhouses and were called **paupers**. They formally lost the right to vote and lived under harsh rules. Families were split up, and paupers were forced to work and wear a distinctive uniform. The architects of the New Poor Law attempted to minimize spending on the sick poor. A small number were treated at home by Poor Law medical officers; others were forced into workhouses alongside able-bodied paupers, or perhaps housed in a separate sick-ward, where they were attended by a visiting practitioner and nursed by fellow inmates. However, in the mid-1860s, a number of groups, including Poor Law medical officers, attacked these conditions and campaigned for the sick poor to be given decent medical care. Following this campaign, legislation was passed that allowed for the creation of separate Poor Law hospitals. Large hospitals were built in London, Birmingham, Leeds, Liverpool and Manchester, while smaller workhouses built separate wards for the sick. They had trained nurses, a large number of beds and vastly improved conditions (Abel Smith, 1964, pp.46–82). In 1892, the male ward in the Stockport Workhouse was staffed by just one nurse and two assistants; by 1900, the ward had one sister, one staff nurse and six trainee nurses (Pickstone, 1985, p.219). These Poor Law hospitals had to take in anyone who could not obtain care by other means. Where the voluntary hospitals dealt with the respectable working class, the Poor Law hospitals took in the chronic sick and the elderly. They provided basic care and were never as well equipped as voluntary hospitals. Steven Cherry has pointed out that while historians have often chosen to emphasize the low standards of care in Poor Law hospitals, it is important to note that the Poor Law was an important provider of hospital care; in the early twentieth century, it provided almost twice as many beds as the voluntary sector.

Over time, local government also played a greater role in the provision of other types of hospital along with many other health services (discussed in Chapter 9). From 1866, local authorities were responsible for the systematic provision of isolation hospitals to deal with infectious diseases, which greatly increased the number of beds available. Under the Local Government Act 1929, they also took over Poor Law infirmaries as municipal hospitals (Cherry, 1992, pp.44–50).

The increased role of local government in hospital provision was not confined to Britain. The introduction of compulsory sickness insurance in the late nineteenth and early twentieth centuries, and the greater municipal provision of health care, resulted in a further proliferation of hospital facilities elsewhere in Europe. Germany led the way in this development, with the introduction of '**policlinics**', dispensaries treating infants, alcoholics, and the victims of tuberculosis and sexually transmitted diseases. After 1895, tuberculosis **sanatoria** were set up in Germany, with patients' costs subsequently covered by insurance schemes.

There was a steady growth in the physical size of institutions. In the early eighteenth century, most hospitals were very small by modern standards (the Allgemeines Krankenhaus and Haslar Hospital were unusually large). The Serafimer Hospital in Stockholm grew from 8 beds in 1765 to 140 beds by 1800 (Brandstrom and Tedebrand, 1993, p.27). Leeds Infirmary, a relatively large voluntary hospital, had only 27 beds by 1771, but 60 by 1780 and 128 by 1802, serving a population of around 200,000. Overall, there was a massive increase in the numbers of hospital beds. By 1800, it was estimated that the total number of beds in voluntary hospitals was approximately 4,000, with half of these in London (Woodward, 1974, p.36). The biggest increase in the provision of hospital beds occurred after the 1860s. As you can see from Table 2.1, in England and Wales between 1861 and 1938 the total number of beds increased four-fold.

Table 2.1 Number of beds in hospitals by type of institution for England and Wales

Hospitals		1861	1891	1911	1921	1938
Teaching	Voluntary	5,291	7,228	8,284	9,584	12,610
General	Voluntary	6,658	15,184	21,651	27,443	45,397
	Public		12,138	40,927	37,840	52,974
	Total	6,658	27,322	62,578	65,283	98,371
Infectious diseases	Voluntary	238	443	160	178	195
	Public		10,314	31,786	41,415	39,256
	Total	238	10,757	31,946	41,593	39,451
Tuberculosis	Voluntary	288	1,075	4,200	7,015	7,848
	Public			1,300[1]	6,531	15,609
	Total	288	1,075	5,500	13,546	23,457
Maternity	Voluntary	139	210	311	462	3,587
	Public				2,463	6,442
	Total	139	210	311	2,925	10,029
Other special	Voluntary	2,008	4,701	6,495	9,521	15,114
	Public				26[1]	5,572
	Total	2,008	4,701	6,495	9,547	20,686
Chronic and unclassified	Voluntary	150	679	2,120	2,347	2,484
	Public	(50,000)[2]	60,778	80,260	83,731	56,015
	Total	50,150	61,457	82,380	86,078	58,499
Total	Voluntary	14,772	29,520	43,221	56,550	87,235
	Public	(50,000)	83,230	154,273	172,006	175,868
Grand total		(64,772)	112,750	197,494	228,556	263,103

[1] Probably understated
[2] The estimated number of sick poor in wards within workhouses
(Pinker, 1966, p.61)

While the number of hospital beds grew, the number of patients treated grew even more rapidly as the length of hospital stays declined. In Britain, the average time spent in hospital declined by one-third between 1861 and 1911. In Norway, the number of hospitals doubled, but the number of admissions tripled, from over 4,500 to around 15,000 (Larsen, 1996, p.78). Hospitals also always treated far higher numbers of outpatients than inpatients. In its first year of operation, Leeds Infirmary treated 89 inpatients and 272 outpatients.

2.4   The changing appearance of the hospital

The late nineteenth century saw the development of a new, specialized hospital architecture that was devised by architects who took a particular interest in building these institutions and was disseminated through books on hospital design. You read earlier how Jacques Tenon argued for the need to make the hospital environment as healthy as possible through careful design. In practice, however, design rarely lived up to Tenon's ideals. Although the architect of the new Allgemeines Krankenhaus in Vienna had tried to make the building as sanitary as possible, there were never enough lavatories, some wards could be entered only by going through other wards, he forgot to include spaces for the staff to sleep, and corridors filled with smoke from the small kitchens scattered throughout the building. The hospital had quickly acquired a bad reputation for being dirty and having high levels of mortality among both patients and staff (Risse, 1999, pp.262–5).

By the nineteenth century, the standard architectural model used for hospitals – an adapted country-house structure, with large blocks or wings arranged around courtyards – was no longer seen as healthy for hospital design. The problems of overcrowding, the predominance of serious cases, more ambitious surgery and the ageing of some of the early hospital buildings were linked to severe outbreaks of infection that came to be known by the term **hospitalism** (Bynum, 1994, pp.132–7). The cause was poorly understood – hospitalism was defined as 'a general morbid condition of the building, or of its atmosphere, productive of disease' (quoted in Porter, 1999, p.375). In the mid-nineteenth century, several investigations into the problems of hygiene and the defects of existing hospital construction were undertaken, led by the architectural journal the *Builder*. Florence Nightingale (1820–1910) became a particularly vocal advocate for a new architecture. The preface to her *Notes on Hospitals* (1863) begins:

> It may seem a strange principle to enunciate as the very first requirement in a Hospital that it should do the sick no harm. It is quite necessary, nevertheless, to lay down such a principle, because the actual mortality *in* hospitals, especially those of large crowded cities, is very much higher than any calculation founded on the mortality of the same class of diseases among patients treated *out of* hospital would lead us to expect. The knowledge of this fact first induced me to examine into the influence exercised by hospital construction on the duration and death-rate of cases received into the wards.

> (Nightingale, 1863, p.iii)

Nightingale's experiences during the Crimean War of 1854–6 helped hone her ideas on hospital organization and the layout, hygiene and ventilation of the sick wards. At Scutari, she had worked in a temporary hospital based in a huge barracks. Drains ran under the buildings, the water supply was inadequate and contaminated, and the soldier patients were laid out in vast halls. Mortality there

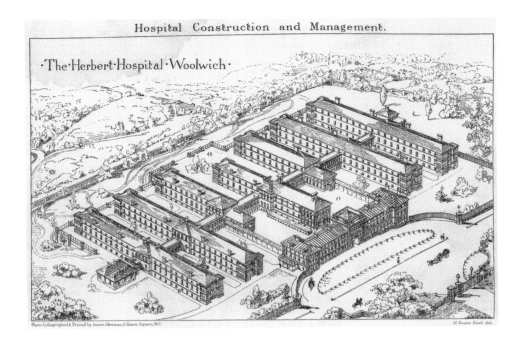

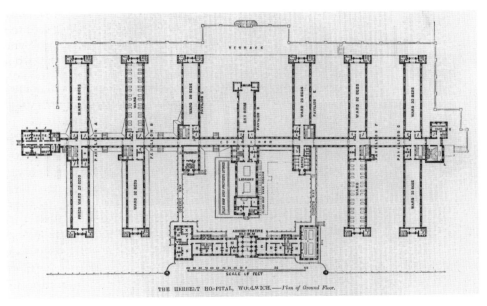

Figures 2.3 and 2.4   The Herbert Hospital, Woolwich (built 1859–64), bird's-eye view and ground plan. This was one of the first pavilion plan hospitals and clearly shows the basic layout. Built under the supervision of Florence Nightingale for the army, it accommodated 658 beds in seven parallel pavilion blocks. The administration block provided a grand entrance to the complex. Wellcome Library, London (Figure 2.3); British Architectural Library, RIBA, London (Figure 2.4)

was always much higher than in a temporary hospital built of small huts at Rentioki (Thompson and Goldin, 1975, pp.154–5). Back in Britain, Nightingale advocated the use of a 'pavilion' design for hospitals in which the wards were housed in separate blocks or pavilions. This was not a new concept – the wards at the eighteenth-century St Bartholomew's Hospital were built in separate blocks, and the Lariboisière Hospital in Paris can also be seen as a forerunner of the pavilion scheme. However, in mid-nineteenth-century pavilion designs, the number of blocks increased and wards were kept well away from any possible source of infection such as the laundry or mortuary, as well as being separated from one another to prevent infection spreading through the hospital (Figures 2.3 and 2.4). Nightingale's ideas predated the germ theory – indeed she always refused to accept that diseases might arise from specific germs but held that all diseases arose from dirt, an extreme view shared by few medical practitioners. In her vision of the ideal hospital, nurses gained a new and vital role in maintaining the highest standards of cleanliness (Figure 2.5). The first reading in this chapter is taken from Nightingale's *Notes on Hospitals*.

You will read more about Florence Nightingale's views on nursing in Chapter 6.

Exercise

Read 'Designing the ideal hospital' (Source Book 2, Reading 2.4).

1   What features are to be avoided in hospital design?

2   How would you sum up Nightingale's principles of good hospital design?

Discussion

1   According to Nightingale, stagnant air around hospital buildings should be avoided at all costs. Air will stagnate in courtyards, in crowded areas of town, and even among trees.

2   A good hospital design ensures that air is able to move freely around the buildings. For this reason, pavilion blocks should be well separated, and should be low buildings – just one or two storeys high. The wards themselves must be capable of thorough ventilation, and thus the ceilings need to be high (but not too high) and the wards not too wide. Hospitals must be equipped with good drains, which do not allow the passage of air back from the sewers into the wards (notice that Nightingale claims this 'bad air' is the cause of fevers). The drains must run well away from the buildings, and must be cleaned. Sinks and toilets are to be kept separate from the wards.

The new pavilion plan was adopted all over Europe by the end of the nineteenth century by hospital administrators eager to see that their institutions reflected the most modern thinking on design (Taylor, 1991). Eppendorf General Hospital in Hamburg, for example, built between 1885 and 1888, was based on a pavilion design with eighty-three separate blocks or buildings, arranged in streets. The spaces between the wards were filled with lawns and flowerbeds. The roomy thirty-bed wards were divided between medical, surgical and infectious cases. Offices,

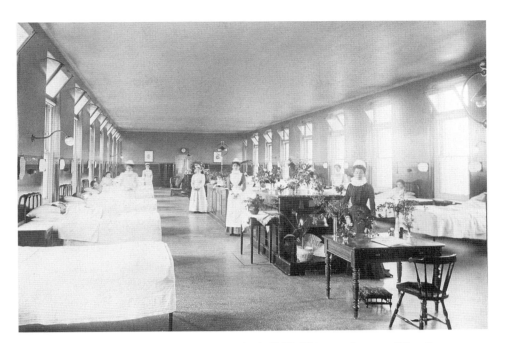

Figure 2.5 York Ward, Portsmouth Hospital, 1902. This ward exemplifies the concern with fresh air and cleanliness in the late nineteenth- and early twentieth-century hospital. Fresh air is admitted through the open windows which run down the length of the ward. The large stove (beside the sister standing in the foreground) also helps to circulate air. Notice the shiny, easily cleaned surfaces – the terrazzo floor and painted walls and ceilings. Like most hospital wards of this time, there is some attempt to make the space look more home-like, with plain furniture, plants and flowers. Some wards even had their own pianos. Wellcome Library, London

kitchens, an ice house, laundry and disinfecting house were built on one corner of the site. In an article published in the British journal the *Hospital*, the Eppendorf institution was described as 'a model hospital' and 'the best example of elaborate arrangements for the restoration of health which yet exists' (Risse, 1999, pp.427–32).

Old hospitals were adapted to take account of these new ideas and to fill the demand for more beds. At the Norfolk and Norwich Hospital, for example, the old building was turned over to administration and new pavilions added to the ends of the building (Taylor, 1997, pp.111–31). The use of the pavilion design, which required very large amounts of land, declined only in the twentieth century, when infection became less of a problem and air conditioning rendered unnecessary the use of large open spaces between wards.

By 1900, the hospital was becoming a complex of specialized spaces dedicated to different aspects of hospital work. In addition to separate wards for medical and surgical cases, and special wards for different types of complaint, large hospitals had several operating theatres, specialist departments to accommodate new equipment like X-ray machines, huge waiting halls to seat outpatients, and nurses'

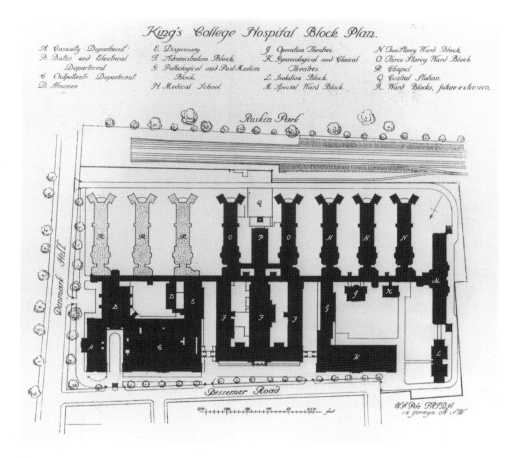

Figure 2.6   King's College Hospital, Denmark Hill, London was built just before the First World War. The plan shows how the pavilion layout could be adapted to accommodate the more complex functions of an early twentieth-century teaching hospital. As well as the central administration block and the six ward pavilions, the site includes a medical school (block H), pathology department (G), electrical department – offering various electrical treatments (B), operating theatres (J and K) and a huge outpatient's department (C). Note also the room set aside for the hospital almoner (D), who would question patients to see if they could afford to pay towards their care and put them in touch with charitable agencies if necessary. British Architectural Library, RIBA, London

homes where staff ate and slept, close to their workplace (Figure 2.6). Hospital staffs were augmented by both trained nurses and growing numbers of junior doctors who were gaining experience on the wards. This increasing complexity reflected the changing role of hospitals – which were now treating more acutely sick patients from a wider section of the population.

2.5   The medical function of hospitals

As described above, in the eighteenth century, hospitals increasingly dealt with the sick, but the sort of care they offered – attendance by local doctors and care by nurses – was no different from the treatment available to the better-off classes in their own homes. In the late nineteenth century, hospitals became centres for high-tech care of the acutely sick from all classes. Medical practitioners were responsible for driving these changes in the function of hospitals. Throughout the eighteenth and nineteenth centuries, practitioners eagerly sought posts in voluntary hospitals. While most received no payment for their services, there were multiple rewards for their efforts. A hospital post brought social prestige – hospital staff enjoyed high status within the local community. It also brought contacts with the hospital's middle- and upper-class subscribers and administrators, who might become a doctor's private patients. Sir Astley Cooper (1768–1841), the esteemed senior surgeon at Guy's Hospital in the early nineteenth century, was reputed to earn as much as £20,000 a year from his private patients, a phenomenally large sum at that time (Plate 8). The hospital also helped practitioners to establish the status of medicine, and to demonstrate their ethos of public service. A hospital position also offered practitioners the chance to see large numbers of patients and thus to hone their medical skills and perform clinical research. By the end of the century, research was crucial to promotion through the ranks of the profession, bringing better hospital positions and teaching posts. So important was a hospital post that some doctors who failed to obtain promotion set up their own specialist institutions. Such ambition drove the boom in the number of specialist hospitals in the nineteenth century. Lindsay Granshaw has described how these hospitals were relatively easy to establish and support, involving little capital expenditure: doctors simply rented part of a house and installed a few beds, a resident matron and perhaps a house surgeon (Granshaw, 1989, pp.199–220).

As you have seen in Chapter 1, at the end of the eighteenth century, hospitals were used increasingly for teaching. Students attended demonstrations, dissections and lectures. More senior students performed many of the routine medical tasks on the ward, treating some patients and dressing wounds. Vienna's Allgemeines Krankenhaus became renowned for its medical education and clinical teaching, with eighty-six of its beds devoted to teaching purposes (Risse, 1992, pp.183–6). At Guy's in London, Astley Cooper carried out his ward rounds accompanied by 'hundreds of students ... listening with almost breathless anxiety to catch the observations which fell from his lips' (quoted in Motion, 1998, p.85). The hospital's place in medical education continued to expand during the nineteenth century. Following the French example, medical education everywhere became more systematic and scientific; medical curricula in universities branched out into more fields of medicine, in what has been referred to as the 'inflation of medical learning'. Clinical teaching on hospital wards became a central aspect of training. Students studying for a medical degree spent a large part of their last years on the wards, and ambitious students stayed on in junior posts to expand their experience. Famous teachers attracted huge numbers of students, which became a source of prosperity for hospital consultants; by the nineteenth century the premium paid by each pupil of an influential London surgeon could be several hundred pounds. For this sum, pupils received individual tuition and influential contacts.

As you read in Chapter 1, the demands for teaching and research meant that practitioners wanted to admit a different class of patient from the traditional

The importance of hospital posts in building the careers of elite practitioners is discussed in Chapter 5.

These changes in medical teaching are discussed in more detail in Chapter 5.

'deserving' sick poor, most of whom suffered from chronic conditions. Rather, practitioners and students were eager to see a wide range of conditions, both acute and chronic, and especially more unusual complaints, regardless of the social background of the patient. Over the course of the century, more cases of acute illness were admitted on the grounds of medical need rather than on the social grounds of being 'deserving'. In the early nineteenth century, practitioners working in hospitals got the chance to deal with more surgical cases, as the victims of urban and industrial accidents (especially railway accidents) were brought to hospitals in increasing numbers. Hospital staff were also able to admit patients through outpatient departments. In most hospitals, the number of outpatients had always been far greater than the number of inpatients, but in the late nineteenth century, there was a steady increase in the number of people attending outpatient departments. In part, this seems to have been fuelled by demand from patients, in part by the hospitals themselves as recovering inpatients were transferred to outpatient departments (Figure 2.7 and Table 2.2). This enormous expansion in outpatient numbers became a feature of all voluntary hospitals. Indeed, the financial crisis that was to engulf hospitals in the late nineteenth century was attributed largely to overdemand by outpatients, many of whom were suspected of not being genuinely deserving cases but well able to pay for their own medical care.

Table 2.2   Inpatient and outpatient admissions to the Huddersfield Dispensary and Infirmary

Date	Population	Outpatients	Inpatients	Outpatients as % of Huddersfield township population	Inpatients as % of Huddersfield township population
1816	c.11,477	1,074	–	9.36	–
1821	13,284	1,518	–	11.43	–
1831	19,035	1,667	69	8.76	0.36
1841	25,068	3,128	192	12.48	0.77
1851	30,880	4,181	187	13.54	0.61
1861	34,877	3,787	176	10.86	0.50
1871	38,654	3,848	230	9.95	0.60

(Marland, 1987, p.105)

In the late nineteenth century, all over the country, medical practitioners gained further influence over admissions as subscribers gradually withdrew from an active role in hospital management, leaving full-time administrators to guide the work of the institutions. Even Keir Waddington, who has made an extensive study of the nineteenth-century London hospitals, admits that it is difficult to pin down exactly why medical practitioners came to take a leading role in directing the function of hospitals. Whatever the reasons, by the 1870s, doctors were sitting alongside governors on hospital committees, and enjoying growing influence. Shifting power relations were not always cordial – there were occasional conflicts

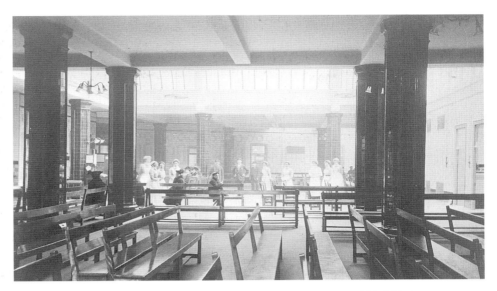

Figure 2.7   Outpatients' hall at St Bartholomew's Hospital, *c*.1908. This is an
example of the huge outpatient waiting halls built in the London teaching hospitals.
Teaching hospitals were particularly eager to find 'interesting' or unusual cases that
could be used to instruct students. As you can see from the staff standing in the
background, such departments were staffed by several doctors – usually junior
doctors – and nurses. By this time, the outpatient department would probably have
been divided according to specialty – with eye cases and women and children seen
separately. Wellcome Library, London

between medical staff and governors, and any innovation from either side was the
subject of negotiation. However, practitioners generally succeeded in persuading
governors to provide the equipment necessary to treat acutely ill patients, and to
employ more medical and nursing staff. This benefited hospitals as a whole.
Teaching hospitals wanted to be seen to be at the cutting edge of medicine, in order
to attract students. Voluntary hospitals also hoped that new and better facilities
would ensure the successful treatment of more patients – and successful hospitals
with low mortality rates were more likely to attract donations from the public
(Waddington, 2000, pp.135–88).

Anaesthesia and **antisepsis** – the use of disinfectants to kill micro-organisms –
also helped to change the face of hospital medicine. Both techniques were used in
patients' homes, but as antiseptic techniques became more complex and doctors
increasingly adopted **aseptic** techniques – the exclusion of germs from the
operating theatre – hospitals, with their specially designed operating theatres,
equipment to sterilize dressings and instruments, and trained theatre nurses,
became the favoured location for surgery. This had an enormous impact on the
workload of hospitals. *A Review of the Surgery of Huddersfield Infirmary for the
Last Twenty-Three Years* (1896), written by the infirmary's honorary surgeon
John Irving, shows how the number of operations in this relatively small West
Yorkshire institution soared from 55 in 1874 to 400 in 1895. This reflected the
introduction of new procedures, particularly in gynaecology and abdominal

The complex
impact of
anaesthesia and
antisepsis on
surgery is
examined in
Chapter 3.

surgery, and minor operations, including the removal of adenoids and tonsils. Irving called for new hospital posts to deal with the workload, with specialist appointments for eye work, abdominal surgery and gynaecology, brain surgery, operations of ear, mouth and throat, as well as general surgery.

New diagnostic technologies were developed in hospitals as part of the shift to understanding disease as a localized phenomenon that could be visualized via physical examination. The most famous example is the invention of the stethoscope by René Laennec, physician to the Necker Hospital in Paris. In 1816, after experiencing difficulties in examining a stout female patient with a suspected heart problem (or perhaps because he felt uncomfortable examining a patient of a different sex and class), Laennec developed a cylindrical device to listen to her chest. The stethoscope did not immediately catch on – George Eliot captured the controversies over its use in her novel *Middlemarch* (1871–2), where Dr Tertius Lydgate (who had studied in Paris) divided the community by his use of the stethoscope. However, it was in general use by the end of the century.

Many of the other tools which opened up the body and improved diagnostic accuracy – microscopes, thermometers, the endoscope (1807) (a device for examining the interior of the body via its orifices), laryngoscope (1829), ophthalmoscope (1851) and sphygmomanometer (a device for measuring blood pressure) (1881) – were small pieces of equipment that could be used both in hospitals and in general practice. Other new medical technologies were so large, expensive and complex to use that they were viable only in hospitals. The design of the electrocardiograph, which recorded the electrical activity of the heart, was refined in hospitals in the early twentieth century. The first electrocardiograph required five technicians to operate it, and although the mechanism became much more compact and simpler to operate by the 1930s, it was still used almost exclusively in hospitals. The use of X-rays was also based mainly in hospitals. In 1895, Wilhelm Konrad Röntgen (1845–1923), professor of physics at Würzburg, gave his first formal lecture on the properties of X-rays: by 1900, the use of X-rays had spread throughout Europe both for diagnosis – to show broken bones and locate foreign bodies – and to treat deep-seated cancers. Similarly, radium treatment for cancers, ultraviolet light therapy (called Finsen light therapy after Niels Finsen (1860–1904), who developed it) used to treat skin complaints and electrical treatments all required specialist facilities that could be provided only through hospitals. By the turn of the century, hospitals also had laboratories to help with the diagnosis of a variety of diseases.

The introduction of diagnostic laboratories is discussed in Chapter 4.

The use of new technology helped to create medical specialties that were housed in separate departments. New areas of medicine established in hospitals around the turn of the century included neurology, cardiology, pathology, dermatology, ophthalmology, gynaecology, paediatrics, and the treatment of ear, nose and throat conditions. These formed the basis for practice in specialist hospitals, but large general hospitals quickly developed their own specialist departments, fearing that they might lose students and patients. St Thomas's Hospital in London opened a throat department in 1882, a skin and ear department in 1884, and a gynaecology department in 1888. In the 1890s, the hospital added departments for dentistry, electrotherapy, X-ray, vaccination and mental diseases.

2.6   The social function of hospitals

These changes in the function of voluntary hospitals, from dealing with the deserving sick poor to treating the acutely sick, brought with them fundamental changes in the social function of the hospital, in the relationships between the institution and the community and between patients and subscribers. As you will realize from your reading in Chapter 1, hospitals were not just about helping the sick poor. The hospital was a medium for exchanges: the poor received care but were used in turn as teaching materials; and practitioners gave their services but gained prestige.

A case study of the Huddersfield Dispensary and Infirmary

The story of the development of the Huddersfield Dispensary and Infirmary, in Yorkshire, is typical in many ways of a middle-sized nineteenth-century voluntary infirmary and shows how such institutions served their local community. The Huddersfield Dispensary was set up in 1814 ostensibly to commemorate the ending of the Napoleonic wars but also to serve political ends – its establishment was driven by anxiety about the considerable distress experienced by the poor of the manufacturing districts in the economic downturn that followed the conflict. Such concerns were not unusual: many hospitals were founded to help heal class divisions. Roy Porter has gone so far as to state that 'the infirmary threw a cloak of charity over the bones of poverty and naked repression' (Porter, 1989, p.152). Peaks in the founding of infirmaries coincided with disorder; there were, for example, periods of concentrated philanthropy following the Jacobite Rising of 1745 and food riots in 1766–7 (Lane, 2001, p.82). John Pickstone has argued, on the basis of his work on the Manchester region in the nineteenth century, that infirmaries served to dampen down social unrest and produce cohesion in society not just between rich and poor but also between the propertied classes themselves. Philanthropy was a common ground where Anglicans and Nonconformists, Whigs and Tories could work together to improve the lot of the poor and raise the profile of their community (Pickstone, 1985, pp.17–19, 75).

The founding of the Huddersfield Dispensary also fulfilled civic ambitions. It was founded partly in response to a feeling that Huddersfield, a rapidly growing and ambitious woollen town, was falling behind other local communities in the provision of medical charity. This was not new: as you have read, hospitals had served a similar role from medieval times. Such ambitions were still present in nineteenth-century town halls: local government officials wanted to preside over towns with the best possible range of services as proof of their civilized status. Pickstone has described the building of hospitals in northern English industrial towns as a way of countering their image as 'frontier towns' with few amenities (Pickstone, 1985, p.142).

Perhaps the people who gained most from hospitals, however, were the subscribers who funded them. The chief supporters of the Huddersfield Dispensary were local manufacturers, who were particularly keen to direct the institution's energies towards curing not only the 'deserving poor' but those actively engaged in local industry 'who have not passed the meridian of Life ...'

(Marland, 1987, p.128). Over 2,000 cases a year were treated here, mostly people suffering from epidemic diseases and accident cases. The dispensary flourished, and within ten years its officers and management committee were pressing for the establishment of a hospital with inpatient wards, again to serve the needs of the local manufacturers – the wards would be used 'more especially for those frequent Accidents arising from the extensive Use of Machinery'. Subscribers often directly admitted their workers for treatment. For employers of labour, it was a cost-effective approach.

The dispensary's medical officers entered into the campaign for a new hospital with great enthusiasm, as can be seen in the next reading which is an extract from the appeal for funds, written by Dr Turnbull, c.1825.

Exercise

Read 'An appeal for funds' (Source Book 2, Reading 2.2). Take careful note of the reasons Dr Turnbull gives for founding a hospital, and then try to work out how these would help subscribers as well as poor patients.

Discussion

Turnbull clearly sets out a case for a hospital to serve the poor of the community: it will provide medical treatment for families who cannot afford care, and thus stop them from falling into debt. However, he describes a hospital that will benefit wealthy members of the community as well. It will increase Huddersfield's civic status – the town will have the same sort of institution as cities in Europe and (perhaps more importantly) as neighbouring Leeds. There are sound financial reasons why a hospital will benefit subscribers: by curing poor workers, it will restore them to their employment (and thus add to the profits of potential subscribers – the local manufacturers who employ them and shopkeepers who sell them goods). By treating workers, the hospital will also ensure that they do not sink into moral decay and come to rely on the poor rates (also paid by wealthier members of the community). The control of epidemic disease will protect the families of subscribers from infection.

In 1831, the Huddersfield and Upper Agbrigg Infirmary finally opened its doors with much ceremony (Figure 2.8). Another important benefit to ordinary subscribers was that, in return for their money, large events such as this, and the infirmary's annual general meetings, offered an opportunity to rub shoulders with the great and the good. In addition, subscribers' names appeared in published lists of donors, displaying their wealth and their concern for the suffering of those less fortunate than themselves. We should not, however, be entirely cynical of subscribers' motives. Well into the nineteenth century, the setting up of hospitals was still fuelled to some extent by religious motivations in a revival of charitable piety. Those most active in the charities contributed a good deal of time and effort as well as money to their chosen cause.

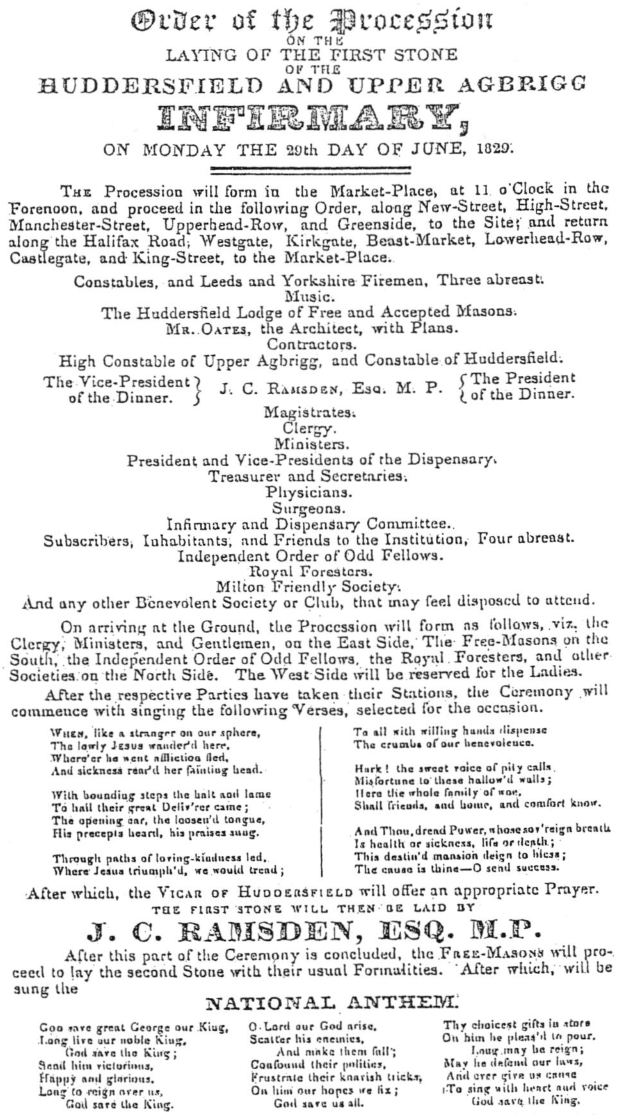

Order of the Procession
ON THE
LAYING OF THE FIRST STONE
OF THE
HUDDERSFIELD AND UPPER AGBRIGG
INFIRMARY,
ON MONDAY THE 29th DAY OF JUNE, 1829.

THE Procession will form in the Market-Place, at 11 o'Clock in the Forenoon, and proceed in the following Order, along New-Street, High-Street, Manchester-Street, Upperhead-Row, and Greenside, to the Site; and return along the Halifax Road, Westgate, Kirkgate, Beast-Market, Lowerhead-Row, Castlegate, and King-Street, to the Market-Place.

Constables, and Leeds and Yorkshire Firemen, Three abreast.
Music.
The Huddersfield Lodge of Free and Accepted Masons.
MR. OATES, the Architect, with Plans.
Contractors.
High Constable of Upper Agbrigg, and Constable of Huddersfield.
The Vice-President of the Dinner. } J. C. RAMSDEN, ESQ. M. P. { The President of the Dinner.
Magistrates.
Clergy.
Ministers.
President and Vice-Presidents of the Dispensary.
Treasurer and Secretaries.
Physicians.
Surgeons.
Infirmary and Dispensary Committee.
Subscribers, Inhabitants, and Friends to the Institution, Four abreast.
Independent Order of Odd Fellows.
Royal Foresters.
Milton Friendly Society.
And any other Benevolent Society or Club, that may feel disposed to attend.

On arriving at the Ground, the Procession will form as follows, viz. the Clergy, Ministers, and Gentlemen, on the East Side. The Free-Masons on the South, the Independent Order of Odd Fellows, the Royal Foresters, and other Societies on the North Side. The West Side will be reserved for the Ladies.

After the respective Parties have taken their Stations, the Ceremony will commence with singing the following Verses, selected for the occasion.

WHEN, like a stranger on our sphere,
The lowly Jesus wander'd here,
Where'er he went affliction fled,
And sickness rear'd her fainting head.

With bounding steps the halt and lame
To hail their great Deliv'rer came;
The opening ear, the loosen'd tongue,
His precepts heard, his praises sung.

Through paths of loving-kindness led,
Where Jesus triumph'd, we would tread;

To all with willing hands dispense
The crumbs of our benevolence.

Hark! the sweet voice of pity calls,
Misfortune to these hallow'd walls;
Here the whole family of woe,
Shall friends, and home, and comfort know.

And Thou, dread Power, whose sov'reign breath
Is health or sickness, life or death;
This destin'd mansion deign to bless;
The cause is thine—O send success.

After which, the VICAR OF HUDDERSFIELD will offer an appropriate Prayer.
THE FIRST STONE WILL THEN BE LAID BY
J. C. RAMSDEN, ESQ. M.P.

After this part of the Ceremony is concluded, the FREE-MASONS will proceed to lay the second Stone with their usual Formalities. After which, will be sung the

NATIONAL ANTHEM.

GOD save great George our King,
Long live our noble King,
God save the King;
Send him victorious,
Happy and glorious,
Long to reign over us,
God save the King.

O Lord our God arise,
Scatter his enemies,
And make them fall;
Confound their politics,
Frustrate their knavish tricks,
On him our hopes we fix;
God save us all.

Thy choicest gifts in store
On him be pleas'd to pour.
Long may he reign;
May he defend our laws,
And ever give us cause
To sing with heart and voice
God save the King.

N. B. Constables will be stationed to prevent the Ground from being occupied by Persons who do not join in the Procession.

MR. BOWER has kindly agreed to form and conduct the Procession.

T. KEMP, PRINTER, NEW-STREET, HUDDERSFIELD.

Figure 2.8   Order of procession at the laying of the foundation stone of Huddersfield Infirmary, 1829. This order of procession encapsulates how a charitable infirmary drew together the middle and upper classes of a town, and local societies and institutions – the ranks of society who not only took a leading role in all sorts of civic matters, but also traditionally supported hospitals. The most important people at the ceremony (who follow the musical band and the architect) are the local member of parliament, magistrates, clergymen and ministers. The medical staff follow the lay governors of the existing Huddersfield Dispensary, and its subscribers (who may well become subscribers to the new infirmary) are also given a prominent position. Notice the religious and patriotic elements of the ceremony

Exercise

Read the first part of 'Rules for the admission and discharge of patients' (Source Book 2, Reading 2.1). Who controls entry to the hospital? Is it the administrators or the medical staff?

Discussion

Clearly, the recommendation from a subscriber is the key to gaining admission to the hospital: this can be seen not only in the content of the extract but in the ordering and detail of the points discussed. By contrast, the medical staff have very little control over the admission of patients – they have powers to admit only a limited number of accident cases. The physical condition of applicants also has little effect on their chances of admission – it is the admitting board that has the authority to decide which of the patients recommended by medical staff should be granted entry. Medical criteria also seem to have little effect on patients' discharge – two months is the standard length of stay. (Note the long list of conditions that are not to be treated in the infirmary.)

Some historians have seen the hospital as a means for middle-class subscribers to impose their morals and standards of behaviour on working-class patients: the sick poor would emerge from hospital not just cured of their physical ills but having learned how to behave, as can be seen in the next reading, which is again taken from the rules and regulations of the Huddersfield Infirmary.

Exercise

Read the last two parts of 'Rules for the admission and discharge of patients' (Source Book 2, Reading 2.1). What do they suggest about the medical condition of patients? Do you agree that rules like these were an attempt to impose codes of behaviour on patients?

Discussion

The rules suggest that patients are not lying ill in bed, but are able to move around. Some of the regulations seem geared to medical concerns, such as requiring patients to obey the medical staff. Others, such as the prohibition on swearing or playing cards and the requirement to attend religious service on Sundays, seem to have no medical function, and thus must be directed towards maintaining moral order within the infirmary. The concern about controlling patients' behaviour just outside the infirmary, in the garden, suggests the administrators' keenness to ensure that outside observers view the hospital as an orderly institution.

Changing social relations

By the late nineteenth century, the network of social relationships mediated through the hospital had altered radically. In Britain, the state had taken over the responsibility of caring for the very poor in infirmaries run by the Poor Law, although funded from rates (effectively a tax on the wealthier classes who had previously funded voluntary hospitals). Voluntary hospitals continued to care for the poor, but subscribers no longer controlled access to hospitals – admission was now made on the basis of medical and training needs, not social criteria. Nevertheless, voluntary hospitals maintained some of their old social functions. New hospitals continued to embody civic pride, with impressive frontages and architectural details such as clocks and towers, but as subscribers ceased to play a leading role in running the hospitals, the grand rooms that had accommodated subscribers' meetings were replaced by more modest offices for administrators. Subscribers still gained social status through their connections with a hospital, and more opportunities to meet their social superiors as hospitals devised new methods of fund-raising. In Huddersfield, the infirmary remained a key focus of charitable enterprise in the town. While the chief sources of revenue continued to be annual subscriptions, donations and legacies, funds were also raised through charitable events such as infirmary balls, concerts, dinners, bazaars and sermons.

In the late nineteenth century, many hospitals faced financial crises as the costs of hospital care rose steeply. From the outset, indeed, the Huddersfield Infirmary was in economic difficulties: the total setting-up cost had been a massive £7,500. More staff than expected had been required to cope with the workload, and running costs were more than £1,500 per annum, twice the estimate of the founders. Thereafter, costs continued to rise, despite the best efforts of shrewd infirmary managers who kept salaries to a minimum, insisted that local suppliers of drugs, foodstuffs and alcoholic beverages, coal and furniture competed for tenders, and most importantly kept subscriptions and other sources of income coming in to the charity's coffers (Figure 2.9). Increasingly high-tech care brought hospitals further financial problems: more specialized treatment facilities, such as operating theatres, elaborate X-ray machines and more nurses, were expensive. At the same time, hospitals were deeply concerned about 'charity abuse' – patients who could afford to pay for their care seeking admission to hospitals or using outpatient departments.

In Chapter 13 you can read more about the entry of middle-class patients to hospitals.

Increasingly, hospitals expected patients to pay towards their care. The established voluntary hospitals were slow to turn to patients as a source of funding, fearing that instituting charges might threaten their charitable status and discourage traditional donors. However, from the 1870s, more and more hospitals provided special facilities for wealthy patients who paid directly for their care. Some hospitals accommodated private patients in general wards; others built private wards or private rooms, which were made as home-like as possible, with more comfortable furnishings than the general wards. Private care was expensive. In the 1880s, accommodation, nursing and basic medical care cost from 1 to 3 guineas (£1.05–£3.15) per week, but in return patients received care and privacy. Private patients were not as a rule used as teaching material. By 1890, half of London's hospitals admitted paying patients. In continental Europe, private

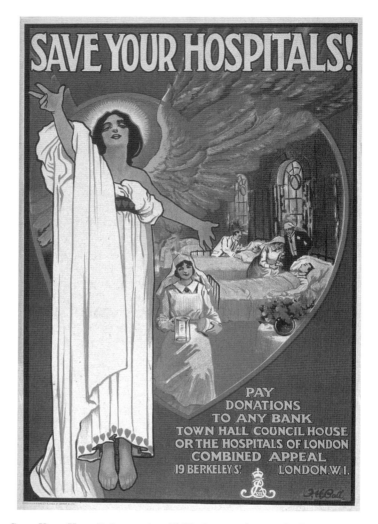

Figure 2.9   Save Your Hospitals, poster, 1922. An angel appeals for funds to support a busy hospital ward, where both a doctor and nurses tend to patients. The stress on 'your' hospital catches the desire that all classes – rich and poor – should feel that they have some collective responsibility to keep hospitals working. The image of the angel may seem odd in a purely secular context, but it carries many positive messages – connotations of mercy and aid to the suffering, a divine status that lifts the appeal above financial squabbles and the increasingly commercial nature of hospitals, and a reference to the important role of churches in philanthropy. Wellcome Library, London

hospitals were founded to give access to hospital care to the better off. In Britain, cottage hospitals in rural areas always encouraged contributions from patients towards the cost of treatment. Sir Henry Burdett (1847–1920), a champion of cottage hospitals, saw them as providing 'against indiscriminate charity relief' and as securing justice for the medical profession, who were now allowed to treat their own private patients in hospital (Granshaw, 1992, p.209).

By the twentieth century, even working-class patients were expected to pay something towards the cost of their care. Hospitals appointed almoners to ascertain the extent to which patients were able to contribute to the hospital. Working-class patients also gained access through contributory schemes such as 'Saturday funds'. Donations, often as little as 1d (0.042p), were collected through workplaces, providing some donors with preferential (if not guaranteed) access to hospitals. The Norfolk and Norwich Hospital Saturday Fund, for example, established in 1919, provided regular donors and their families with free hospital treatment so long as they had been referred for treatment by their general practitioner and held a voucher from their fund secretary. In some areas, the working classes became major supporters of hospitals. In the 1920s, well over half of the Norfolk and Norwich Hospital's patients belonged to the scheme, and receipts made a crucial contribution to the institution's finances. Across England and Wales, the income derived from contributory schemes rose from around 4 per cent in the 1900s to almost 30 per cent in the 1930s. Overall, contributory schemes, pay beds and contributions towards the costs of care provided an ever larger slice of hospital incomes (Cherry, 1997, p.319).

These changes meant that by 1900, voluntary hospitals had subtly altered their status, from charities serving poor patients and wealthy subscribers to institutions that combined some charity work with the selling of medical services directly to the rich and indirectly to the working classes through contributory schemes.

2.7 Gateways to death? Critical views of nineteenth-century hospitals

Although we now think of hospitals as institutions that provide, or should provide, first-class care, a number of historians have questioned whether the care provided in eighteenth- and nineteenth-century hospitals really benefited patients. Commentators, particularly Michel Foucault, have argued that patients paid for their care by surrendering control over their bodies. In his book *The Birth of the Clinic* (1973), Foucault described how medical practice began to embody what he termed the 'clinical gaze': practitioners saw their patients as clinical objects showing signs of pathology rather than individual subjects with complex histories. As you have seen in Chapter 1, Foucault and Jewson have argued that the modern hospital effectively silenced the patient. The 'objective' technological measurements of temperature or pulse and the medical case history replaced the 'subjective' testimony of patients, leaving them powerless to discuss their case or treatment.

Did patients feel the same in the nineteenth century? It is difficult to prove that hospital staff did or did not ignore the feelings of their patients. Judging by their writings, some practitioners appear to have had a callous attitude. Friedrich Benjamin Osiander (1759–1822), professor of obstetrics at the university hospital in Göttingen, declared in 1794, 'The hospital is not here to serve the patients, but the patients to serve the hospital':

> [T]he pregnant and delivering women who are admitted to our hospital are regarded, as it were, as living manikins, with which everything is done that is useful for the students and midwives and that facilitates the labour

of childbirth (always however with the greatest protection for the health and life of the patients and their children).

(quoted in Schlumbohm, 2001, p.73)

On the other hand, in the early nineteenth century the medical student and poet John Keats graphically described his repugnance at seeing the suffering of patients on the wards at St Thomas's and Guy's hospitals in London. At this period, Astley Cooper's attitude to hospital patients was described as being marked by 'a tenderness of voice and expression, and with an interest so clearly depicted in his manner, that he at once acquired [their] confidence, respect and gratitude' (Cooper, 1843, vol.2, p.78).

It is equally hard to discover if patients felt powerless during their time spent in hospital. There are very few accounts of hospital life from the patient's perspective. One that does survive was written by Margaret Mathewson, who was admitted to the Royal Infirmary in Edinburgh with an infection in her shoulder and used as the subject of a clinical lecture. We need to be cautious in using Mathewson's diary, however, as it was written for a specific purpose – as a testament to her Christian faith – and so gives a rather partial picture of hospital life. The next reading is made up of extracts from her detailed account of the routine of ward life, including a reminder that the introduction of anaesthesia did not alter the pain and discomfort experienced after operations (indeed, the side effects of chloroform added to post-operative discomfort).

Exercise

Read 'The patient's experience' (Source Book 2, Reading 2.3). How does Mathewson feel about her care, and about being used as a subject for clinical teaching?

Discussion

Mathewson actually describes little of her own feelings. She does, however, record her great fear at the prospect of being the subject of a clinical lecture, and her terror at discovering the plan for the operation on her shoulder. However, she records no resentment towards the doctors for this, or for the fact that they keep her waiting unnecessarily when she is not used in that day's clinical teaching, or for the great pain they inflict while dressing her wound. Mathewson may feel powerless but she seems to have no expectation of any power – she neither questions nor complains about any aspect of her treatment, or even the assumption that she will work preparing dressings and bandages. We might speculate that Mathewson wishes to present a picture of Christian submission to her sufferings or, as Foucault and Jewson suggest, that she sees herself participating in a sort of unwritten contract. In return for causing discomfort and fear, Lister might be able to save her arm.

Other research by historians suggests that patients' experiences of, and feelings towards, hospitals varied quite markedly. Some patients so resented hospital rules and regulations that they discharged themselves. Such resentment was more likely to occur in the larger hospitals, which became massive 'medicalized' institutions, and was less common in smaller ones with only a handful of inpatient beds and where doctors' access to patients was limited. In such hospitals, the charitable imperative remained paramount, with social rather than medical considerations dictating admissions.

Another criticism levelled at nineteenth-century hospitals was that far from curing patients, they were likely to kill them. In the 1970s, Thomas McKeown, a professor of social medicine (and therefore inclined to associate good health with social conditions rather than with medical treatment), claimed that nineteenth-century hospitals 'positively did harm'. However, in 1974, John Woodward set out a comprehensive challenge to McKeown's conclusions. The final reading for this chapter is an extract from the conclusion to Woodward's book, *To Do the Sick No Harm*.

Exercise

Read 'Gateways to death?' (Source Book 2, Reading 2.5).

I   Why does Woodward dismiss the evidence of high hospital mortality, and what sources does he use to prove his thesis?

2   Does anything in Woodward's account make you doubt these figures?

Discussion

I   Woodward argues that claims of very high mortality in nineteenth-century hospitals are based on false evidence. In the first place, he states, there has been a misrepresentation of hospitals' procedures for the admission, segregation and refusal of patients suffering from infectious diseases. Second, he argues that statistics have been misread, by contemporary as well as modern commentators. High rates of surgical mortality in the early nineteenth century are assumed to mean that mortality in the earlier period was even higher, and Florence Nightingale simply used an invalid method to arrive at her mortality figure of 90 per cent. Woodward himself uses mortality figures issued by the hospitals themselves in their published reports, and finds that mortality varied between individual hospitals, ranging from 2 to 10 per cent.

2   In his discussion of the reasons for the variation in mortality between institutions, Woodward points out that the hospitals – which depended on charitable contributions for their existence – had a strong interest in keeping the mortality statistics as low as possible in order to emphasize the value of the institution. They would therefore refuse admission to patients who were likely to die, and some hospitals specialized in treating non-life-threatening conditions. Even so, Woodward concludes that hospitals successfully treated large numbers of patients.

2.8   Conclusion

By the twentieth century, patients saw the hospital as the main provider of specialized care. This was an enormous shift in perception from the eighteenth century, when hospitals were seen largely as places of shelter and succour. From being marginal in health care, they became the focus of expertise and high-tech equipment. For doctors, hospitals became the places where they were taught, where they saw many of their patients and where they gained experience. They represent the pinnacle of medical achievement.

While it is easy to see massive changes between 1800 and 1900, strong continuities between nineteenth-century hospitals and their predecessors should not be overlooked. The shift to providing high-quality medical care was not a nineteenth-century phenomenon but was firmly rooted in the eighteenth century. By isolating the sick, medieval leper and plague hospitals had served to protect other citizens from infection, just as fever and cholera hospitals would in the nineteenth century, and infectious disease hospitals and tuberculosis sanatoria in the twentieth. The idea of using hospitals to alleviate the condition of the poor and to dampen down discord was a motivation for hospital-building before the eighteenth century and well into the nineteenth century. In the nineteenth century, the hospital continued to have a welfare function: patients were still admitted on social grounds, because they were poor and needy as well as ill. It could even be argued that this kind of multi-functionalism survives into the twenty-first century, as hospitals still serve a welfare role, sheltering the weak and elderly where other facilities are not provided. This mixing of welfare and medical functions is one of the themes you might like to consider as you work through material on hospitals in later chapters. What were the purposes of hospitals, and what did hospitals actually do?

References

Abel Smith, B. (1964) *The Hospitals, 1800–1948: A Study of Social Administration in England and Wales*, London: Heinemann.

Borsay, A. (1999) *Medicine and Charity in Georgian Bath: A Social History of the General Infirmary, c.1739–1830*, Aldershot: Ashgate.

Brandstrom, A. and Tedebrand, L.-G. (eds) (1993) *Health and Social Change: Disease, Health and Public Care in the Sundsvall District 1750–1950*, Umea: Umea Demographic Database, University of Umea.

Bynum, W.F. (1994) *Science and the Practice of Medicine in the Nineteenth Century*, Cambridge: Cambridge University Press.

Cherry, S. (1992) *Medical Services and the Hospitals in Britain, 1860–1939*, Cambridge: Cambridge University Press.

Cherry, S. (1996) 'Change and continuity in the cottage hospitals c.1859–1948: the experience in East Anglia', *Medical History*, vol.36, pp.271–89.

Cherry, S. (1997) 'Before the National Health Service: financing the voluntary hospitals, 1900–1939', *Economic History Review*, vol.2, pp.305–26.

Cooper, B.B. (1843) *The Life of Sir Astley Cooper, Bart*, 2 vols, London: John W. Parker.

Foucault, M. (1973) *The Birth of the Clinic*, New York: Pantheon.

Granshaw, L. (1989) 'Fame and fortune by means of bricks and mortar: the medical profession and specialist hospitals in Britain' in L. Granshaw and R. Porter (eds) *The Hospital in History*, London: Routledge, pp.199–220.

Granshaw, L. (1992) 'The rise of the modern hospital in Britain' in A. Wear (ed.) *Medicine in Society*, Cambridge: Cambridge University Press, pp.197–218.

Jones, C. (1989) *The Charitable Imperative: Hospitals and Nursing in Ancien Régime and Revolutionary France*, London: Routledge.

Lane, J. (2001) *A Social History of Medicine: Health, Healing and Disease in England, 1750–1950*, London: Routledge.

Larsen, O. (1996) *The Shaping of a Profession: Physicians in Norway, Past and Present*, Canton: Science History Publications.

Loudon, I. (1981) 'The origins and growth of the dispensary movement in England', *Bulletin of the History of Medicine*, vol.55, pp.322–42.

Marland, H. (1987) *Medicine and Society in Wakefield and Huddersfield 1780–1870*, Cambridge: Cambridge University Press.

Marland, H. (1990) *Sickness, Charity and Society*, Doncaster: Waterdale, in association with Doncaster Library Services, occasional paper no.3.

Motion, A. (1998) *Keats*, London: Faber.

Nightingale, F. (1863) *Notes on Hospitals*, London: Longman, Green, Longman, Roberts & Green.

Pickstone, J.V. (1985) *Medicine and Industrial Society: A History of Hospital Development in Manchester and its Region, 1752–1946*, Manchester: Manchester University Press.

Pinker, R. (1966) *English Hospital Statistics 1861–1938*, London: Heinemann Educational.

Porter, R. (1989) 'The gift relation: philanthropy and provincial hospitals in eighteenth-century England' in L. Granshaw and R. Porter (eds) *The Hospital in History*, London: Routledge, pp.149–78.

Porter, R. (1999) *The Greatest Benefit to Mankind: A Medical History of Humanity from Antiquity to the Present*, London: Fontana.

Risse, G.B. (1986) *Hospital Life in Enlightenment Scotland: Care and Teaching at the Royal Infirmary of Edinburgh*, Cambridge: Cambridge University Press.

Risse, G.B. (1992) 'Medicine in the age of Enlightenment' in A. Wear (ed.) *Medicine in Society: Historical Essays*, Cambridge: Cambridge University Press.

Risse, G.B. (1999) *Mending Bodies, Saving Souls: A History of Hospitals*, Oxford: Oxford University Press.

Schlumbohm, J. (2001) 'The pregnant women are here for the sake of the teaching institution: the lying-in hospital of Göttingen University', *Social History of Medicine*, vol.14, pp.59–78.

Taylor, J. (1991) *Hospital and Asylum Architecture in England 1840–1914*, London: Mansell.

Taylor, J. (1997) *The Architect and the Pavilion Hospital: Dialogue and Design Creativity in England 1850–1914*, London: Leicester University Press.

Thompson, J.D. and Goldin, G. (1975) *The Hospital: A Social and Architectural History*, New Haven: Yale University Press.

Van der Velden, H. (1996) 'The Dutch health services before the compulsory health insurance, 1900–1941', *Social History of Medicine*, vol.9, pp.49–68.

Waddington, K. (2000) *Charity and the London Hospitals, 1850–1898*, Woodbridge: Boydell.

Woodward, J. (1974) *To Do the Sick No Harm: A Study of the British Voluntary Hospital System to 1875*, London: Routledge & Kegan Paul.

Source Book readings

Rules and Regulations of the Huddersfield and Upper Agbrigg Infirmary, 1834, Huddersfield Public Library, Kirklees District Archives and Local Studies Department, B.362, pp.16–20 (Reading 2.1).

W. Turnbull, *An Appeal on Behalf of the Intended Hospital at Huddersfield*, Kirklees Central Library, Local History, Tomlinson Collection, *c.*1825, pp.1–3 (Reading 2.2).

M. Goodman, *Lister Ward*, Bristol: Adam Hilger, 1987, pp.36–7, 49–50, 58–9, 64–5, 67, 78–80, 84 (Reading 2.3).

F. Nightingale, *Notes on Hospitals*, London: Longman, Green, Longman, Roberts & Green, 1863, pp.32–6, 43–4 (Reading 2.4).

J. Woodward, *To Do the Sick No Harm: A Study of the British Voluntary Hospital System to 1875*, London: Routledge & Kegan Paul, 1974, pp.123–36, 139–40, 142 (Reading 2.5).

3

The Emergence of Modern Surgery

Thomas Schlich

Objectives

When you have completed this chapter you should be able to:

- describe the occupational changes in surgery that turned it from a separate craft into a specialist field within the medical profession;

- understand the development of surgical concepts of disease and the body and their role in changing the outlook of modern medicine;

- describe the major developments in surgical techniques;

- understand the relationships between professional, conceptual and technical changes in surgery;

- explain how these developments have been interpreted and presented by historians.

3.1   Introduction: modern surgery as a historical issue

Modern surgery as we know it has come into being during the last 200 years. In 1800, surgeons were in the process of shedding their artisan status as they began routinely to acquire formal training in medical theory and practical skills. They were breaking away from the barbers and bloodletters, the occupations with which they had traditionally been grouped. Surgeons' field of activity was restricted to the body surface: they dealt with lesions and injuries, often in emergency situations. Major operations such as the amputation of limbs or the removal of stones from the bladder were excruciatingly painful and had low survival rates. Surgeons performed these operations in patients' homes or hospital wards, wearing their everyday clothes.

By 1930, surgery had reached its golden age. Surgeons were not only acknowledged as doctors and scientists, but they were even considered to be modern heroes. The operating theatre had become the glittering centre of the modern hospital, a place where miracles could happen. Surgeons now operated on all parts of the body, including the thorax and the skull, repairing bones, removing tumours and restoring complicated internal body structures. They were consulted about the treatment of a wide range of diseases, internal and external, and their spectacular successes outshone all other branches of medicine. In short, surgery had become the most important but least questioned technology of body manipulation.

What had happened during this time? How did modern surgery become a prestigious and important field of activity? Until recently, historians saw the rise of surgery as a story of technical progress. According to this narrative, surgery succeeded simply because great surgeons invented new techniques to solve a growing number of medical problems. The history of surgery consisted of a series of pioneering operations. This enumeration of surgery's technical achievements implicitly privileges technology and individual achievement as the driving forces of surgical history. Examples of this effect are Roy Porter's passages on the history of surgery in *The Greatest Benefit to Mankind* (Porter, 1999, pp.597–627).

Historiography is discussed in detail in the introduction.

However, the **historiography** – historians' understanding of the subject or period – has moved on, and they have looked at different aspects of the history of surgery. Historians have linked the changes in surgical practice to conceptual and professional changes (Gelfand, 1980; Lawrence, 1992). They have also elucidated the underlying rationale of surgical techniques such as psycho-surgery (Pressman, 1998) or organ transplantation (Schlich, 1998), and have emphasized connections between surgery and other developments in modern societies (Cooter, 1993; Gilman, 1999; Schlich, 2002). In doing so, they have put forward proposals for a restructuring of the narrative of the history of surgery (Tröhler, 1993).

To counteract the implicit technological bias that underlies the traditional way of telling the story, I have deliberately chosen to discuss technical aspects at the end of this chapter, even though the development of new techniques was important in shaping other areas of the history of surgery. In the first part of the chapter, I look at the professional dimension and examine how surgeons entered the medical profession; the second part is devoted to a study of the parallel development of surgical concepts; and in the final part I look at how the developments in these first two dimensions went hand in hand with changes on the technical level.

In addition to presenting the essential facts of what happened to these three aspects of surgery, I discuss the importance of different types of historical explanation and examine how professional, conceptual and technical developments were interwoven and interdependent. Did technical progress elevate the professional position of surgeons, or was it the other way round? Were new concepts of body and disease the reason why new surgical techniques were developed? Or was the newly acquired technical competency the basis of new concepts of body and disease?

3.2 Profession

Masters and apprentices: surgery as a craft

The high status that surgeons enjoy today is of relatively recent origin. In the medieval west, physicians and surgeons belonged to separate occupational groups with separate fields of responsibility. Surgeons had the status of craftsmen: they were organized in guilds and were often linked with other crafts, such as barbers, apothecaries and grocers. Their sphere of work was basically the treatment of the exterior of the body. This included all kinds of procedures, from shaving and bloodletting to applying ointments and pulling teeth. A representative list of the tasks performed by ordinary surgeons in eighteenth-century Paris includes:

> treating cuts, bruises, ulcers and other superficial lesions, lancing boils and abscesses, excising skin tumours, removing foreign bodies from wounds and body orifices, reducing nonstrangulated hernias with trusses and external manipulations, setting fractures, reducing dislocations, treating venereal diseases, and applying external medications to a wide variety of visible ailments.
>
> (Gelfand, 1980, pp.39–40)

Only a few of the several hundred Paris master surgeons performed major operations such as amputations, removal of bladder stones, trepanation (the removal of bone from the skull, probably to relieve pressure on the brain), eye surgery and, most difficult, operations on strangulated hernias. (A non-strangulated hernia happens when a piece of tissue or part of an organ protrudes through the lining of the body cavity. It retains a blood supply and can be physically manipulated back into place. In a strangulated hernia, the blood supply to the protruding tissue or organ is cut off. This means it cannot be dealt with by manipulation and is very dangerous.) Operative surgery thus mostly dealt with problems close to the body's surface. Operations were resorted to only in emergency situations or for conditions that were extremely painful and debilitating.

But not all surgeons kept within the official boundaries of their craft: many did not restrict themselves to external treatment and unofficially practised internal medicine as well. Being much more numerous, and therefore more accessible, than physicians, surgeons played a central role in the provision of general health-care services in most of Europe until the second half of the nineteenth century. Physicians, who were fewer in number and charged higher fees, were an elite group enjoying the relatively high status of university-educated scholars. They regarded surgeons not as colleagues but as subordinates whose proper function consisted in following their orders in the performance of manual procedures. Learned physicians likened their relationship with surgeons and apothecaries to that of a general marshalling his soldiers or an architect supervising masons and carpenters. Characteristic of the superior attitude physicians adopted towards surgeons was a remark attributed to Guy-Crescent Fagon (1638–1718), premier physician to Louis XIV (1643–1715). In 1701, the surgeon Georges Mareschal (1658–1736) operated on Fagon for bladder stone. When the surgeon proffered advice on the post-operative regimen, the physician replied, 'I needed your hand, but I do not need your head' (Gelfand, 1980, p.42).

Although they found their social peers among artisans, not all surgeons were of low status, as some historians tend to portray them. A few surgeons were quite wealthy and thoroughly conversant with the theory of medicine (Sander, 1989).

Students and professors: surgery as a medical specialty

During the late seventeenth and eighteenth centuries, across most of northern Europe, surgeons gained in economic and political power. The wide range of procedures once carried out by surgeons was split up, as surgery was dissociated from barbering and its traditional trade links. In London, for example, the Company of Surgeons split from the barbers in 1745. At the same time, surgical training went through radical change. Traditionally, surgeons were equipped for practice by an apprenticeship lasting several years. An apprentice would follow his master in his work, gradually picking up the skills of surgery. In the late eighteenth century, apprenticeship was supplemented and eventually replaced by formal training at hospitals, public lectures and private anatomy schools, where students were taught courses in surgery, physiology, pathology, midwifery, and the diseases of women and children. New surgical schools were established by the state and old ones expanded. The Paris surgical school at Saint-Côme had a new amphitheatre built in 1691 when it became clear that the old building of 1615 could no longer accommodate the crowds of 700–800 young surgeons wishing to attend the public demonstrations. The construction, which was completed in 1695, was magnificent and stunned contemporaries (Gelfand, 1980, p.33) (Figure 3.1).

Chapter 5 explores the ways in which the training of physicians also changed at this time.

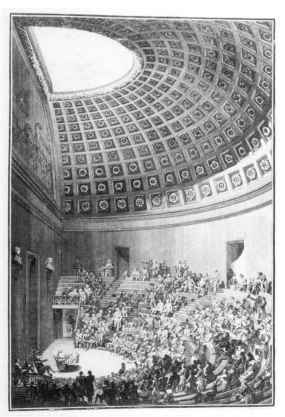

Figure 3.1   Main amphitheatre of the Paris college of surgery, as depicted by the architect Jacques Gondoin (1780). Wellcome Library, London

As a result of these changes, a surgeon's education increasingly resembled that of a physician, with its emphasis on lectures and book-based learning. Let us consider the consequences of the new pattern of training for surgery as a profession. Previously, surgical education had been organized in an essentially private arrangement between teacher and pupil. Apprentice surgeons were educated by a single master who taught his pupils whatever he knew. The existence of surgical schools, by contrast, made the content as well as the form of education a matter of collective consensus. A common education presupposes, first, the existence of a body of theoretical knowledge that is recognized as being necessary to competent practice, and second, which is equally important, sufficient professional coherence and organization to standardize that knowledge and present it to large groups of students. Training at large institutions required the surgical community to agree on uniform standards for entry into practice (Gelfand, 1980, p.83).

In principle, surgery had two possible institutional frameworks by which it might become a liberal profession: it could remain separate and autonomous, or it could merge with medicine. In the early stages, the first path was followed in most European university centres, with the creation of surgical schools. Before long, however, the military need for practitioners with the skills of both physicians and surgeons led Enlightenment monarchs to found schools that taught both medicine and surgery. In 1724, Frederick William I of Prussia (1786–97) founded a Collegium Medico-Chirurgicum in Berlin. Similarly, the Josephinum, established in Vienna in 1781, was a comprehensive, lavishly endowed school of medicine and surgery controlled by surgeons. Related institutions were set up in Dresden, St Petersburg and Copenhagen (Gelfand, 1980, p.154).

In France, surgery and medicine were officially united in the 1790s when the state established three medical schools (*écoles de santé*) in Paris, Montpellier and Strasbourg, bringing together medical and surgical training. The Paris school was famous and much admired. Visiting foreign students and doctors, like Joseph Frank, a young German doctor who was in Paris in 1802, considered the 'reunion of medical and surgical instruction' to be one of the outstanding innovations of the revolutionary medical school (Gelfand, 1980, p.167).

You may find it helpful to refer to the map of German states (Plate 3) throughout this chapter.

In other countries, the shift from artisan to university-trained surgery happened more gradually. In the German-speaking lands (Plate 3), the traditional trade of the barber-surgeon persisted parallel to university-based surgery until it was abolished in the course of the nineteenth century (Sander, 1989, p.11). In the south German kingdom of Württemberg, for instance, laws were gradually implemented to restrict barber-surgeons' range of activities so that they were eventually no longer able to provide their traditional wide range of health-care services and thus lost their professional niche. By the end of the nineteenth century, the trade of barber-surgeon had almost died out.

One option for those affected by such regulations was to gain additional qualifications. In Württemberg, many barber-surgeons rose to the status of surgeon or physician. One historical study discovered that 137 barber-surgeons in nineteenth-century Württemberg acquired additional qualifications to allow them to practise internal medicine. No less than one in ten barber-surgeons' sons acquired a degree and rose to the status of doctor (Gross, 1999, p.235).

The changing qualifications acquired by the Palm family reflect broader changes in medical licensing that are discussed in Chapter 5.

I would like to illustrate this process of transition by looking at the Palm family of southern Germany. Figure 3.2 shows seven generations of medical practitioners in the course of almost three centuries. At the top of the family tree you can see Jakob Christoph Palm, who was a barber-surgeon in the first half of the eighteenth century in Schorndorf, a small town in the kingdom of Württemberg. He passed on the trade to his son Johann Leonhard. His grandson, Wilhelm Friedrich Palm, set up practice as a municipal surgeon in the imperial city of Ulm in 1797. Subsequently, he wished to extend his practice to include medicine as well, and in 1812 he was admitted to take the state medical examination without having passed the usual university exam. His son, Johannes, worked as an apprentice to his father from 1808 to 1813. Like his ancestors, he passed through the traditional apprenticeship training, but he then did something that was new in his family: in May 1816, after a period as military doctor in the Württemberg army, he matriculated in medicine and surgery at the University of Tübingen. Lacking the required academic education in classical languages and philosophy, however, he was denied admission to the medical examination. In September and October 1818, he passed the university's exams in surgery and obstetrics, and took his doctorate in surgery. In the following year, he set up practice in his home town as surgeon and obstetrician. Once in Ulm, he increasingly took to treating internal as well as external diseases. This awakened the suspicion of local physicians, who forced the authorities to prohibit him from practising internal medicine. Subsequently, he made another effort to acquire a medical degree, but was once more denied the qualification by the Württemberg Ministry of the Interior because of his lack of a classical education. Meanwhile, the conflict with the doctors in Ulm had intensified. Palm was reported for unlicensed practice and spent three weeks in prison. After several attempts, he was finally admitted to the medical exam in Stuttgart, which he passed in July 1822. After Johannes, the Palm family was to produce another three generations of university-trained practitioners. This medical dynasty would end only with Karl Hans F. Palm, whose son was killed in an Allied bombing raid in March 1945 (Gross, 1999, pp.227, 249).

By the late nineteenth century, the fierce competition between doctors and surgeons, illustrated by the career of Johannes Palm, had died away. Now, surgeons were highly trained and highly regarded specialists with their own clear-cut field of activity inside the medical profession. They went to university or medical school to study medicine, and they embarked on additional training to specialize in surgery only after taking their medical exams, in the same way that other doctors specialized in fields such as paediatrics or dermatology. During this additional training, they learned to master the sophisticated techniques required of modern surgeons in large hospitals, under the supervision of experienced surgeons. These changes in the professional set-up were accompanied by a corresponding transformation on the conceptual level.

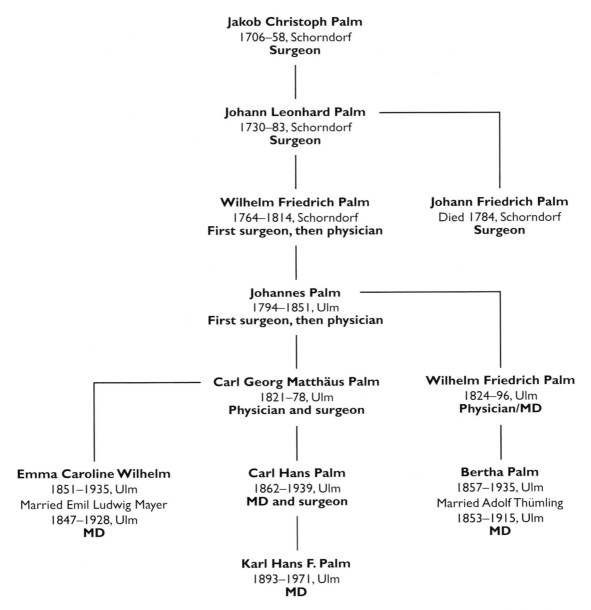

Figure 3.2 The Palm family. Translated and adapted from Gross (1999), p.249. By permission of Franz Steiner

3.3   Concepts

Inside-out: the surgical viewpoint

One of the reasons why surgeons had originally restricted themselves to minor operations and emergencies was the risk involved in major surgery, which could result in serious blood loss, functional impairment or infection (Wangensteen and Wangensteen, 1978, pp.3–18). Traditionally, historians of medicine believed that the limitations of surgical technique explained why surgery was restricted to such a small range of operations. Of equal importance, however, is the fact that the curing of diseases by surgery did not make sense within the concepts of the body prevailing at that time. This is difficult for modern readers to grasp. Today, we have got used to the idea that surgeons can open up the body and alter its interior structure in order to cure some medical conditions. But in the eighteenth and well into the nineteenth centuries, the body was seen as a functional whole interacting with its external environment. People believed that diseases were caused by disruptions in the balance of humours, resulting from the sick person's way of life or some other environmental factor. Diseases could be treated by changing the environment or lifestyle, or by restoring the humoral balance through vomiting, purging and bloodletting. How could this balance be restored by opening up the belly and cutting out some little part of the intestine, as today's surgeons routinely do in cases of appendicitis? Such a notion would have been regarded as absurd.

Before the use of surgery could expand, a new rationale had to emerge that would allow violation of the body's integrity. As the medical historian Christopher Lawrence has stressed, even the simplest surgical practices employ a theory of the body and of disease. Extracting a tooth, he explains, 'implies a theory of the local origin of pain and the relative harmlessness of removing a body part' (Lawrence, 1992, p.15). Modern surgeons view the body as a composite of organs and tissues with particular functions. Disease can affect these at the structural or functional level, and surgery can cure these problems by removing the diseased structures or restoring function.

This localistic approach required surgeons to turn the way they thought about the body inside-out – or, more accurately, outside-in. Traditionally, the diagnosis and treatment of diseases had been guided by signs on the exterior of the body – the red skin that accompanied inflammation, the swelling of tumours and so on. When surgeons – and later physicians, too – tried to understand internal diseases, they started to think of the same processes that occurred on the outside of the body happening on the inside as well. They borrowed familiar categories and terms to describe these processes, and spoke of inflammations, abscesses, ulcers, gangrene and tumours.

This approach not only provided the conceptual basis of modern surgery, it also changed medicine as a whole: surgeons, who were used to thinking of disease as localized anatomical change, taught physicians to use the same localistic approach. In 1781, the permanent secretary of the French Royal Society of Medicine, Félix Vicq d'Azyr (1748–94), advised all medical students to learn to think like surgeons:

> Surgery in effect teaches us by the theory of external inflammations about the nature and course of internal inflammations and suppurations. He who knows how gangrene occurs externally and what it does ... will be the only one to understand the ravages this diseases can cause when, hidden in the viscera, it attacks the organs essential to life.
>
> (quoted in Gelfand, 1980, p.155)

In the first reading for this chapter, Christopher Lawrence reviews research into this new way of thinking about the body. He uses as his starting point an important article by the historian Owsei Temkin, who emphasized surgery's role in the emergence of modern medicine (Temkin, 1951).

Exercise

Read 'Surgery and medicine' (Source Book 2, Reading 3.1). When exactly does Lawrence see a new, more surgical way of thinking about the body and disease emerging?

Discussion

Lawrence sees Temkin's argument as an important step forward in understanding the history of surgery, one which drew attention to the changing ways of 'seeing' and thinking about the body and disease. Temkin thought that this new way of thinking about disease emerged in the late eighteenth century, and was linked to the rise in status of surgeons. Lawrence shows how new research has fleshed out Temkin's claim that there was a coming together of medical and surgical thinking from the late eighteenth century. However, historians have also recognized different stages in the development of surgical ideas. In the eighteenth century, practitioners like Giovanni Battista Morgagni and Alexander Monro secundus described the local manifestations of diseases. However, while the character of a disease was dictated by the place where it occurred (so, for example, all lung diseases were in some way related), the body was still thought of as a holistic entity in which all the parts and functions were intimately related. Disease might appear in the lungs, but it had fundamental effects throughout the body. Localized disease could therefore still be treated with generalized therapy. Historians are divided as to whether or not there is a strong continuity between late eighteenth-century and nineteenth-century thinking. Where Foucault sees continuity, Maulitz suggests that the crucial break with old ways of thinking came in the early nineteenth century when Bichat argued that diseases affected specific tissues, and only those tissues. Since some tissues – skin, or skeletal muscle – were found throughout the body, disease might appear to affect the whole body while actually it was still localized within a specific type of tissue.

Cutting out the disease: pathological anatomy and resective surgery

Attempts to understand disease by observing structural change formed the basis of pathological anatomy which, as you discovered in Chapter 1, became the key science for medicine in the nineteenth century. In many places in the second half of the eighteenth century – France, Germany, the Baltics, Russia, Italy, Britain and America – surgeons and physicians correlated the signs and symptoms they found in the living patient with the structural changes they saw in post-mortem examination, when they used the techniques of surgery to dissect the bodies of patients who had died and find exactly where disease had been located. In the early nineteenth century, it was in Paris above all that this approach to medical practice flourished. Xavier Bichat, who started his career as a surgeon, abandoned the idea that organs – such as the kidney, or heart – were the sites of disease. Instead, he claimed that diseases affected specific tissues. These might be located in one organ, or – like the lymph glands – might be spread throughout the body. Bichat therefore brought together the surgical notion of disease with medical concepts of general, or systemic, pathological change. As a result, pathology became the common foundation for the unified art of healing (Maulitz, 1993, pp.173–8).

The localized theory of disease was radically revised by the work of Rudolf Virchow of Berlin (Figure 3.3). Taking up the idea that the bodies of animals and plants are made up of cells, Virchow proclaimed that cells can originate only from other cells.

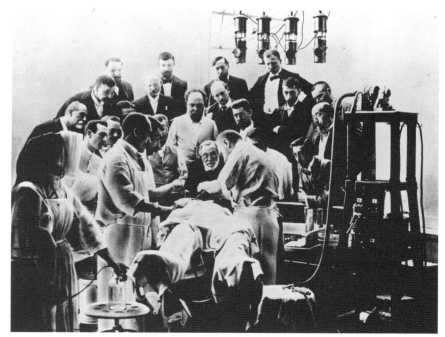

Figure 3.3   The renowned pathologist Rudolf Virchow showing his interest in surgery while attending an operation in Paris in 1900. This image is emblematic of the relationship between surgery and pathology. Bildarchiv Preußischer Kulturbesitz, Berlin. Wellcome Library, London

He therefore reduced disease processes to the cellular level: now, the real seat of disease was no longer the organs or the tissue as such, but the cells. Virchow's *Cellularpathologie,* published in 1858, became the cornerstone of mainstream medical theory for decades. His ideas gave surgery a new rationale: if the body is divided into independent microscopic elements, surgeons can cut out the diseased cells without compromising the function of the rest of the body. Surgical intervention became the therapeutic implementation of cellular pathology.

Accordingly, in the nineteenth century, surgeons sought ever more sophisticated ways to treat disease by cutting it out of the body. This kind of surgery is called resective surgery, resection meaning the surgical removal of an organ or structure. The German surgeon Theodor Billroth (1826–94) epitomized the resective approach. Like other surgeons of the day, Billroth had had a basic training in pathology. He carefully followed the work of Virchow and his successors in the 1860s on the origins of tumour cells, hoping that cellular pathology would provide new, more scientific, surgical techniques. His expectations were realized when cellular pathology provided the tools to differentiate between malignant tumours and other kinds of pathological tissue formation (Maulitz, 1993, pp.182–3). Billroth pioneered many types of resective surgery for cancer. He developed different ways of removing the stomach and parts of the intestines and then restoring the continuity of the system, and performed his first successful elective operation on the stomach, a partial resection of the organ for gastric cancer, in 1881 (Wangensteen and Wangensteen, 1978, p.142). (An elective operation is one planned in advance – as opposed to emergency surgery.) In the USA, William S. Halsted (1852–1922), who had trained with Billroth, devised radical mastectomy, an operation in which the breast, all the lymph nodes in the nearest armpit, and the muscles of the chest wall are removed. It remained the most frequently applied treatment for breast cancer for many years.

The resective approach to surgery demonstrates neatly how surgery and medicine interacted. Medicine adopted a localistic approach from surgery and developed a new understanding of disease as pathological change of tissues and cells. This in turn served as the basis for resective surgery. These developments also link the conceptual changes with the transformation of surgery in the professional dimension. By including the surgical point of view in medical education, physicians gained a new and productive approach to disease; learning medicine helped surgeons to see the body in a way that made surgery on the body's interior possible. This interaction continued when a new type of surgery emerged alongside resective surgery.

A new strategy: from resection to reconstruction

One of those who became particularly proficient at removing diseased structures was the Swiss surgeon Theodor Kocher (1841–1917). Among other achievements, he developed a technique for the resection of goitre. Goitre is the name for a pathological enlargement of the thyroid gland and can be life-threatening. Initially, the operation to remove a goitre was very dangerous: between 1860 and 1867, Billroth performed the operation on twenty patients, eight of whom (40 per cent) died. In Kocher's hands, resection of goitre became a safe procedure. By 1909, he had performed 4,000 resections and the mortality rate had fallen from 14 per cent to 0.7 per cent (Tröhler, 1993, p.994).

However, even after successful removal, goitres tended to regrow, so that patients had to submit themselves to the complicated operation several times. Kocher therefore resorted to a more radical solution and started to remove the whole thyroid gland. At that time, the role of the gland in the body was completely unknown. However, the normal function of the gland became apparent as a consequence of Kocher's operations. After removal of their thyroid gland, patients developed a characteristic clinical picture which included physical weakness, loss of intelligence, swollen hands and feet, a puffy face and anaemia – in short, all the symptoms we associate today with impaired thyroid function.

Kocher's first reaction to the unexpected consequences of his operation was to try to reverse the removal of the gland. In July 1883, he transplanted thyroid tissue from one patient's goitre to another patient who was suffering from the effects of total thyroid removal. This was the first modern organ transplantation – an attempt to cure a complex internal disease by replacing an organ.

Though Kocher was not particularly happy with the effect in this case, it was the starting gun for the development of research into organ transplantation and the concept of organ replacement. Kocher's operation was immediately used as a physiological experiment: researchers performed thyroidectomies on animals, meticulously documenting the results and then checking their findings by reinserting the organ. The same technique was adapted to a number of other organs and diseases, and the observed symptoms were defined as specific disease entities. They were often equated to some disease that was already known, such as diabetes, which was redefined as a lack of the function of a particular portion of the pancreas. Surgery therefore not only elucidated the function of certain organs and tissues but also helped to bring about the better understanding and treatment of a number of hitherto mysterious diseases.

Though the original transplant technique was subsequently replaced by better methods of substituting the gland's function, thyroid transplantation became the prototype of all other organ transplants. The principle was applied to other organs, such as the pancreas, testes and ovaries. In 1905, in New York City, Alexis Carrel (1873–1944) and C.C. Guthrie (1880–1963) carried out the first heart transplant in a dog. In 1906, in Lyon, Mathieu Jaboulay (1860–1930) performed the first kidney transplant in a human being (Schlich, 1998).

By 1900, the principle of organ replacement was generally accepted, and research into its clinical application gave rise to a new branch of surgery, transplant surgery. It seemed to be only a question of time before all diseased organs and tissues could be replaced, and surgeons sought new techniques to make this possible. The peak of technical perfection was reached by the French-American Alexis Carrel, who in 1912 won the Nobel Prize for his work on blood vessel surgery and organ transplantation. The technical perfection of his surgery made Carrel aware that transplants from one individual to another were often unsuccessful – but not as a result of the surgery itself. He experimented by grafting a dog's kidney from its original site to the neck, and found that the organ survived for an unlimited period of time as long as it remained within the same animal. However, if he performed exactly the same operation but transferred the kidney to a different dog, the transplanted organ invariably died. Apparently, the tissues of individuals of the same species possessed a unique biological identity. Surgeons and scientists described and analysed this phenomenon, and some even suggested that the immune system was responsible for the 'rejection' of foreign tissues. As they were unable to overcome this obstacle, however, transplant surgery was abandoned in the 1920s and was not taken up again until 1945.

With the emergence of organ transplantation, a new generation of surgeons turned away from the local and structural approach and started once again to look at the body as an integrated system. Instead of cutting out the disease, they attempted to reconstruct the original structures and functions of the body. This type of surgery can be called physiological or reconstructive surgery (Tröhler, 1993, p.984). For these surgeons, physiology, not pathological anatomy, was the key to understanding disease. They went beyond observation and description of life phenomena, and tried actively to intervene in living organisms to control their body functions (Pickstone, 2000).

The development of physiology is described in Chapter 4.

The next reading is taken from *An Introduction to the Study of Experimental Medicine*, first published in 1865, by Claude Bernard (1813–78), a pioneer of experimental physiology.

Exercise

Read 'Surgery and experimental medicine' (Source Book 2, Reading 3.2). How does Bernard use surgery in his work?

Discussion

Bernard uses surgery to isolate and then selectively to sever a precise group of nerves in order to prove his hypothesis about the role of these nerves in controlling temperature. In this case, Bernard's results required him to reconsider his original ideas. Thus, surgery is a tool by which he can make very precise changes to the function of living organisms and then observe the results.

Like pathological anatomy, experimental physiology had its roots in a surgical approach to the body and its functions. As you have seen, physiologists' active intervention into animals' bodies was often achieved by surgical means. The activist impulse to intervene in the organism, the operative facility and practical knowledge of gross anatomy, as well as the instruments and the language used, all point to the surgical background of that science (Lesch, 1984).

3.4 Technique

Historians of surgery used to claim that anaesthesia and antisepsis revolutionized surgery. As you have read in Chapter 2, anaesthesia and antisepsis revolutionized the function of hospitals, but the history of their introduction is far from simple. A much more complicated, and more sophisticated, picture emerges if we ask about the conditions in which innovation occurred and spread. Technical innovations, such as anaesthesia, antisepsis and asepsis, need an appropriate context in which to be generated, appraised and disseminated (Lawrence, 1993, p.982). The factors you have looked at in the preceding sections – the existence of a surgical profession with an established body of theoretical knowledge based on a new perception of the body and its pathology – were crucial to the development and introduction of technical innovations during the second half of the nineteenth century. At the same time, anaesthesia, antisepsis and asepsis changed the character of operative surgery beyond recognition. These new techniques made possible the successful and comprehensive application of the concepts of resective and reconstructive surgery.

The extension of surgery did not rely on anaesthesia or antisepsis. Resective surgery within the abdominal cavity, for instance, had long been associated with high rates of infection, but began long before these technologies were available. In 1809, the American Ephraim McDowell (1771–1830) first successfully removed a large cyst on an ovary. Without the use of anaesthetics, he operated on 47-year-old Jane Crawford, removing nearly 7 kilograms of dirty gelatinous substance from her cyst. The patient not only survived but lived for a further thirty-one years. McDowell later published an account of his operation and of two other successful operations to remove ovarian cysts; both were performed on black women (Wangensteen and Wangensteen, 1978, pp.227–9). By the middle of the century, the operation was performed regularly in England by Charles Clay (1801–93) in Manchester, and by the distinguished London surgeon Thomas Spencer Wells (1818–97), whose one-thousandth ovariotomy, in 1880, was the occasion of congratulatory editorials in the British press (Wangensteen and Wangensteen, 1978, pp.230–2).

Another daring operation that was developed before the advent of anaesthesia and antisepsis under the conditions of the American frontier was the repair of vesico-vaginal fistulae. This is an artificial connection between the bladder and the vagina that is usually caused by complications in childbirth. It is extremely debilitating for its victims. In 1845, in Alabama, James Marion Sims (1813–83) attempted an operation to repair the condition on a number of slave women who had to bear the hour-long operation without anaesthesia. His thirtieth attempt, in 1849, was successful, and subsequently Sims became famous for his method of repairing a lesion then generally regarded as untreatable (Wangensteen and Wangensteen, 1978, pp.239–41). American conditions proved favourable for this sort of innovation; there, the medical profession was less regulated, and, at least in the southern states, surgeons could practise on slaves. As was to be expected, such operations met with a mixed reception. Critics regarded them as being carried out for the sake of scientific curiosity and surgical practice, and equated them with vivisection (Porter, 1996, pp.227–8).

A redistribution of power: anaesthesia

Such extensive operations became much easier with the introduction of anaesthesia. Prior to this, speed was the order of the day, and the only way to minimize pain, shock and loss of blood. Amputation, one of the few major operations that was frequently performed at the time, is a famous (or infamous) case in point. Surgeons measured in seconds the time they needed to amputate. Benjamin Bell (1749–1806), a distinguished surgeon of the Edinburgh Royal Infirmary, could divide all but the bone in a thigh amputation in six seconds. When Robert Liston (1794–1847), of University College Hospital in London, amputated, it was said that 'the gleam of his knife was followed so instantaneously by the sound of sawing as to make the two actions appear simultaneous'; he was able to amputate a thigh, close the wound and complete the dressing in a mere three and a half minutes (Wangensteen and Wangensteen, 1978, pp.36, 455).

Speed was no longer significant, however, once the problem of pain was solved. Doctors had always used analgesics, including alcohol, opium or soporific drugs, to dull pain. But anaesthesia – an expression coined in 1846 by the American writer Oliver Wendell Holmes (1809–94) to indicate the effects of ether – was not introduced systematically into surgical practice until the 1840s. Among its many inventors was William E. Clarke, a practitioner from Rochester, New York, who in 1842 extracted a tooth under ether. The use of ether as a surgical anaesthetic was also tested by a Boston dentist, William T.G. Morton (1819–68). On 16 October 1846, at the Massachusetts General Hospital in Boston, Morton administered ether while the surgeon John Collins Warren (1778–1856) removed a tumour from the neck of a young man (Figure 3.4).

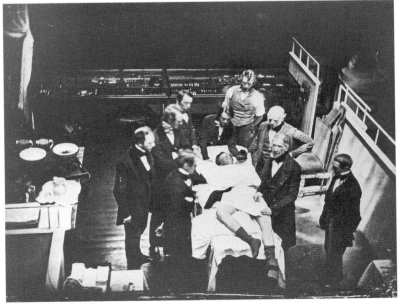

Figure 3.4   An early operation under anaesthesia, *c.*1847, Massachusetts General Hospital. Whole-plate daguerrotype, attributed to Southworth and Hawes, Boston. John Collins Warren in foreground, right centre. Wellcome Library, London

You will explore the professional issues around the introduction of ether anaesthesia in Chapter 5.

The use of ether as an anaesthetic spread quickly. On 21 December 1846, Liston amputated the diseased thigh of a patient under ether. According to a witness, the surgeon entered the crowded amphitheatre saying, 'We are going to try a Yankee dodge today, gentlemen, for making men insensible.' The patient, a 36-year-old butler, was brought in on a stretcher. The ether was applied. 'Time me,' said Liston when he was given the signal that the patient was ready. When the operation was over, the recorded time taken to sever the limb was between 25 and 28 seconds. Within five minutes the patient, who had already been wheeled out of the operating room, was asking when the operation would take place (Wangensteen and Wangensteen, 1978, pp.282–3). We do not know if Liston was simply too accustomed to operating at breakneck speed or if he did not trust the new technique sufficiently to change his habitual way of performing the operation. The new anaesthetic technique was taken up with great rapidity: it was tried on 22 December 1846 in Paris, on 23 January 1847 in Bern, Switzerland, on 6 February in Berlin, and on 8 March in The Hague, Holland (Tröhler, 1993, p.986). Several related innovations then followed, such as the introduction of new agents for inhalation anaesthesia (including chloroform), and techniques for the local application of anaesthetics into the skin or spine to block particular parts of the nervous system (Pernick, 1985, p.237).

Despite its rapid uptake, anaesthesia was not accepted unconditionally. A number of reasons were brought forward against the indiscriminate use of anaesthetics. Some were strictly medical, such as consideration of the risk involved: according to the pharmaceutical knowledge of the day, ether administered in the quantities required to produce anaesthesia was poisonous, and patients frequently suffered from side effects such as nausea, as Margaret Mathewson described in the reading in Chapter 2. After chloroform was introduced as an anaesthetic agent in 1848, reports of sudden death from cardiac arrest began to fill the medical and popular press, contributing to the view of nineteenth-century hospitals as 'gateways to death'. Some doctors feared that anaesthesia might impair wound-healing, an idea based on the observation that painless wounds often did not heal well. Pain seemed to be a sign of life and so was equated with healing and recovery. Other concerns were social. It was obvious to contemporaries that anaesthesia would reshape the power relations in medical practice. (As you have read in Chapter 1, in the nineteenth century practitioners had already gained power over their patients by developing new techniques of physical examination and devising a technical language that patients could not follow.) Critical voices warned against the surgeon's increased power over the unconscious patient, which might induce him to perform extensive and unnecessary operations (Pernick, 1985, pp.35–76).

Exercise

Look at the cartoons in Figure 3.5, which were published in a French satirical magazine shortly after the introduction of anaesthesia, and at Figure 3.6, an engraving entitled *Furor Operativus*, from around 1875. What do these artists see as the consequences of anaesthesia? Who will it be good for? Will society benefit? Can we take these images seriously as historical sources?

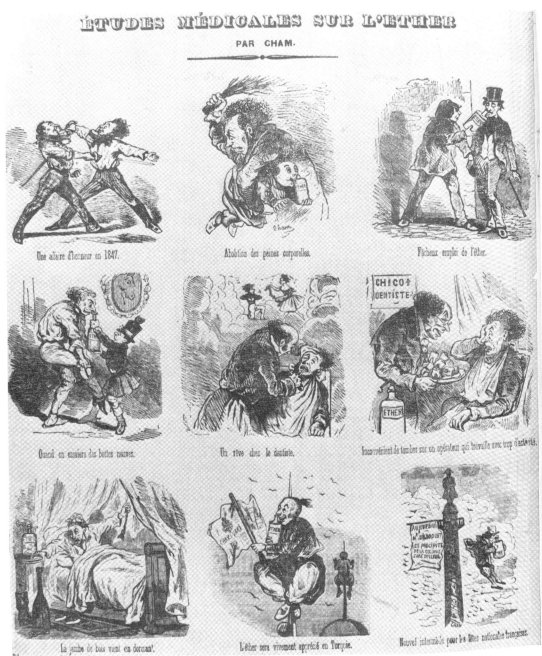

Figure 3.5   This series of cartoons, 'Medical studies on ether', by Cham, 1847, purports to illustrate some of the implications of the abolition of pain through anaesthesia. From: 'A duel in 1847'; 'Abolition of corporal punishment'; 'Unfortunate use of ether'; 'When one tries on new boots'; A dream at the dentist's'; 'It is difficult to stop an over-enthusiastic practitioner'; 'The wooden leg comes while sleeping'; 'Ether will be greatly appreciated in Turkey'; 'New interlude for national bank holidays'. Reproduced from the *Journal of the History of Medicine and Allied Sciences* (October 1946), vol.1, p.610. By permission of Oxford University Press

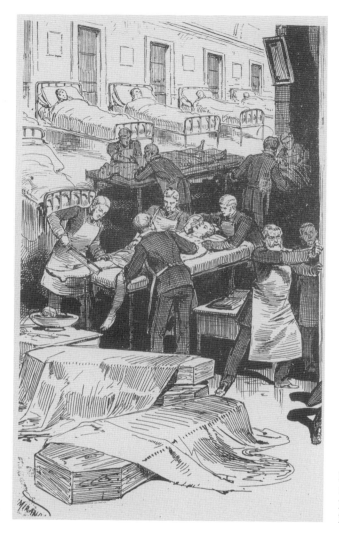

Figure 3.6 *Furor Operativus* by Fernando Miranda, *c.*1875. Bettmann Archive/Corbis

Discussion

Even though they were published with a satirical purpose in mind, the images would work only if the public recognized the issue and 'got the joke', so we can be fairly certain that they do reflect the views of some people at the time. They represent anaesthesia as a very mixed blessing: it spares individuals the pain of dentistry and of putting on a new pair of boots. However, the loss of consciousness also brings a loss of control – allowing the thief to steal a wallet, the dentist to remove too many teeth or – in the very grim image in Figure 3.6 – enabling surgeons to operate while patients pay the price with their lives. The abolition of pain also threatens to upset the moral structure of society: corporal punishment or the duel can no longer deter antisocial behaviour.

So perhaps it was not so irrational, after all, to be somewhat apprehensive about this innovation. However, anaesthesia undoubtedly made surgery more acceptable to both patients and practitioners, which contributed to the central position it gained within medicine and society.

But did surgeons really put their own professional interest before that of their patients? The next reading is from Martin S. Pernick's book on surgery in America, *A Calculus of Suffering: Pain, Professionalism and Anesthesia in Nineteenth-Century America*, one of the very few detailed studies of surgical practice. Although it describes American practice, early research suggests that the European experience was similar.

Exercise

Read 'The impact of anaesthesia' (Source Book 2, Reading 3.3).

1   Try to sum up how Pernick's account differs from contemporary accounts of the arrival of anaesthetics. What evidence does he find for an explosion in the number of operations?

2   Does he agree that practitioners undertook 'experimental' operations, causing unnecessary deaths?

Discussion

1   Pernick presents a much more complex picture of the impact of anaesthesia on surgical practice than the contemporary accounts suggest. Contemporary accounts suggest a blanket increase in surgery, not all of which is necessary for the patient's recovery. Pernick's data show that there was a sudden increase in the number of operations at the Massachusetts General Hospital. However, the increase was not spread across all patient groups. Not all patients were routinely given anaesthetics – women, children and native-born Americans (i.e. not immigrants) were more likely to receive them. The growth in the number of operations was greatest among those groups who were most likely to receive anaesthetics. Anaesthesia thus brought about a sort of levelling up, where the groups of patients previously thought too weak or too sensitive to stand surgery could be operated on.

Pernick argues that we should not leap to the conclusion that this was just the result of the availability of anaesthetics. Historians have to factor into their calculations a general increase in hospital patients. They have to consider how anaesthesia allowed surgeons to perform different types of operation – more complex surgery to save a limb rather than simply amputation. Pernick suggests that a growing number of industrial accidents also pushed up the numbers of patients requiring surgery. He questions the validity of historical judgements about whether operations performed in the late nineteenth century were 'necessary' or 'unnecessary'. As he points out, an untried operation performed on a dying patient can be interpreted as an unnecessary intervention or as a heroic effort to save a life.

2   Pernick suggests that there is evidence that the availability of anaesthesia did make some practitioners more willing to try experimental procedures. However, he also finds some evidence of patients demanding dangerous surgery and practitioners refusing to operate. Overall, he suggests that 'experimental' operations increased to a smaller extent than those of more established, successful procedures. He argues that according to statistics, although the data are less than perfect, mortality rates from surgery did not increase with the arrival of anaesthetics. Rather, the greater numbers of victims of serious accidents – who received surgery as a last resort – helped to push up the number of deaths.

But all this does not mean that anaesthesia led to the rise of modern surgery in any simple way. The historical evidence shows that surgeons had already created a range of complicated operations before the advent of anaesthesia, many of which required a protracted period at the operating table. And even after anaesthesia had become available, surgeons did not always use it (Lawrence, 1992, p.25). Most importantly, surgery on internal organs became a rational therapeutic option not because of anaesthesia but because of the change in medical concepts discussed above. Perhaps one can even conclude, with Christopher Lawrence, 'so great was the determination [of surgeons] to invade [the body] by the 1840s that, in retrospect, the invention of technologies to facilitate this invasion seems inevitable' (Lawrence, 1992, p.25).

Anaesthesia changed the nature of surgery, and the design and function of hospitals. From the late nineteenth century, large hospitals had more than one purpose-built operating theatre. Anaesthesia also changed the character of the operating theatre: 'Eliminating the wild, disorderly pre-anaesthetic scenes of screaming and brutality made possible the eventual emergence of the controlled, efficient, rationalized modern operating room, in which the quiet is broken only by the rhythmic whoosh of the anaesthetist's air bag' (Pernick, 1985, p.235). Anaesthesia also allowed the introduction of antisepsis and the eventual control of surgical infection: 'The hyperhygienic rituals of modern aseptic surgery would be inconceivable in a world where a struggling, convulsed patient still had to be wrestled to the table and where every second of delay was an eternity of pain' (Pernick, 1985, p.237).

A revolution in cleanliness: antisepsis, asepsis

The other central technology in this context is antiseptic and aseptic surgery, which helped to make surgery safer. In the early nineteenth century, amputation of the thigh, for example, often had a mortality of 45 to 65 per cent. Rates reported by individual surgeons and clinics varied greatly, partly through variations in the type of patient and in the reasons for amputation, but also because of the different levels of attention paid by each surgeon to hand-washing, preparation of the operation site, instruments and dressings (Wangensteen and Wangensteen, 1978, pp.49–50).

Until the mid-nineteenth century, even some distinguished surgeons paid little attention to such things. An American student visiting Guillaume Dupuytren's clinic at the Hôtel-Dieu in Paris reported, 'The French students ... were a very dirty, ill-dressed set ... But indeed M. Dupuytren was no better. He wore a dirty white apron, superfluously protecting a dirtier pair of trousers, a greasy threadbare coat, and well-worn carpet shoes' (Wangensteen and Wangensteen, 1978, p.50). Though such a retrospective description is probably influenced by a desire to contrast past surgery with later aseptic cleanliness (and probably anti-French sentiments too), it fits in with many other eyewitness accounts of the time. Another surgeon recalled that in 1861, 'We operated in old blood-stained and often pus-stained coats ... with undisinfected hands ... we used undisinfected instruments ... and marine sponges which had been used in prior pus cases and only washed in tap water' (Wangensteen and Wangensteen, 1978, p.487) (Plate 6).

Between 1860 and 1890, surgery underwent a revolution with regard to cleanliness. During these years, many surgeons introduced new routines to help avoid wound infection. As early as 1848, Ignaz Semmelweis (1818–65) of Vienna had noted that the fever that often affected women after childbirth could largely be prevented if the doctors and students who examined the women scrubbed their hands and nails in soap and water, and then in chlorine water. But his observations had no influence on surgical practice. Independently, around mid-century, a school of 'cleanliness and cold water surgery' was established in London by Thomas Spencer Wells, whose ovariotomy operations were described earlier. Wells washed with cold water, used fresh towels when operating, closed incisions with metallic thread, and admitted only those spectators who testified in writing that they had not been in an autopsy room for seven days. Starting in the 1860s, a number of surgeons harnessed cleanliness, the isolation of the operating field and chemical purification into an integrated system that enabled them to perform internal surgery with greater safety (Lawrence, 1992, p.26). However, such techniques varied between individual surgeons: the standardized surgical routine of today was devised only in the following half-century.

Traditionally, much of this development is attributed to one person, namely Joseph Lister (1827–1912) (Porter, 1999, pp.370–4). Lister's method was based on antisepsis – the killing of any infective agents present in the wound and in the environment by use of disinfectants such as carbolic acid. This was not a completely new idea: antiseptic agents like turpentine or alcohol had been occasionally administered to wounds for a long time; carbolic acid was known to fight the odour of decomposition and was widely used as a disinfectant. Some surgeons also employed carbolic acid to fight putrefaction in wounds. Its effect, however, was never systematically appraised and propagated, nor was its use developed into a comprehensive system supported by scientific arguments (Wangensteen and Wangensteen, 1978, pp.301–22).

This task fell to Joseph Lister. Lister's technique consisted of disinfecting the wound, the surgical instruments, the surgeon's hands and, for a time, even the air around the operation, using a machine to spray a fine mist of carbolic acid (Figure 3.7). He started developing his antiseptic technique against putrefaction of wounds in 1865 while regius professor of surgery in Glasgow. His first trial took place on 12 August 1865 on an 11-year-old boy whose left leg had been run over by a cart. Lister dressed the boy's compound fracture of the tibia with lint soaked in linseed oil and carbolic acid. At the time, compound fractures often led to extensive wound suppuration, forcing the surgeons to amputate the affected limb. Lister kept the dressing in place for four days, covering it with tinfoil to prevent evaporation. The wound healed perfectly, and the boy walked out of the Glasgow Infirmary six weeks later.

In 1867, Lister published three articles explaining his new techniques by reference to Louis Pasteur's germ theory. According to Pasteur (1822–96), germs were present throughout the environment and could lead to fermentation in certain foodstuffs. Lister claimed that in a similar process germs got into wounds, where they lived on dead tissue and caused putrefaction. (You will learn more about Pasteur's work on micro-organisms in Chapter 4.)

Lister tried to prove his case using statistics. According to his reports in 1864 and 1866, sixteen of his thirty-five patients undergoing amputation (46 per cent) had died, whereas in 1867–9, when he applied his antiseptic techniques, it was only six out of forty (15 per cent) (Tröhler, 1993, p.989). But this did not convince all of his colleagues. Some surgeons criticized Lister's concentration on local wound treatment and complained that his drill of antiseptic procedures was complicated and cumbersome. Others pointed to widespread experience which suggested that wounds often healed better when left clean and open than when they were soaked continually in disinfectant fluid. His critics claimed that simpler methods, with more emphasis on cleanliness, would bring about the same or even better results.

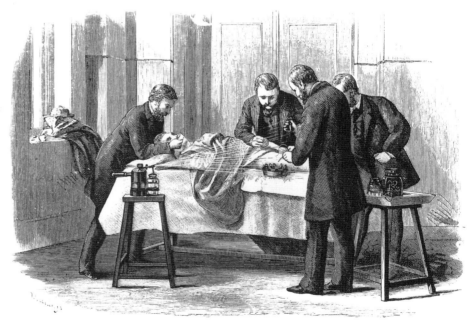

Figure 3.7   Use of the Lister carbolic acid spray. Bridgeman Art Library, London

Quantitative arguments were presented by both promoters and critics of antisepsis, but no statistics finally proved the greater efficacy of one method of treating wounds over another. Comparison was complicated by the fact that all surgeons, including Lister, constantly modified their techniques in an endeavour to achieve better results (Lawrence and Dixey, 1992, p.157). During the second half of the nineteenth century, various surgeons took up, dropped or modified Listerian techniques (Lawrence and Dixey, 1992, p.175; Worboys, 2000, pp.73–107, 150–92). In 1868, Theodor Kocher, for instance, described above in the context of his operations on goitre, became one of the first continental surgeons to apply Lister's methods, but he used a modified form of the technique only for selected cases and as one component in a more general effort to create hygienic conditions for surgery (Tröhler, 1984, pp.27–30).

By the 1880s, surgeons were developing a variety of antiseptic and aseptic routines to make surgery safe. Many of these techniques amounted to what came to be called 'asepsis'. Where antisepsis sought to kill any germs already present, aseptic techniques tried to prevent any contamination with infectious agents. Everything that would touch the wound, including the surgeon's hand, was painstakingly washed and disinfected. Instruments and surgeons' gowns were sterilized with heat. The introduction of asepsis as a sophisticated and standardized system is most often dated to 1877 and attributed to the German surgeon Ernst von Bergmann (1836–1907). Aseptic surgery required a complete redesign of operating theatres, with the use of glass and other impermeable surfaces throughout. Students who had observed operations were now excluded from the space and admitted instead to special closed viewing galleries.

Gradually, the modern aseptic ritual of sterilized gowns, masks and rubber gloves was created. In 1897, Johann von Miculicz-Radecki (1850–1905) of Breslau claimed that speaking during operations enhanced droplet infection – a term coined by him – and that this risk could be markedly diminished by wearing face masks. Surgeons began to wear cotton or silk gloves during their operations, and in 1890 the American surgeon William S. Halsted introduced rubber gloves for use in the operating theatre (Wangensteen and Wangensteen, 1978, pp.7–9).

These new techniques were increasingly justified by the emerging science of bacteriology. In the late 1870s, Robert Koch (1843–1910) gave what was to become aseptic surgery a new scientific basis. In his work on wound infection, he cultured and identified bacteria and demonstrated convincingly that they caused suppuration. According to Koch, identifiable species of bacteria caused distinct disorders, one of these being wound infection. All the well-known problems such as putrefaction, suppuration and wound fever could thus be seen as the result of the invasion of living host tissue by infective bacteria. Bacteriology therefore furnished objective criteria for evaluating the efficacy of the measures taken to prevent or to fight surgical infection, and some scientifically oriented surgeons in Germany and Switzerland, such as Bergmann, Kocher and Mikulicz-Radecki, even set up their own bacteriological laboratories in their clinics.

Even Lister reinterpreted his ideas over time: he no longer blamed airborne agents for the putrefaction of dead tissue; he abandoned the carbolic spray; and he laid more stress on asepsis instead of antisepsis. Eventually, antisepsis and asepsis came to be viewed as a single doctrine, with Lister as its prophet. As Lawrence and Dixey claim, there was undeniably a major transformation, 'a revolution even, in surgery between the late 1860s and the 1890s, but it is possible to see it not as deriving from a single sudden innovation engineered by a small group (the Listerians) but as the accumulation of many small deviations from intellectual and practical routine among the surgical community *as a whole*' (Lawrence and Dixey, 1992, p.207).

At the end of this transformation a surgical operation looked much as we know it today, with a team of surgeons and operation-room personnel clothed in sterilized gowns, wearing rubber gloves and face masks, and moving in a highly disciplined manner. In Figure 3.8 you can see Kocher operating in 1912 with Halsted watching. The scene looks almost like a modern operating theatre apart from the fact that the surgeons do not wear face masks.

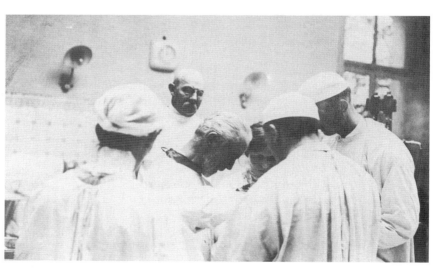

Figure 3.8   Theodor Kocher during an operation in 1912. William S. Halsted of Baltimore attends the operation as a guest. Despite his emphasis on rigid asepsis in general, Kocher did not believe in the benefit of the face mask. Wellcome Library, London. By permission of Professor Ulrich Tröhler

A sophisticated technology of the body: further transformations

Even after the introduction of major technical innovations such as anaesthesia and asepsis, surgeons continued to improve their techniques. Surgical techniques to repair and alter body structures grew ever more sophisticated. The discovery of X-rays by Wilhelm Konrad Röntgen in 1895 facilitated surgical diagnosis and the planning of operations, revealing changes in the body's structure that were otherwise hidden from the physician's view. The longer operating times and calmer conditions allowed by anaesthesia facilitated intricate procedures in the innermost parts of the body. The notion came to be accepted that gentle operating technique with meticulous attention to the control of blood loss and conservation of body tissues gave better post-operative results. Techniques to reconstruct blood vessels and to maintain the continuity of organ cavities such as the bowel were refined. In the last quarter of the nineteenth century, great masters of surgery designed new devices and operations that bore their names, for example the 'Kocher clamp' or the 'Billroth I operation'. In their efforts to make surgery safer, surgeons also turned their attention to pre- and post-operative care. They started to set up more precise criteria for indications to operate, and to document and evaluate the results of treatment.

All this made surgery less dangerous and more reliable than ever before, as figures such as the decline in death rates from Kocher's goitre operations, quoted above, show so convincingly. Surgery was no longer a last resort; instead, it became a realistic therapeutic option and an attractive alternative to other strategies of treatment. The new character of surgery is nicely exemplified in the removal of the gall bladder and the appendix, both of which started to become common in the 1880s. Surgeons removed these organs on a routine basis in order to prevent life-threatening situations. Being truly elective interventions, these procedures contributed much to making surgery an unquestioned part of modern life (Porter, 1996, p.232).

The marked change in the number and type of operations is reflected in the records. In Chapter 2, you read about the increased number of operations performed in hospitals in the late nineteenth century. Lister's notebooks report no abdominal surgery up to 1893; but the abdominal surgery practice of William Watson Cheyne (1852–1932) at King's College Hospital in London increased steadily in the decade between 1902 and 1912, from fewer than one in twenty cases to around one in six (Porter, 1996, p.232). The rapid expansion of operative surgery can also be seen in textbooks. The first edition of Kocher's *Chirurgische Operationslehre* [Textbook of Operative Surgery] in 1892 was 200 pages long; its fifth German edition of 1907 comprised nearly 1,100 pages, of which the longest section was devoted to new techniques and operations. Nearly half of the book treated new fields such as abdominal and thoracic surgery, and surgery of the nervous system including the brain and spinal cord (Tröhler, 1993, p.993).

Just as surgery provided a valuable tool with which to perform physiological experiments, anaesthesia and antisepsis also contributed to the performance of fundamental research. The next reading shows the first two pages of a lecture Kocher gave in 1909 when he was awarded the Nobel Prize for Medicine.

Exercise

Read 'Surgery and research' (Source Book 2, Reading 3.4).

1   In what context does Kocher want his work to be seen?

2   What significance does the Nobel laureate assign to surgery within medicine?

3   How does he describe the role of the new techniques of anaesthesia and antisepsis for the creation of new knowledge about the body?

4   What type of surgery does his work represent?

Discussion

1   Kocher starts by referring to a number of great scientific breakthroughs and mentions the names of individuals who were regarded by 1909 as scientific heroes: Pasteur, Lister and Koch. By placing his work in this context, Kocher is

suggesting that his own research is on the same level as their historic achievements.

2   In experiments using surgical techniques, on the physiological functioning of organs, he sees a vital means by which the organism's workings in health and disease might be understood. Anaesthesia and antisepsis are prerequisites for physiologists to gain new knowledge about the body's function unaffected by the influences of pain or infection. (This is a good example of how contemporaries understood that the development of surgical techniques was intertwined with the production of scientific knowledge.)

3   The kind of surgery described by Kocher is clearly no longer the type of resective surgery that focused on cutting out diseased structures.

4   Its objective is to reconstruct the body's functions, and in this sense it belongs to reconstructive surgery.

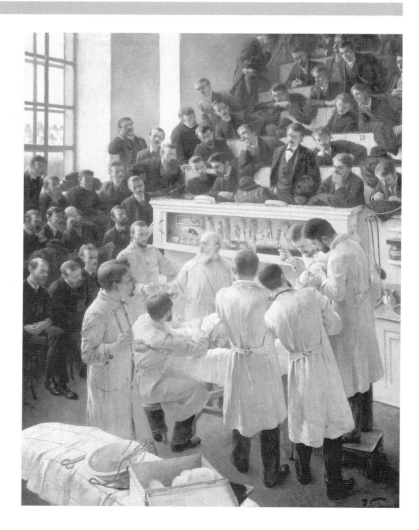

Figure 3.9   Theodor Billroth at work in the Allgemeines Krankenhaus in Vienna. Painting by Adalbert Seligmann, 1891. Österreichische Galerie Belvedere, Vienna

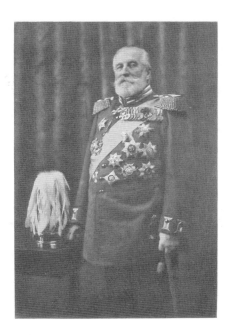

Figure 3.10   His Excellency Ernst von Bergmann, MD, medical corps brigadier, privy councillor, professor and head of Berlin's first surgical clinic in the Ziegelstrasse. By permission of Universität Zürich, Medizinhistorisches Institut und Museum

Kocher was the first surgeon to receive a Nobel Prize, reflecting the surgeon's new status within medicine. The 1891 painting of Theodor Billroth, shown in Figure 3.9 (and on the cover of this book), bears witness to this attitude. Successful surgeons such as Ernst von Bergmann, depicted in Figure 3.10, attained a social prestige equal to that of the greater nobility, industrial magnates and generals (Mörgeli, 1999, p.208). The rising social status of the surgeon was closely linked to technical advances, which allowed them to operate on structures in all body cavities, including abdomen, chest and brain. In turn, these successes further strengthened the surgical point of view on the conceptual level.

Specialization

With the expansion of surgery, some of its practitioners started to specialize in particular fields, reflecting a wider trend for specialties to develop in many areas of medicine. Some specialties were organized around particular technologies. Modern eye surgery (ophthalmology) was founded by Albrecht von Graefe (1828–70) in Berlin. At the centre of the new specialty was the ophthalmoscope, a diagnostic device introduced by the physiologist Hermann von Helmholtz (1821–94) in 1851, which allowed doctors to see the condition of the inside of the eye. The field quickly became established and by 1880 all twenty-seven medical faculties in the German-speaking lands except Jena had chairs of ophthalmology. Similarly, ear, nose and throat surgery emerged on the basis of the newly introduced laryngoscope (1854–5), which allowed observation of the interior of the larynx (voice-box), and the otoscope (1860), which allowed doctors to see into the ear. Other specialties were founded by appropriating specific areas of activity. Orthopaedic surgery, for instance, was originally concerned with congenital deformities of bones and joints. It became a surgical specialty in the nineteenth century when it extended its territory to developmental anomalies and to disabilities due to age, infections or injuries of the skeletal system. Gynaecological surgery took its origin partially from learned physicians' involvement in obstetrics, and in particular when obstetric surgery was opened up due to the introduction of the Caesarian section operation in the last two decades of the nineteenth century.

You will discover more about the process of professionalization in Chapter 5.

The development of specialties resembles the professionalization of medicine on a smaller scale. Both processes are characterized by self-organization, self-regulation and monopoly of a particular field of activity. There are a number of indicators for successful specialization, among them the publication of journals, the establishment of specialized societies with extensive jurisdiction on matters of training and qualification, and a formalized and officially recognized training and qualification. On the institutional level, departments, clinics and chairs at the universities and medical schools were another sign that a field had become a specialty (Tröhler, 1993, pp.1008–24).

The processes of specialization are explored again in Chapter 12, in the context of the First World War.

Specialization is by no means the result of a logical or natural progression. The sense in which it is dictated by the development of knowledge or technique is complex. Today in English-speaking countries, treatment of recent bone fractures is the task of orthopaedic surgeons, whereas, in the German-speaking world, the field is assigned to general surgery (Schlich, 2002, pp.10–19, 158–9). Often, fields of responsibility were disputed. In the past, both general surgeons and gynaecologists wanted to treat breast cancer. The outcome of these struggles depended on a number of factors that had nothing to do with the nature of the contended field. Frequently, it was the political power of the groups involved or the influence of individual leaders that tipped the balance. Sometimes, the logic of administrative organization in a particular country determined which fields emerged as specialties. As medical historian George Weisz found, the reason to specialize at all may be seen not so much as a reaction to the rapid expansion of knowledge but rather in 'a new collective desire to expand medical knowledge that initially prompted doctors to specialize' (Weisz, 2003, p.539).

Solving problems with the scalpel: the attractiveness of the technological fix

The twentieth century became the century of surgery, as surgery became the 'technological fix' to solve all sorts of problems – not all of them medical. The attractiveness of the technological fix of surgery led to excesses. In the first half of the twentieth century, various types of operation that were later deemed to be useless were performed on a routine basis, such as the fixing of 'misplaced' organs. Others were performed in numbers that today seem irrational, such as tonsillectomies in children with sore throats or hysterectomies for women suffering from menopausal problems (Tröhler, 1993, pp.1002–3).

In addition, ever more social or cultural problems were redefined as medical problems and thus made amenable to a surgical solution. A case in point is transplantation of the testis as a 'cure' for homosexuality and, its female counterpart, ovary transplants to stop 'deviant' behaviour (Schlich, 1998, pp.132–77). In the 1930s, psycho-surgery was used to correct deviant behaviour in cases that seemed to resist other therapies. The Portuguese surgeon Antonio Caetano Egas Moniz (1874–1955) introduced lobotomy for chronic schizophrenia in 1936 and was awarded a Nobel Prize in 1949 (Pressman, 1998). Plastic surgery was devised to improve physical appearance and counteract appearance-based discrimination.

It is obvious that surgery reflects a modern tendency to prefer a technological fix to other strategies: liposuction instead of diets, liver transplants instead of treatment for alcohol addiction, brain surgery instead of psychotherapy, trauma surgery instead of safe driving, and – to put it polemically – war surgery instead of diplomacy. Some of these technological solutions, such as lobotomy, have fallen into disgrace; others have seen an enormous expansion since the second half of the twentieth century, such as the paragon of elective surgery – cosmetic surgery (Gilman, 1999). Traumatology is another successful branch of modern surgery that has experienced an expansion in response to the risks societies are ready to accept in industry, traffic and sports (Schlich, 2002). As these examples indicate, surgery is often involved in decisions about the way we live and how we organize society. Typically, the cultural, social and conceptual implications of surgery have become invisible: 'In surgery', Christopher Lawrence rightly claims, 'the fiction that medicine has nothing to do with politics reached its purest expression. Surgical intervention could be represented as the inevitable, scientific solution, in comparison to which alternative solutions seemed inferior' (Lawrence, 1992, p.32).

3.5   Conclusion: the rise of modern surgery

Contrary to all appearances, the development of surgery was by no means natural or self-evident. Nor was it in any simple way the result of technical progress. Many people tend to think that technical innovation has driven the whole process because the story of modern surgery is presented as a sequence of technical innovations. Told in this way, the history of modern surgery is a history of progress, the story of the 'rise' of surgery. A different picture emerges when the focus is broadened to examine the professional, conceptual and technical dimensions and their influences on one another. Seen from this perspective, the surgical point of view is not a timeless, absolute and value-free way of describing the body and disease. It is only a partial perception, one possible way of seeing the world, shaped by the professional, cognitive and technical interests of those who were involved in creating this particular form of bodily knowledge (Lawrence, 1992, p.21).

References

Cooter, R. (1993) *Surgery and Society in Peace and War: Orthopaedics and the Organization of Modern Medicine, 1880–1948*, Basingstoke: Macmillan.

Gelfand, T. (1980) *Professionalizing Modern Medicine: Paris Surgeons and Medical Science and Institutions in the Eighteenth Century*, Westport and London: Greenwood.

Gilman, S.L. (1999) *Making the Body Beautiful: A Cultural History of Aesthetic Surgery*, Princeton: Princeton University Press.

Gross, D. (1999) *Die Aufhebung des Wundarztberufs: Ursachen, Begleitumstände und Auswirkungen am Beispiel des Königreichs Württemberg, 1806–1918* [The Abolition of the Trade of Surgery, Causes, Conditions and Consequences: The Example of the Kingdon of Württemberg], Stuttgart: Franz Steiner.

Lawrence, C. (ed.) (1992) *Medical Theory, Surgical Practice: Studies in the History of Surgery*, London: Routledge.

Lawrence, G. (1993) 'Surgery traditional' in W.F. Bynum and R. Porter (eds) *Companion Encyclopaedia of the History of Medicine*, vol.2, London: Routledge, pp.961–83.

Lawrence, C. and Dixey, R. (1992) 'Practising on principle: Joseph Lister and the germ theories of disease' in C. Lawrence (ed.) *Medical Theory, Surgical Practice: Studies in the History of Surgery*, London: Routledge.

Lesch, J.E. (1984) *Science and Medicine in France: The Emergence of Experimental Physiology, 1790–1855*, Cambridge: Harvard University Press.

Maulitz, R.C. (1993) 'The pathological tradition' in W.F. Bynum and R. Porter (eds) *Companion Encyclopaedia of the History of Medicine*, vol.1, London: Routledge, pp.169–91.

Mörgeli, C. (1999) *The Surgeon's Stage: A History of the Operating Room*, Basel: Editiones Roche.

Pernick, M. (1985) *A Calculus of Suffering: Pain, Professionalism and Anesthesia in Nineteenth-Century America*, New York: Columbia University Press.

Pickstone, J.V. (2000) *Ways of Knowing: A New History of Science, Technology and Medicine*, Manchester: Manchester University Press.

Porter, R. (1996) 'Hospitals and surgery' in R. Porter (ed.) *The Cambridge Illustrated History of Medicine*, Cambridge: Cambridge University Press, pp.212–45.

Porter, R. (1999) *The Greatest Benefit to Mankind: A Medical History of Humanity from Antiquity to the Present*, London: Fontana.

Pressman, J.D. (1998) *Last Resort: Psychosurgery and the Limits of Medicine*, Cambridge: Cambridge University Press.

Sander, S. (1989) *Handwerkschirurgen: Sozialgeschichte einer verdrängten Berufsgruppe* [Barber Surgeons: The Social History of a Suppressed Occupational Group], Göttingen: Vandenhoeck & Ruprecht.

Schlich, T. (1998) *Die Erfindung der Organtransplantation: Erfolg und Scheitern des chirurgischen Organersatzes, 1880–1930* [The Invention of Organ Transplantation: Success and Failure of Surgical Organ Replacement, 1880–1930], Frankfurt and New York: Campus.

Schlich, T. (2002) *Surgery, Science and Industry: A Revolution in Fracture Care, 1950s–1990s*, Basingstoke: Palgrave Macmillan.

Temkin, O. (1951) 'The role of surgery in the rise of modern medical thought', *Bulletin for the History of Medicine*, vol.25, pp.248–59.

Tröhler, U. (1984) *Auf dem Weg zur physiologischen Chirurgie: Der Nobelpreisträger Theodor Kocher 1841–1917* [Towards Physiological Surgery: The Nobel Laureate Theodor Kocher, 1841–1917], Basel, Boston and Stuttgart: Birkhäuser.

Tröhler, U. (1993) 'Surgery, modern' in W.F. Bynum and R. Porter (eds) *Companion Encyclopaedia of the History of Medicine*, vol.2, London: Routledge, pp.984–1028.

Wangensteen, O.H. and Wangensteen, S.D. (1978) *The Rise of Surgery: From Empiric Craft to Scientific Discipline*, Folkestone: William Dawson.

Weisz, G. (2003) 'The emergence of specialization in the nineteenth century', *Bulletin of the History of Medicine*, vol.77, no.3, pp.536–75.

Worboys, M. (2000) *Spreading Germs: Disease Theories and Medical Practice in Britain, 1865–1900*, Cambridge: Cambridge University Press.

Source Book readings

C. Lawrence, 'Democratic, divine and heroic: the history and historiography of surgery' in C. Lawrence (ed.) *Medical Theory, Surgical Practice: Studies in the History of Surgery*, London: Routledge, 1992, pp.20–3 (Reading 3.1).

C. Bernard, *An Introduction to the Study of Experimental Medicine*, New York: Dover, 1957, pp.168–9 (Reading 3.2).

M.S. Pernick, *A Calculus of Suffering: Pain, Professionalism and Anesthesia in Nineteenth-Century America*, New York: Columbia University Press, 1985, pp.208–21 (Reading 3.3).

E.T. Kocher, 'Concerning pathological manifestations in low-grade thyroid diseases', Nobel lecture, 17 December 1909, *Nobel Lectures, including Presentation Speeches and Laureates' Biographies: Physiology or Medicine 1901–1921*, London: Elsevier, for the Nobel Foundation, 1967, pp.330–1 (Reading 3.4).

4

The Rise of Laboratory Medicine

Deborah Brunton

Objectives

When you have completed this chapter you should be able to:

- understand that laboratories were used for a wide range of functions – research, teaching, diagnosis and the production of therapies;

- describe how laboratory medicine transformed the understanding of the body and disease by the end of the nineteenth century;

- appreciate that the laboratory had a limited impact on medical practice until the twentieth century;

- explain why some practitioners resisted the introduction of laboratory medicine into medical practice.

4.1   Introduction

In Chapter 1 you read about Nicholas Jewson's analysis of the changes in medicine in the late nineteenth century. 'Laboratory medicine' represented a fundamental shift away from the established view of the body and disease. Where hospital medicine saw disease as a collection of symptoms in life, which related to changes in body structure discovered at post-mortem examination, laboratory medicine sought to explain the structure of the body at the cellular level and to describe its function as a complex series of dynamic processes. Within this medical cosmology, the laboratory usurped the hospital as the locus of research, and the laboratory scientist claimed a greater authority than the clinical practitioner. The diagnosis of particular infectious diseases now relied on tests on tissue samples performed at the lab bench, not simply on the subjective analysis of patterns of symptoms.

At the time Jewson published his article 'The disappearance of the sick-man from medical cosmology, 1770–1870' (1976), few historians would have questioned *how* the laboratory acquired this central role within medicine. In an era when 'high-tech', scientific medicine seemed to supply an endless stream of new theories and better therapies, the laboratory was assumed to have won its place simply on the grounds of utility. Since the 1970s, however, that faith in scientific medicine has waned. Sociologists of science have argued that all knowledge, including knowledge discovered in the lab, is socially constructed; in other words, it is influenced by social, political and economic processes. Sociologists of health have suggested that the price of 'high-tech' cures has been patients' loss of control over their body and therapy. In the 1980s, AIDS proved that medical science was not all-powerful.

In this more sceptical climate, historians of medicine since the 1980s have asked *why* the laboratory acquired its prestigious position within medicine. They have shown that laboratories flourished in particular political and cultural circumstances. Knowledge generated in the laboratory was not immediately embraced by all. In the face of opposition from some practitioners who saw it as a threat to their established knowledge and skills, researchers had to demonstrate the value of this new understanding. Practical results, however, did not immediately flow from the laboratory.

This chapter explores the rise of laboratory medicine from 1830 to 1930. It reassesses when and how the laboratory transformed medical theory and practice, and explores the ways in which historians have written about the history of the laboratory.

4.2   What is a laboratory?

Many historians speak of 'laboratory medicine' as if it were a monolithic entity. In fact, this is really a convenient shorthand. As you will see, laboratory medicine has covered many different areas of medical knowledge, and the laboratory itself has had a range of functions. If you look carefully at Jewson's paper, you will see that he uses 'laboratory medicine' to mean both new knowledge discovered in the laboratory at the end of the nineteenth century and diagnosis carried out in the laboratory. However, the functions of the lab were (and are) even wider than he suggests.

The first laboratories were constructed to carry out research. From the seventeenth century, a few wealthy amateur scientists had rooms in their homes where they conducted chemical experiments. Private laboratories such as these (small areas in the home where practitioners carried out research that was often linked to their practice) continued to exist into the twentieth century. From the eighteenth century, laboratories began to find a place in public institutions. Universities and medical schools built chemistry laboratories where staff could conduct research. These labs also had a teaching function: here, staff prepared the experiments they used to illustrate lectures (which were mainly attended by medical students) and to teach research skills to a few favoured students (Fenby, 1989, pp.29–32).

The growth of laboratory teaching is discussed in more detail below.

In the nineteenth century, research and teaching functions were separated. Special teaching laboratories first appeared in the 1800s. At first, these were small spaces in which a few students were systematically taught how to analyse chemicals or use microscopes. By the middle of the century, all medical students were expected to undergo some laboratory training, and by 1900, much of their early training was spent moving between the lecture room and the laboratory.

At the same time, university and medical-school staff and their senior students conducted research in separate, well-equipped laboratories either within the university or in research institutes. At the end of the nineteenth century, institutions dedicated to medical research and separate from universities were established across Europe. The Pasteur Institute was founded in Paris in 1888, the Institute for Infectious Diseases was established in Berlin in 1891 and the Institute for Experimental Medicine in St Petersburg was created the following year. The British Institute of Preventative Medicine (later renamed the Lister Institute) was founded in London in 1893 (Weindling, 1992a, pp.170–1). In the twentieth century, research labs were also set up by pharmaceutical companies to find new drugs, to produce vaccines and anti-toxins used to treat diseases, and for quality control – to test the potency of products. In Germany, many of these pharmaceutical labs had close connections with universities and research institutes.

At the end of the nineteenth century, laboratories were set up to provide an additional function – diagnostic testing. Local government and hospital laboratories provided diagnostic services to practitioners inside and outside institutions, identifying infectious diseases, analysing body fluids and diagnosing cancerous tumours. Public-health laboratories also checked the quality of foodstuffs sold in shops.

Laboratories, then, were used for a wide range of activities – research, teaching, drug production, testing and diagnosis. These varied functions were reflected in the physical spaces of the laboratory.

Exercise

Look at the photographs in Figures 4.1–4.10. Note the differences between these different types of laboratory, but think too about what they have in common. What features defined all these spaces as 'laboratories'?

Teaching laboratories

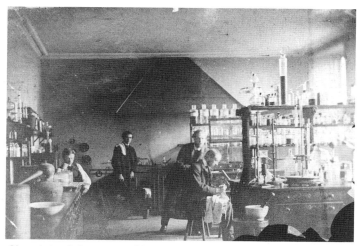

Figure 4.1   Chemistry laboratory, Glasgow University, 1864. A very early photograph of a chemistry laboratory. The lab was created in 1831, when it was reckoned to be 'one of the best and most complete of its time'. However, the space looks rather small: only a few students could have worked here. The room contains arrays of benches, each of which has a set of chemicals, as well as a variety of pieces of apparatus for distilling chemicals, and a large mortar and pestle. University of Glasgow/SCRAN

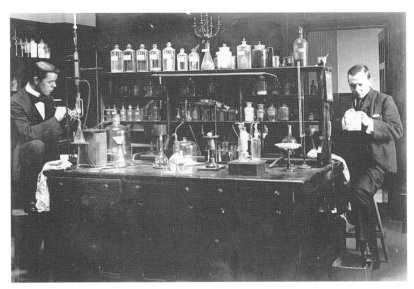

Figure 4.2   Chemistry laboratory, Glasgow University, 1894. This was one of the larger laboratories built on Glasgow University's new campus at Gilmorehill in 1870. The benches and equipment are remarkably similar to those used thirty years earlier. Bottles of chemicals still dominate the picture, although the equipment for analysing and synthesizing chemicals looks rather more sophisticated. University of Glasgow/SCRAN

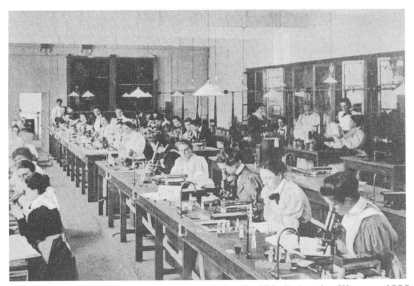

Figure 4.3   Physiology laboratory, London School of Medicine for Women, 1899. This photograph clearly shows the arrangement of space and equipment in a large late nineteenth-century teaching laboratory. The students sit at long benches, each with an identical set of equipment – in this case a microscope and the materials needed to view and prepare slides. (Note that this is a very different set of skills from those taught in a chemistry laboratory.) Good lighting is provided throughout the room. At the side and back of the lab, you can see the demonstrators who helped the students with their work. Wellcome Library, London

Specialist laboratories

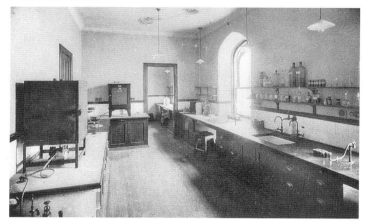

Figure 4.4   Research laboratory, Royal Victoria Dispensary, Edinburgh, *c*.1913. Founded in 1887, the Royal Victoria Dispensary was the first dispensary in Britain set up especially to deal with tuberculosis patients. This laboratory, along with the rest of the dispensary, was installed in a set of flats in Spittal Street, Edinburgh. Although described as a research laboratory, it was highly specialized in its functions: workers probably spent much of their time cultivating specimens of tuberculosis bacteria. The lab therefore contains a limited amount of equipment: benches, sinks and some chemicals. The large box in the left foreground is an incubator in which bacteriological specimens were grown. Lothian Health Services Archive/SCRAN

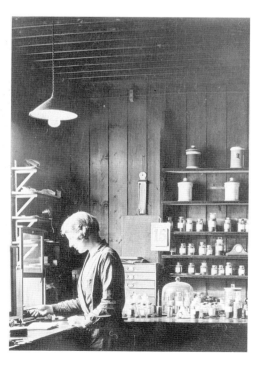

Figure 4.5   Miss Cairns at the chemical explosives works, Roslin, *c*.1910–20. Many laboratories were established within factories, where workers could monitor the quality of the chemicals or pharmaceuticals produced. Although this lab was within an explosives factory, it gives a good idea of the small scale of the facilities and the rather simple equipment required for routine testing within industry. By courtesy of the National Museums of Scotland/SCRAN

Size isn't everything

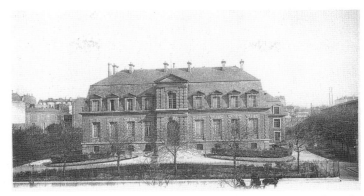

Figure 4.6   The Pasteur Institute, Paris, 1888. The institute was built in Paris in 1888 both to honour the work of Louis Pasteur and to provide a base for his further research. It occupied a site of 11,000 square metres and included research laboratories, staff accommodation, a small ward for clinical research, laboratories for teaching advanced courses in microbiology and, eventually, Pasteur's tomb. © Institute Pasteur/Wellcome Library, London

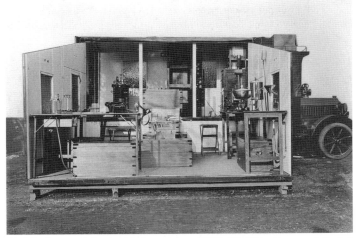

Figure 4.7   Mobile bacteriological laboratory, 1912–13. This tiny mobile laboratory contains many of the standard pieces of equipment seen in other pictures – benches and a sink (with a water pipe) in the left foreground. It also contains sterilizers on the bench on the right. Mobile labs such as this were used in the First World War to identify diseases and infections among sick and wounded soldiers. Wellcome Library, London

The research laboratory

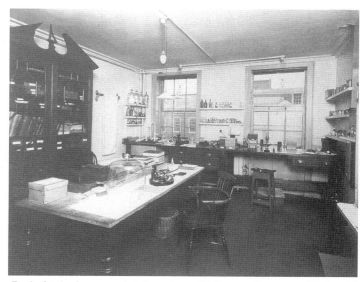

Figure 4.8   Pathological research laboratory, Wellcome Bureau of Scientific Research, 1926. The Burroughs Wellcome Drug Company set up laboratories in 1894 and had one of the largest research facilities of any British pharmaceutical firm in the early twentieth century. However, this pathology laboratory in the 1920s still has very simple equipment – chemicals for staining preparations and microscopes. Note the large bookcase – in a research lab, workers would need to consult books and journals to help with their investigations. Wellcome Library, London

Scientists at work

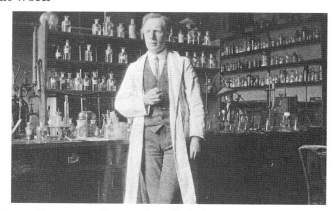

Figure 4.9   George Barger, professor of medical chemistry, Edinburgh University, c.1920. This photograph shows the modern archetype of the scientist: Barger is shown in his laboratory against the background of a bench crowded with chemicals and equipment. He wears the white coat that we now associate with both scientists and doctors. Barger was one of the pioneers of medical chemistry (later called biochemistry), and introduced the subject to the curriculum at Edinburgh University. Lothian Health Services Archive/SCRAN

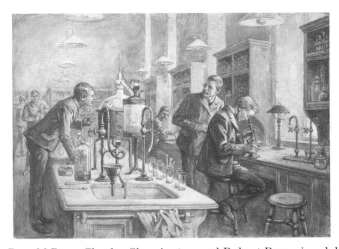

Figure 4.10   Ronald Ross, Charles Sherrington and Rubert Boyce in a laboratory at the Liverpool School of Tropical Medicine, 1899. At this time, tropical medicine was just emerging as a specialist area of study into the causes of diseases that hampered development in European colonies in Africa and Asia. This drawing shows two of the most eminent men in the new field. Ronald Ross (1857–1932) had discovered the role of the mosquito in transmitting malaria in 1897, while Rubert Boyce (1863–1911) was instrumental in setting up the Liverpool School and worked on yellow fever. Charles S. Sherrington (1857–1952) is best known as a physiologist for his work on the role of reflexes in coordinating function. This is a research laboratory yet the equipment, again, is relatively simple – microscopes and glassware. The identity of the three men is revealed by their location. The artist gives a sense of dramatic enquiry by posing the figures in animated discussion in the midst of their work at the laboratory bench. Wellcome Library, London

Discussion

These photographs show how the physical space of the laboratory varied in size, location, layout and equipment. In part, this variation was a reflection of function: a lab used for product testing required different facilities and equipment from one used for teaching. All the laboratories nevertheless share one feature: the presence of specialist equipment – chemicals, microscopes and balances. These were used by researchers to observe biological and chemical phenomena, and to perform experiments. The equipment defined the laboratory; it turned a space – whether in a purpose-built research institute, a room in an Edinburgh flat, or a van – into a laboratory.

4.3   Transforming knowledge

Just as you should not think of 'the laboratory' as a monolithic institution, the medical knowledge that emerged from research laboratories in the nineteenth and early twentieth centuries was not a coherent whole. Rather, it covered a number of separate fields: the minute structure and function of the healthy and diseased body; the effects of drugs on the body's **physiology**; and the results of infection by micro-organisms. Research in these quite distinct fields went on simultaneously, developing in distinct ways. This research revolutionized medical practitioners' understanding of the body, of disease and of therapeutics. In 1800, the body was understood in terms of its structure: researchers worked on uncovering the detailed anatomy of the healthy body and on pathological anatomy – the structural changes brought about by disease. Laboratory medicine completely revised this understanding by bringing fundamental new insights into the structure and, especially, the function of the body. There is room here for only a brief overview of the discoveries made in laboratory medicine. You can read a fuller account in Roy Porter's *The Greatest Benefit to Mankind* (1999), pp.320–47, 428–54, 534–82, or in the relevant essays in Bynum and Porter, *Companion Encyclopaedia of the History of Medicine* (1993): 'Microscopical tradition', vol.1, pp.102–19; 'Physiological tradition', vol.1, pp.120–52; 'Biochemical tradition', vol.1, pp.153–68; 'Pathological tradition, vol.1, pp.169–91; 'Immunological tradition', vol.1, pp.192–204; and 'Drug therapies', vol.2, pp.915–38.

As you read in Chapter 1, the earliest form of new knowledge associated with the laboratory was revealed by the microscope. From the 1830s, thanks to technical improvements to the instrument, practitioners were able to explore minute structures within the body – the study of histology. In 1839, Theodor Schwann realized that animal tissues, like plant tissues, were made up of cells, and that all cells were derived from other cells. Over the next decades, helped by new techniques such as the use of chemicals that selectively stained different parts of the cell, researchers uncovered the structure of a wide range of cells. Johannes Purkyně (1787–1869) and others, for example, uncovered the unique structure of nerve cells, with their long, thread-like processes that form networks throughout the body, and Jacob Henle (1809–85) revealed long, looping cells within the kidney. Researchers also began to explore disease at the cellular level. In 1858, Rudolf Virchow developed the doctrine that all diseases were the result of abnormal changes in cells, and studied the growth of cancerous tumours.

The most important developments in medical knowledge came in revelations concerning the function of the living body, the study of physiology, which flourished after 1850. Medical practitioners had long been interested in how the body worked, but until the nineteenth century they had few means of investigating the function of organs and tissues in the living body. From the 1830s, researchers began to use the microscope, and to devise experiments to explore the processes going on within the body. In 1847, a group of German researchers declared that the body operated by the same physical laws as the rest of the world and could be investigated through chemical and physical analysis. Across Europe, in Germany, France, Britain and Russia, researchers began to measure and experiment on the body in new ways. They subjected body fluids to chemical analysis. Using new surgical techniques (discussed in Chapter 3), they experimented on animals and humans, analysing changes in the pressure and flow of body fluids, measuring changes in body temperature, isolating and stimulating tissues and glands to investigate their functions, and exploring the chemical and nervous pathways by which the body's functions are coordinated.

Physiological researchers explored every system of the body, but the nervous system proved a particularly fruitful area of research. For the first time, experiments allowed researchers to uncover the function of the different parts of the nervous system. By selectively stimulating different nerves, researchers revealed that not all nerves perform the same functions. They discovered that there are three separate systems of nerves – motor (controlling conscious movement), sensory (responding to stimuli in the outside world) and autonomic (controlling functions below the level of consciousness – such as the working of the digestive system). Researchers discovered that brain function is localized; experiments in which the surface of the brain was stimulated, or in which parts of the brain were surgically removed, showed that specific areas process different types of information, such as movement, vision and balance. They also explored how nerves communicate by electrical impulses, and in 1848 Hermann von Helmholtz measured the speed of the nerve impulse. Researchers discovered the role of reflexes – nervous responses originating in the spine rather than the brain (a sort of nervous 'short-cut') – which are used in coordinating movement and other body functions. Ivan Pavlov (1849–1936) showed in his famous experiment that reflex responses can be learned: a dog that had learned to associate the ringing of a bell with food would salivate when the bell was rung, even if no food was presented.

A second major area of physiological research was on the body's digestion and **metabolism**. Laboratory workers explored how food is broken down, waste products secreted and body function maintained at steady rates. Claude Bernard, one of the pioneers of physiology, worked on many aspects of digestion and his research established a number of the fundamental tenets of physiology. His work on the liver in 1848 demonstrated that the body is capable of building up, as well as breaking down, complex molecules. Even when animals were fed on a sugar-free diet, the liver was able to synthesize glycogen (a form of starch), which was stored and then broken down into sugars when required by the body. Bernard also showed that the body is able to regulate its own internal environment; for example, it could maintain a constant internal temperature, a concept later named 'homeostasis' (Lesch, 1984, pp.197–224). In Germany, around the same time, Karl Ludwig (1816–95) discovered that the kidneys produce urine, by filtering out waste products and water from the blood under the high pressure generated by the unique structure of the kidney's cells.

By the twentieth century, physiology had divided into sub-disciplines. New areas of research emerged in different ways. **Endocrinology**, the study of the chemical messengers produced by the body to regulate physiological activity, emerged as a new field of research following a crucial discovery in 1902. Ernst Starling (1866–1927) and William Bayliss (1860–1924), working at University College London, showed that the intestines secrete a substance that stimulates the pancreas – a quite separate organ – to begin secreting digestive juices. This unknown substance, which they called 'secretin', was the first **hormone** to be identified. Other hormones identified during the next few decades include adrenaline (produced by the adrenal glands, which regulates blood pressure), insulin (produced in the pancreas, which regulates the level of sugars in the blood) and the sex hormones (which regulate reproduction). **Biochemistry**, another important sub-discipline of physiology, was born from an existing research tradition. Medical practitioners had been investigating 'animal chemistry' – the chemistry of body fluids, especially the products of metabolism and digestion – since the early nineteenth century. In the early twentieth century, biochemical research coalesced around a few major problems – the nature of proteins, metabolic processes and nutrition. Between 1912 and 1930, as a result of studies on diseases known to be caused by diet deficiency, the vitamins A, B1, B2, D and E were identified.

Laboratory research also provided new understanding of the causation of certain diseases through the study of bacteriology. By 1860, Louis Pasteur had shown that fermentation and putrefaction arose from organisms present in the air. This work later inspired surgeons to investigate the role of micro-organisms in causing wound infections (discussed in Chapter 3). In 1878, Pasteur demonstrated that some diseases, including anthrax, were also the result of the action of micro-organisms. In 1882, Robert Koch identified the bacteria responsible for tuberculosis – the first time that a specific disease had been shown to be caused by a bacterium. He followed up this triumph by identifying the cholera bacterium in 1883. Thereafter, until 1900, the organisms responsible for diseases were identified at the astonishing rate of one per year: Koch's students discovered the agents responsible for diphtheria, typhoid, pneumonia, leprosy, plague and syphilis. This new understanding of the agents responsible for disease was made possible by simple improvements in experimental techniques. Richard Julius Petri (1852–1921) introduced the now ubiquitous shallow glass dishes that bear his name, and Koch devised the technique of growing bacteria on solid gels rather than in liquid broth. These changes allowed researchers to see the characteristic colour and shape of colonies of bacteria.

As well as working on disease causation and disease processes, laboratory researchers explored the effects of drugs on body function, a field known as **pharmacology**. This was another area of research with a long tradition. In the early nineteenth century, practitioners studying the ways in which poisons act on the body had sometimes employed the extremely dangerous technique of consuming a small amount of the drug and noting the symptoms. Robert Christison (1797–1882), a distinguished Edinburgh professor and expert on poisons, almost killed himself during one such experiment. Realizing that the poison was taking effect and that he was dying, he is alleged to have shouted from the window to a medical colleague who happened to be passing. The colleague rushed in and forced him to drink soapy water, which made him vomit up the poison. In the 1840s, using animals as experimental subjects, Bernard showed that poisons affect very specific areas within the body. Curare (the poison used on blowpipe arrows), for example, acted only at the point at which a nerve met a muscle. By the mid-nineteenth century, developments in the chemical industry supplied new knowledge about the structure of molecules, and thus how drugs interact with the cells of the body. Paul Ehrlich (1854–1915) devised the theory that is the basis for the design of modern chemical drugs: that the molecules of the drug can act only when they lock on to a special receptor on the surface of a particular type of cell. Ehrlich's idea opened up the possibility of 'magic bullets': drugs that would target microbes within the body, leaving all other cells unharmed (Bynum and Porter, 1993, vol.2, pp.915–38).

In addition to producing new knowledge, the work of laboratory researchers affected medicine in other, fundamental ways. The success of laboratory research led to the reorganization of the research process. In the mid-nineteenth century, researchers worked independently, often with limited facilities, exploring a wide range of topics. Bernard, for example, spent much of his research working in the basement of the College de France. Using his surgical skills, and an ability to design simple and elegant experiments, he worked not only on liver function and the action of poisons, but on the nervous control of heat within the body. By the 1870s, research was increasingly based in large institutes, where a number of workers carried out coordinated and systematic programmes of investigation. The historian Daniel Todes has called Pavlov's institute a 'knowledge factory'. There, a stream of medical graduates worked for short periods on specific problems within Pavlov's overall project to explore the function, integration and control of the digestive system (Todes, 1988). (His famous experiment on reflexes was just a tiny part of that programme.)

Laboratory research also changed the nature of medical knowledge. In the early nineteenth century, symptoms were described in qualitative terms: patients were 'feverish'; they had a raised pulse-rate; or their urine was a particular colour. These were subjective accounts, in which clinical signs were detected by the physician's sense of touch or sight. In laboratory medicine, body function was measured: information was gathered accurately and objectively. Body temperature and blood pressure were measured, and urine was subjected to chemical analysis. In short, medicine was turned from an art into a science. This new quest for objectivity was reflected in the development of new equipment. Some machines were quite simple – the clinical thermometer measured temperature, and the spirometer measured the capacity of the lungs. Others were more complex. The archetypal piece of physiological equipment was the kymograph, devised in the 1840s by Ludwig. This transmitted changes in pressure in an artery to a pen, which produced a trace on a revolving drum. The kymograph thus made a direct, permanent and visual record of a transitory physiological phenomenon. It spawned a range of related devices, including the myograph (to measure muscle contraction) and the polygraph (to measure the pulse in arteries and veins). In the twentieth century, a new generation of machines traced out levels of electrical activity in the body; these included the electroencephalogram (EEG), used to plot the electrical activity within the brain, and the electrocardiograph (ECG), to trace the action of the heart. The graphs they produced became 'proof' of otherwise invisible physiological functions (Chadarevian, 1993; Frank, 1988, pp.211–94) In 1895, one researcher summed up:

> As modern civilisation is impossible without railway lines, the telegraph, and the telephone, so today research in physiology, pharmacology, or pathology are inconceivable without the use of the graphical method ...

Now the mere assertion could no longer suffice, one wanted to see it 'supported by a curve'.

(Chadarevian, 1993, p.273)

Researchers also established new standards of proof by which discoveries could be accepted by communities of researchers. The best example of this is the set of rules devised by Koch for identifying the bacteria associated with diseases, known as 'Koch's postulates'. These required that:

1   the organism suspected of causing a particular disease could be discovered in every instance of the disease;

2   when extracted from the body, the germ could be grown in the laboratory and maintained for several generations;

3   when this culture was injected into animals, it should induce the same disease observed in the original source;

4   the organism could then be retrieved from the experimental animal and cultured again.

This new knowledge of the body changed the way in which practitioners thought about disease. Practitioners began to interpret symptoms as the manifestation of an underlying disruption of physiological processes. Bacteriological discoveries meant that infectious diseases were no longer identified by a characteristic pattern of symptoms, but by the presence of bacteria. In the first reading for this chapter, Andrew Cunningham explores the circumstances surrounding the identification of the bacteria that causes plague.

Read 'Laboratory knowledge' (Source Book 2, Reading 4.2).

1   According to Cunningham, what were the steps that led to the discovery of the bacteria?

2   How well does Cunningham's account fit with Jewson's description of laboratory medicine?

1   Cunningham describes how the first step taken by the two rival investigators is to set up laboratories, which sound like very simple affairs with minimal equipment. Thereafter, they follow Koch's postulates, which set out a strict research programme. Both consistently find a micro-organism in the bodies of many plague victims. This organism is cultured in the laboratory (notice that the two descriptions of the bacteria vary slightly). When injected into laboratory animals, the organism produces the symptoms of plague. After this, both researchers feel confident that when they publish their findings their results will be accepted by the scientific community.

2   Cunningham's account fits well with Jewson's description of laboratory medicine as being divorced from the patient's bedside and the work of practitioners. No patients appear in Cunningham's account – the dead victims of plague supply the tissue samples, and everything else is done by the researcher.

It is tempting to think that laboratory medicine completely changed medicine. Nineteenth-century researchers frequently drew a clear distinction between the type of work performed in the laboratory and work carried out in the hospital, in order to emphasize the novelty of their work: whereas the hospital or bedside was the site for qualitative and subjective observation, in the laboratory, they claimed, researchers and students could conduct experiments, singling out one particular chemical reaction within the body, or the function of one organ, and producing objective observations and quantitative measurements. While many historians, including Jewson, have accepted this distinction, there were strong continuities between laboratory medicine and hospital medicine. In the early nineteenth century, researchers in pathological anatomy presented their work as 'scientific': they were engaged in carefully observing the effects of disease on body function (in life) and structure (after death). Laennec's stethoscope is now thought of as a diagnostic tool but it was originally devised as a way of augmenting pathologists' understanding of disease. It allowed practitioners to trace the progress of disease, which was then confirmed at autopsy (as you have read in the translation of Laennec's case in Chapter 1) (Warner, 1995, p.187). Many laboratories were built within hospital medical schools, and laboratories geared to diagnostic procedures were a feature of hospitals in the early twentieth century.

The acceptance of new ideas

As you have read in Chapter 1, some practitioners questioned the new medical knowledge emerging from the laboratory. They wondered whether researchers really saw the body's minute structure through the microscope, or whether they saw optical phenomena produced by the microscope itself. Others doubted whether the bacteria identified by Koch were really the sole cause of infectious disease. However, the doubters were the minority, and the findings of laboratory researchers were rapidly accepted by most medical practitioners. This may be seen in the speed with which these ideas, and the processes of laboratory research, were adopted into medical teaching and the requirements for medical licences. Medical qualifications are an important marker of the acceptance of new knowledge: they defined the knowledge that students were expected to acquire in order to become competent practitioners.

You will read more about how education and licensing defined the medical profession in Chapter 5.

The first formal courses taught in the laboratory were in chemistry. In Glasgow, Thomas Thomson (1773–1852) set up a practical chemistry class in 1807. From 1824, Justus von Liebeg (1803–73), professor of chemistry at the University of Geissen, trained students in a range of techniques and then supervised their specified research projects (Porter, 1999, pp.322–5). In the 1830s, teachers in France, Britain and Germany set up classes in which students could learn how to use the microscope (La Berge, 1994, pp.296–362). These classes were all fairly small. Laboratory teaching for the entire body of medical students was first established in university medical faculties in the German states in the 1840s and 1850s, initially in chemistry and later in physiology, pathological anatomy and pharmacology. These novel courses attracted hundreds of students from across Europe and America (Bonner, 1995, pp.231–64).

In the second half of the nineteenth century, courses in laboratory sciences became a standard part of medical training. In France, large-scale laboratory teaching was instituted in the 1860s and 1870s. In Britain, the large medical schools in London and Edinburgh introduced laboratory teaching to the medical curriculum from the 1870s. Students began their training in laboratories, learning the basic sciences of chemistry, zoology and botany, before moving on to study medical subjects, including physiology, pathology, histology and pharmacology and finally completing their training with clinical studies on the hospital wards. Students were required to attend laboratory classes to obtain a medical licence. In the German states, laboratory studies were made part of the licensing requirements from 1858. In France, laboratory work was required for a licence in 1878, while some British licensing authorities required attendance at laboratory classes as part of their requirements for qualification from the early 1870s.

Why did medical practitioners embrace the new laboratory sciences? Why were students so eager to take courses in the laboratory, and teachers so willing to offer them? Some idea of the possible reasons for this acceptance can be found in Claude Bernard's *Introduction à l'étude de la médecine expérimentale* [An Introduction to the Study of Experimental Medicine], written in 1865. This is a polemical work which presents an ideal vision of medical education rather than a picture of teaching in France at the time.

Exercise

Read 'The power of the laboratory' (Source Book 2, Reading 4.1).

I   What role does Bernard see for the hospital and the laboratory in teaching and practice?

2   What are the implications of Bernard's vision for senior hospital staff, who constituted the elite of the medical profession?

Discussion

I   Bernard argues that the laboratory has to be at the centre of both teaching and medical practice. The laboratory is the source of knowledge of the body and of disease: it produces the newest and therefore the most complete knowledge, built on past researches but free of the false theorizing of past generations, and verified by experiment, not merely by observation. All medical students should be trained there in experimental skills (this is the 'pinnacle' of their studies), and all practitioners should have their own laboratory to help them investigate cases encountered in their practice. The hospital still has a role in training, which is complementary, but subservient, to the laboratory. In hospitals, students can observe disease phenomena, but only in the laboratory can they perform experiments to help them understand the physiological processes underlying those phenomena.

2   Bernard does not explicitly discuss the effects of this vision for the laboratory on the profession. Clearly, he accords a new and greater value to laboratory teaching within medical education. By downplaying the role of the hospital in teaching and the production of knowledge, he is granting greater authority to the scientist over the clinician. He also makes clear that the clinician cannot challenge the conclusions drawn from laboratory research – only other scientists, trained to the same standard and with the same knowledge of the scientific literature, can judge the veracity of laboratory work.

In the past, historians accepted the arguments made by Bernard and his fellow researchers: that practitioners accepted the new laboratory medicine because it offered a deeper understanding of the body and promised more effective therapies. More recently, though, historians looking at the impact of the laboratory on practice have found that few new therapies emerged before 1900 (as you will explore later in this chapter). They have suggested a range of other reasons – professional, educational, social and political – for its acceptance.

For a more detailed discussion of the changing status of medical practitioners at this time, see Chapter 5.

Some historians have argued that the laboratory served an important rhetorical function. At a time when practitioners felt that they did not enjoy the public respect owed to a profession, they used the new knowledge discovered in the laboratory to project an image of their occupation as 'scientific', progressive, rational and objective. They hoped that the association of medicine with science would bring it a new authority and help to improve the social standing of practitioners (Warner, 1995, pp.169–70, 179–83).

Work on the introduction of laboratory teaching in the German-speaking universities suggests that new courses were instituted not simply to teach new, practical knowledge. In the next reading, you will see that even though the German state governments had a reputation for being generous patrons of laboratory science, researchers nevertheless had to make a good case for new laboratories.

Exercise

Read 'The rationale for the laboratory' (Source Book 2, Reading 4.3).

1   What arguments do the three researchers use to persuade the authorities of the need for a new physiology institute?

2   How do these compare with Bernard's arguments?

Discussion

1   Remarkably, all three applicants put forward different reasons to found new research institutes. Purkyně's claim is based simply on the status of physiology as a new science. He argues that physiology is now a distinctive body of knowledge, with its own methodology. It is separate from anatomy and the other sciences,

and therefore deserves a position similar to that of the older sciences within the university, with its own facilities for teaching and research. Schultz, by contrast, makes a case for a physiological institute for pedagogical reasons, using educational theories current at this time. He sees a close link between teaching and research: professors should be engaged in research, and students should learn by experimentation rather than by acquiring facts from books. Physiology is particularly suited to this approach. It is concerned with life, and is not a 'dead' science. The only candidate to argue that training in physiology will be of practical use to students in the practice of medicine is Budge. Notice, however, that he argues that the skills of observation learned at the laboratory bench – not just the knowledge – will prove useful.

2   These three documents are therefore all in some ways at odds with Bernard's essay. Where Bernard argues that a knowledge of physiology is crucial to medical practice, providing students with an understanding of how the body functions in health and disease, these German professors see physiology as a subject worthy of study in its own right, or as a vehicle for teaching skills.

Historians have also argued that the rise of laboratory teaching in the German states owed much to its social context; in other words, that a particular set of cultural, political and economic circumstances favoured the creation of new research institutes and posts for researchers. In the 1840s, the twenty-eight German-speaking universities that were generously funded by state governments placed a high value on *Wissenschaft* – a search for knowledge. This in turn placed a high value on research, and created the expectation that university staff should be researchers as well as teachers. As you saw in the previous reading, it also emphasized that students should seek knowledge for themselves, and should not simply absorb facts from textbooks. In the mid-nineteenth century, universities engaged in fierce competition to employ the most distinguished scholars who would add to the prestige of the institution and thereby attract large numbers of fee-paying students, and to this end they provided new research and teaching facilities.

The eagerness of university staff and administrators to pursue laboratory teaching also reflected broader changes in German culture. The 1840s saw a fundamental restructuring of German society. The power of the old elite who held their position through birth and social connections was increasingly threatened by the rise of the middle classes. This conflict underpinned the revolutions of 1848, when all over Europe reformers attempted, but failed, to replace old autocratic regimes with more liberal governments. The growing middle classes held very different values from the aristocracy: they valued talent, hard work and initiative, and believed that merit rather than social standing should become the criterion for advancement. Science would help to advance the nation-state by increasing industrial production, and a scientific education would train the population for life in the modern world (Lenoir, 1992, pp.14–71; Tuchman, 1993, pp.3–13).

The importance of favourable social and political circumstances for the establishment of laboratory teaching is underlined by a comparison of the

German states with France. In France, the success of hospital teaching in the early nineteenth century (which had previously attracted students from across Europe) had led to a split between teaching in the hospital and teaching in the medical school. Neither institution was willing to introduce laboratory sciences into its part of the curriculum, and consequently few teaching laboratories had been established by 1870. However, in the aftermath of their defeat in the Franco-Prussian War in 1871, French educationalists looked to copy methods of teaching from their German victors. The medical curriculum was reformed, and funding was provided for laboratory teaching.

States also supported laboratory research for political reasons. By the end of the nineteenth century, the research laboratory had become a means by which national superiority might be demonstrated, and France and Germany competed to have the best scientists and the best research facilities. In the years after the Franco-Prussian War, France and Germany held up Pasteur and Koch, and their respective university research systems, as proof of the brilliance of French or German science. (This echoed a personal rivalry between Koch and Pasteur.) Koch manipulated these sentiments to obtain his own research institute. In 1890, he pointed out to the Prussian government that the state had no facilities to match the grand new Pasteur Institute in Paris, and that German researchers were in danger of falling behind their French counterparts. The government duly provided most of the funding for a new research institute (Weindling, 1992a, pp.174–8).

In Britain, by contrast, laboratory medicine never acquired such national prestige. The introduction of large-scale laboratory teaching was hampered by an active anti-vivisection movement, described in Chapter 1, and by a lack of funding. Medical schools in Britain did not enjoy state support: they were essentially commercial enterprises. Teaching laboratories were expensive investments, and initially only the large London medical schools could afford to provide and equip such facilities. Some of the smaller provincial medical schools did not acquire laboratory facilities until the 1890s. Britain's main research institute, the Lister Institute, struggled to find support from private individuals. It was not until 1913 that the British government established the Medical Research Council. The MRC's labs became famous for pioneering controlled clinical trials, research on rickets (a deficiency disease) and the effects of the workplace on health, as well as for providing new therapeutic agents such as insulin and vitamin B.

However, even in Britain, the medical laboratory served political ends. In the first decades of the twentieth century, the laboratory offered British government administrators a model for the reform of medical services to make them more efficient. Just as teams of researchers in a laboratory cooperated in solving problems, so the different arms of medical services – GPs, clinics and hospitals – could be made to cooperate in the treatment of patients. The laboratory would play a key role in this process, helping to diagnose and categorize patients into groups that required similar treatment and to sort out more complex cases that required specialist treatment. It also promised to reveal which patients were likely to benefit most from expensive new treatments (Sturdy and Cooter, 1998, pp.439–42).

4.4   Transforming practice

While laboratory research undoubtedly revolutionized understanding of body function and disease, its impact on medical practice is less clear-cut. Laboratory medicine did lead to improved techniques of diagnosis, but research produced few new therapies until the twentieth century. Even when new diagnostic methods and new therapies did become available, practitioners did not rush to adopt them.

The laboratory in diagnosis

Different fields of laboratory research offered a range of new diagnostic techniques. Bacteriological research into the identity of disease-causing micro-organisms provided practitioners with a new and accurate means of diagnosing cases of infectious disease. By the 1890s, specimens from patients suspected of suffering from tuberculosis or diphtheria were routinely cultured to confirm a diagnosis made on the basis of symptoms (Worboys, 2000, pp.211–16, 252–7). Laboratory equipment used to explore physiological function in the healthy body was applied to reveal underlying physiological dysfunction and thus to diagnose disease. The electrocardiograph, for example, which was devised to explore the function of the heart, became a standard piece of hospital equipment used to diagnose heart conditions. It also helped to establish cardiology as a new specialty. Hospitals began to set up small biochemistry laboratories to analyse blood and urine samples taken from patients suffering from physiological diseases such as anaemia or diabetes. In new pathology departments, histological analyses were performed to check whether or not tissues removed during surgery were cancerous (Howell, 1995).

In his article, Jewson assumes that clinical practitioners simply accepted that laboratory scientists – with their new and detailed knowledge of body function – possessed a special authority. Research on British medicine around the turn of the century, however, shows that there was conflict between the two groups, with some practitioners resisting the introduction of laboratory methods of diagnosis. Christopher Lawrence has shown how a group of elite London clinicians built their careers around a model of a gentleman practitioner, broadly educated, versed in the classics and with finely honed clinical skills. Such practitioners relied on attracting patients from the upper classes who shared this type of education and outlook. Far from being scientific reductionists inclined to see their patients simply in terms of diseased organs, these clinicians, like the eighteenth-century practitioners described by Jewson, saw the patient as a sick man, suffering from a unique and individual case of a disease, its course affected by lifestyle and environment. They prided themselves on their skills in clinical diagnosis based on observation and simple physical examination. Not surprisingly, they saw no value in bringing to the bedside the skills and knowledge acquired in the laboratory. One of the staff of St Bartholomew's Hospital was reported to have told his students, 'When you enter my wards your first duty is to forget all your physiology. Physiology is an experimental science and a very good thing no doubt in its proper place. Medicine is not a science, but an empirical art' (quoted in Lawrence, 1999, p.426). Science was equated with specialism, and specialism with a narrow

You will explore the work and identity of elite practitioners in the next chapter.

approach that might lead the practitioner to overlook clinical signs (Lawrence, 1985).

Resistance such as this was typical of a particular cohort of practitioners. Later generations of practitioners who had received training in laboratories as part of their medical degree were more willing to accept that there was a role for science at the bedside. In 1908, Thomas Horder (1871–1955), a distinguished clinician and a member of the London elite, wrote:

> Though the days are past when the student entering the wards often received the superfluous advice to 'forget his physiology', the physiologist is still regarded a little suspiciously at the bedside. Perhaps he is in part himself to blame for that, for he is sometimes inclined to forget that observations made in the laboratory are not infallible, and are not necessarily more correct than clinical evidence ... [P]hysiology can only come to the aid of medicine with becoming modesty, and without overweening dogmatism. There is no finality about either.
>
> (Lawrence, 1999, p.428)

Horder and other practitioners of his generation tried to strike a balance between the role of science and the clinical art. For them, observation still laid the groundwork for diagnosis. Measurement could then ascertain the severity of the condition. For example, a practitioner should be able to diagnose anaemia by observation and questioning: a blood count could measure the severity of the case and help to guide treatment. At all times, the laboratory and the bedside should be linked. The clinician should perform diagnostic tests, and thoroughly understand the implications of the results. Students and practitioners should not become so immersed in the specialized disciplines of the biomedical sciences that they lost sight of the patient as a person (Lawrence, 1999). There is good evidence that by the early twentieth century general practitioners working among the middle classes used laboratory tests to help their diagnosis. Similarly, the development and marketing of small 'kits' containing all the equipment necessary to perform simple analyses of blood and urine suggests that some general practitioners applied to their practice the skills learned in the medical-school laboratory.

Research has suggested that other practitioners were equally cautious about pathological examinations carried out in the laboratory. The next reading, by L.S. Jacyna, is taken from his case study on the role of the pathologist in Glasgow Western Infirmary, 1875–1910.

Exercise

Read 'The role of the laboratory in the hospital' (Source Book 2, Reading 4.4). How do practitioners use the laboratory in their practice, and how does their use of the laboratory compare with that of the elite practitioners described by Lawrence?

Jacyna's account is about the use of a different sort of laboratory science: where Lawrence's practitioners are using physiological measurements, to judge the severity of cases, Jacyna's practitioners want a diagnosis based on a tissue sample. However, the Glasgow practitioners seem to share the London elite practitioners' feeling that the proper role of the laboratory should be strictly limited, and should come after an initial diagnosis has been made: the lab is used to confirm the cancerous nature of a tumour, or to decide which of the possible diagnoses of inflammation, tuberculosis and so on is correct. While practitioners accept that the laboratory has the technology, and that the pathologist has special skills which they lack, they do not immediately use the laboratory for diagnosis; nor do they use it to determine the course of treatment. The laboratory therefore has a strictly limited role – to refine or confirm an existing diagnosis. It assists practitioners in their clinical practice when dealing with a limited number of conditions.

While clinicians might be suspicious of the laboratory, practitioners working in laboratories actively promoted their skills as a means of serving local medical communities, and thus helping to build a niche for the laboratory. In Sheffield, for example, the established medical school added laboratories to its other teaching facilities in the 1890s. These were primarily intended to attract students, who might otherwise go to better-equipped schools for their training. However, the laboratories also provided services to the local medical community. The bacteriology laboratory conducted tests for local hospitals and the local authority, identifying cases of infectious disease. The physiology laboratory worked with local hospitals in carrying out research into occupational diseases linked to local industries, and into goitre – enlargement of the thyroid glands – which was prevalent in the area. The laboratory staff acquired a prominent position among local practitioners, and were seen as experts on particular conditions. General practitioners were therefore willing to refer on more difficult cases to these local experts, who could provide better diagnosis (Sturdy, 1992).

New therapies

As you have discovered, by the 1860s, medical practitioners firmly believed that the new understanding of the body and of disease processes produced in the laboratory would lead to better treatment. Bacteriology perhaps held the greatest promise. Between 1879 and 1885, Pasteur had developed **vaccines** to treat anthrax and rabies. He developed weakened strains of the bacteria, which, when injected into infected animals, proved to be an effective therapy. At this time, the role of the body's immune system in dealing with infection was unknown: Pasteur assumed that the weak bacteria stimulated the body's response to fight off stronger disease bacteria, and thus to cure infections. While these new treatments brought Pasteur great public acclaim, anthrax and rabies were not common diseases. The success of his work prompted researchers to devise other vaccines to treat a wide range of diseases. In 1890, Koch announced a significant breakthrough – a vaccine to treat tuberculosis, then one of the major causes of death. However, tuberculin, a solution of glycerine containing a weakened strain of tuberculosis bacteria, proved to be a spectacular failure. (Ironically, it was discovered to be an effective test for the diagnosis of early tuberculosis.)

Research continued undaunted. By the 1920s, Almroth Wright (1861–1947) had set up what amounted to a production line for new therapeutic vaccines in laboratories at St Mary's Hospital, London. His laboratory turned out a string of vaccines intended to stimulate the body's natural disease-fighting responses. It produced vaccines against:

> boils, pneumonia, bronchial colds, influenza, gonorrhoea, sore throats, intestinal troubles, tuberculosis, and even cancer. There were also 'Anti-catarrh vaccine' and 'Anti-catarrh (Public Schools) vaccine' – the difference between them (apart from their packaging and price) was said to be only their strength.
>
> (Chen, 1992, p.255)

Vaccines were developed using a standard process. Bacteria were collected from patients, identified and cultured. They were then harvested, killed and added to a liquid medium to make the vaccine. The vaccines were sold by Parke, Davis and Company, a large pharmaceutical firm.

As with the introduction of new diagnostic techniques, not all practitioners embraced these new therapies. Some medical men, whose reputations were based on careful clinical skills, feared that the laboratory researcher who made vaccines would threaten their practice. The final reading for this chapter is taken from an article by Michael Worboys on the debate over vaccine therapy and laboratory medicine in Edwardian Britain.

Exercise

Read 'The impact of vaccine therapy' (Source Book 2, Reading 4.5). Does Worboys think that the laboratory scientists posed any real threat to the practice of the clinicians?

Discussion

Worboys argues that the clinicians had little to fear from the laboratory scientists led by Almroth Wright. The fact that the scientists made grandiose claims for the efficacy of vaccines, which had the potential to overturn the authority of elite practitioners, meant that few elite practitioners supported the use of therapeutic vaccines. Those practitioners who did express their support for the use of vaccines were young and on the margins of the profession: none were members of the still powerful old elite. The weakness of the scientists' position can be seen in the rapid waning in popularity of vaccines, as opponents challenged their efficacy and other practitioners became more sceptical of their therapeutic value.

Therapeutic vaccines met with mixed success, but although ultimately discredited they briefly appeared to show that the laboratory would live up to its promise of creating new and better therapies.

Serum therapy was more successful. Researchers realized that in some infectious diseases the symptoms were produced by a toxin released by bacteria, not by the bacteria themselves. In 1890, Emil Behring (1854–1917) discovered that diphtheria, a serious and sometimes fatal disease affecting children, could be cured by injecting patients with serum (the fluid in which the red cells were carried) from animals infected with the disease. The serum neutralized the effects of the toxin. Diphtheria antitoxin, as the substance was named, was in use by 1895 and helped to save the lives of thousands of children. Other sera followed, to treat tetanus, plague and cholera (Weindling, 1992b, pp.73–82).

While bacteriology had begun to deliver some new treatments by the 1890s, other areas of research failed to produce therapies until the twentieth century. In the field of pharmacology, developments in organic chemistry in the 1840s allowed pharmaceutical companies to produce more potent forms of old drugs by isolating the active ingredients from plant drugs, such as morphine (from opium) and aspirin (from willow bark). Research had also given practitioners a better understanding of the action of drugs in the body. However, the first drug to emerge from pharmacological research was Salvarsan, an effective treatment for syphilis, a debilitating and fatal disease. In 1907, Paul Ehrlich tested over 600 arsenic compounds for their therapeutic properties. Number 606 – later named Salvarsan – proved the most effective and it came into use after 1910. In 1914, Neosalvarsan, a related compound with fewer side effects, was introduced. Salvarsan opened up the prospect of other new therapies, but further 'magic bullets' proved elusive. The next effective chemical drug did not appear until 1935, when Prontosil was developed to treat streptococcal infections.

In the 1920s, research into the causes of metabolic diseases such as diabetes led directly to treatment. From the late nineteenth century, practitioners knew that diabetes was associated with some malfunction of the pancreas. Later, it was shown that a substance produced by the islets of Langerhans – small patches of special tissue within the pancreas – was required to digest carbohydrates. However, insulin, the substance produced by the islets, was not isolated until 1921, by Fred Banting (1891–1941) and Charles Best (1899–1978). The following year, they tried injecting diabetic patients with insulin with spectacular success, and the therapy was quickly put on the market. Similarly, work on deficiency diseases such as rickets, beriberi and pernicious anaemia, caused by the absence of a specific vitamin in the diet, quickly led to effective treatment.

4.5   The public's view of laboratory medicine

For laboratory medicine to flourish, in an age when the vast majority of patients paid directly for their care, the public had to be convinced of its merits. The same is true for the rhetorical value of 'scientific medicine': practitioners would raise their status by claiming that medicine was scientific only if the public valued 'science'. The public perception of medical science in Europe has yet to be studied in detail by historians, but research on American attitudes at the end of the nineteenth century suggests that the public did respect 'science', although exactly what was regarded as being 'scientific' was rather vague. The American public certainly embraced the products of laboratory research. In the 1880s, marketing men used the findings of bacteriology to sell cleaning products on their power not only to remove dirt and smells but also to kill 'germs'. Manufacturers even appealed to customers by using scientists' names for their products, such as 'Pasteur's Marvellous Disinfectant'. There was no actual connection between the product and Pasteur's research – in fact, it proved not to kill germs – but his name was invoked to give the product greater value (Tomes, 1998, pp.76–112).

There is some evidence that European consumers were equally enthusiastic about new therapies developed in the laboratory. At the turn of the century, 'gland therapy' briefly became fashionable. In 1889, Charles Edouard Brown-Sequard (1817–94), a respected researcher who had worked on the autonomic nervous system, injected himself with extracts of guinea pig and dog testicles and claimed that they improved his overall health and vigour. Well-off patients in Europe and America clamoured for injections of animal hormones until the therapy was shown to be worthless. As you have seen, at least some sections of the public also embraced therapeutic vaccines. A positive response to scientific medicine is evident in hospital fund-raising campaigns, which often stressed the institution's high-tech equipment. Fund-raising films from the 1920s and 1930s, for example, showcased the work of hospital laboratories, where white-coated technicians cultured specimens, or demonstrated new technologies such as the electrocardiograph and X-ray equipment. Clearly, hospitals felt that the public wanted to see how 'scientific medicine' brought better care.

Perhaps the most spectacular proof of the public's support for the laboratory was the founding of the Pasteur Institute in Paris in 1888, described above. Pasteur attained celebrity status in July 1885 when he announced the successful treatment, using an experimental vaccine, of a 9-year-old boy who had been bitten by a rabid dog (Plate 10). Plans for a research institute to provide Pasteur with research facilities and to celebrate his achievements were first mooted in March 1886. Donations large and small poured in from members of the public all over France. This, plus a subsidy from the French government and the profits from the sale of the rabies vaccine, brought in a total of nearly 2 million francs (Weindling, 1992a, pp.172–3). However, not everyone had faith in science. As you read in Chapter 1, in Britain especially, the anti-vivisection movement questioned the methods used in laboratories to obtain knowledge.

4.6   Conclusion

There is no doubt that the laboratory did eventually transform medicine. The fact that it performed a number of functions meant that its impact was felt in different ways in different aspects of medicine. Research developed in the laboratory revolutionized medical theory between 1830 and 1930. The picture of the body that focused on structure was replaced by a picture of the body as a dynamic system in which health was a reflection of complex, integrated physiological processes. This new knowledge was conveyed to a new generation of practitioners through new teaching methods involving experiments at the lab bench. As you have seen, however, the new knowledge emerging from the laboratory had only a marginal impact on medical practice until the 1920s. Before that time, although diagnosis was improved, few new drug therapies were available to practitioners. The laboratory also affected medicine in less obvious ways, by changing the organization of research and the standards of proof for new theories.

Jewson's suggestion that laboratory medicine altered the structure of authority within the medical profession – that the clinician had to bow to the superior knowledge of the scientist – is refuted by the material presented here. Clinicians certainly feared that the laboratory would devalue their skills and knowledge, but they found an accommodation with it, using the lab to back up their diagnostic skills.

References

Bonner, T. (1995) *Becoming a Physician: Medical Education in Britain, France, Germany and the United States, 1750–1945,* Oxford: Oxford University Press.

Bynum, W.F. and Porter, R. (1993) *Companion Encyclopaedia of the History of Medicine*, 2 vols, London: Routledge.

Chadarevian, S. de (1993) 'Graphical method and discipline: self-recording instruments in nineteenth-century physiology', *Studies in the History and Philosophy of Science*, vol.24, pp.267–91.

Chen, W. (1992) 'The laboratory as business: Sir Almroth Wright's vaccine programme and the construction of penicillin' in A. Cunningham and P. Williams (eds) *The Laboratory Revolution in Medicine*, Cambridge: Cambridge University Press, pp.245–92.

Fenby, D.V. (1989) 'The lectureship in chemistry and the chemistry laboratory: University of Glasgow, 1747–1818' in F.L.R. James (ed.) *The Development of the Laboratory: Essays on the Place of Experiment in Industrial Civilisation*, Basingstoke: Macmillan, pp.32–6.

Frank, R.J. (1988) 'The tell-tale heart: physiological instruments, graphic methods, and clinical hopes, 1854–1914' in W. Coleman and F.L. Holmes (eds) *The Investigative Enterprise: Experimental Physiology in Nineteenth-Century Medicine*, Berkeley: University of California Press, pp.211–94.

Howell, J. (1995) *Technology in the Hospital: Transforming Patient Care in the Early Twentieth Century*, Baltimore: Johns Hopkins University Press.

Jewson, N.D. (1976) 'The disappearance of the sick-man from medical cosmology, 1770–1870', *Sociology*, vol.10, pp.225–44.

La Berge, A. (1994) 'Medical microscopy in Paris, 1830–1855' in A. La Berge and M. Feingold (eds) *French Medical Culture in the Nineteenth Century*, Amsterdam: Rodopi, pp.296–326.

Lawrence, C. (1985) ' Incommunicable knowledge: science, technology and the clinical art in Britain 1850–1914', *Journal of Contemporary History*, vol.20, pp.503–20.

Lawrence, C. (1999) 'A tale of two sciences: bedside and bench in twentieth-century Britain', *Medical History*, vol.43, pp.421–49.

Lenoir, T. (1992) 'Laboratories, medicine and public life in Germany 1830–1849: ideological roots of the institutional revolution' in A. Cunningham and P. Williams (eds) *The Laboratory Revolution in Medicine*, Cambridge: Cambridge University Press, pp.14–71.

Lesch, J.E. (1984) S*cience and Medicine in France: The Emergence of Experimental Physiology, 1790–1855*, Cambridge: Harvard University Press.

Porter, R. (1999) *The Greatest Benefit to Mankind: A Medical History of Humanity from Antiquity to the Present*, London: Fontana.

Sturdy, S. (1992) 'The political economy of scientific medicine: science, education and the transformation of medical practice in Sheffield, 1890–1922', *Medical History*, vol.36, pp.125–59.

Sturdy, S. and Cooter, R. (1998) 'Science, scientific management and the transformation of medicine in Britain', *History of Science*, vol.36, pp.421–66.

Todes, D. (1988) 'Pavlov's physiology laboratory', *Isis*, vol.88, pp.204–46.

Tomes, N. (1998) *The Gospel of Germs: Men, Women and the Microbe in American Life*, Cambridge: Harvard University Press.

Tuchman, A.M. (1993) *Science, Medicine and the State in Germany: The Case of Baden, 1815–1871*, Oxford: Oxford University Press.

Warner, J.H. (1995) 'The history of science and the sciences of medicine', *Osiris*, vol.10, pp.164–93.

Weindling, P. (1992a) 'Scientific elites and laboratory organisation in *fin de siècle* Paris and Berlin' in A. Cunningham and P. Williams (eds) *The Laboratory Revolution in Medicine*, Cambridge: Cambridge University Press, pp.170–88.

Weindling, P. (1992b) 'From medical research to clinical practice: serum therapy for diphtheria in the 1890s' in J. Pickstone (ed.) *Medical Innovations in Historical Perspective*, Basingstoke: Macmillan, pp.72–83.

Worboys, M. (2000) *Spreading Germs: Disease Theories and Medical Practice in Britain, 1865–1900*, Cambridge: Cambridge University Press.

Source Book readings

B. Claude, *An Introduction to the Study of Experimental Medicine*, translated by H.C. Greene, New York: Dover, [1865] 1957, pp.142–3, 145–9 (Reading 4.1).

A. Cunningham, 'Transforming plague: the laboratory and the identity of infectious disease' in A. Cunningham and P. Williams (eds) *The Laboratory Revolution in Medicine*, Cambridge: Cambridge University Press, 1992, pp.209–44 (Reading 4.2).

L.S. Jacyna, 'The laboratory and the clinic: the impact of pathology on surgical diagnosis in the Glasgow Western Infirmary, 1875–1910', *Bulletin of the History of Medicine*, 1988, vol.62, pp.384–406 (Reading 4.3).

R.L. Kremer, 'Building institutes for physiology in Prussia, 1836–1846: contexts, interests and rhetoric' in A. Cunningham and P. Williams (eds) *The Laboratory Revolution in Medicine*, Cambridge: Cambridge University Press, 1992, pp.72–109 (Reading 4.4).

M. Worboys 'Vaccine therapy and laboratory medicine in Edwardian Britain' in J. Pickstone (ed.) *Medical Innovations in Historical Perspective*, Basingstoke: Macmillan, 1992, pp.84–103 (Reading 4.5).

5

The Emergence of a Modern Profession?

D e b o r a h   B r u n t o n

Objectives

When you have completed this chapter you should be able to:

- describe the main changes in the training, practice, behaviour and status of medical practitioners in Europe during the nineteenth century;

- describe the main characteristics of a modern profession;

- assess the historical evidence and decide whether the nineteenth-century medical profession is the same as a modern profession, or whether it is characterized by unique features.

5.1   Introduction: professionalization or reform?

In the late eighteenth and nineteenth centuries, fundamental and sweeping changes took place in medical training and practice. Apprenticeships, which were once the most common form of medical training, gradually disappeared, and a university education became the norm for all practitioners. Responsibility for licensing practitioners shifted from the old medical guilds and colleges to the state and then back into the hands of medical men. The last remnants of the division of practitioners into physicians, surgeons and apothecaries were swept away. Instead, medical men were split into general practitioners and consultants. At the same time, medical practitioners developed a new collective identity, seeing themselves as members of a single occupation, with common interests and conforming to common standards of behaviour. A clear differentiation emerged between members of the regular and orthodox profession, who had gone through recognized forms of training, and those who were considered **irregular healers** and **unorthodox practitioners**.

While historians agree that the practice of medicine was transformed between 1800 and 1900, they have interpreted these changes in two ways. The first interpretation originates in the 1970s, when historians of medicine began to describe these changes as a process of professionalization. This might seem an odd idea because medicine, along with the law and the church, had been described as a profession since medieval times. Physicians, lawyers and clergymen were all seen as professional men since they required a university education to practise. However, historians argue that until the nineteenth century, medicine was not a profession in the modern sense. Only physicians went to university; surgeons and apothecaries, who made up the vast majority of medical practitioners, trained through apprenticeships, a form of education associated with trade.

This interest in the development of the medical profession was inspired by the work of sociologists on the essential characteristics of modern professions. These rather abstract concepts are listed below. They are easier to grasp if you think of them in relation to modern doctors.

- The possession of a body of highly specialized knowledge: we expect our doctors to have a deep knowledge of disease, acquired through a long training in medical school. A doctor's qualifications prove that he or she has completed this training to the standards required of the profession.

- Professional unity and a strong ethos of public service: we do not expect doctors to compete with one another for patients by advertising their services or by offering cut-price practice. We do expect practitioners to cooperate when caring for patients, and to always work for their patients' best interests.

- A monopoly of practice: only members of the medical profession can call themselves doctors. We distinguish between orthodox medical practitioners and those who offer alternative forms of medical treatment by calling them practitioners of 'complementary' or 'alternative' medicine.

- Professional autonomy: medical practice is based on highly specialist knowledge, which is not shared with the general public. Therefore, only doctors can judge whether other doctors are trained to a suitable standard and are competent to practice.

- High social status: doctors earn relatively high salaries and also enjoy a special social respect.

Sociologists and historians of medicine concluded that the modern profession emerged in the middle of the nineteenth century, between about 1840 and 1880. They described the transformation of medical practice as 'professionalization', whereby practitioners sought to improve their social standing, increase their incomes and acquire a new status as experts. In these terms, the development of the profession benefited practitioners, bringing about a 'collective social mobility' (Parry and Parry, 1976).

However, more recently, historians have challenged the merit of these studies and have put forward a second interpretation of the nineteenth-century changes in medicine. Some have pointed out that much of the work of sociologists and the early research by historians focused on the medical professions in America and Britain and that the experience of practitioners in continental Europe was markedly different. Other historians have cast doubts on the whole approach. By focusing on the characteristics of modern professions, they argue that socio-logically inspired studies have overemphasized these features and thus have produced a skewed picture. As part of the movement to study 'history from below', these historians have tried to view change from the perspective of participants – particularly that of ordinary general practitioners. From this viewpoint, changes in nineteenth-century medicine are not a smooth progression towards the creation of a profession. Rather, the period was one of upheaval, with many unconnected changes, and with some practitioners gaining power and status at the expense of others.

In this chapter, I reassess these interpretations of change in nineteenth-century medicine. I use the sociologists' model of the modern professions as a structure, and examine in turn each of the main characteristics as it relates to nineteenth-century medicine in Britain and the rest of Europe.

5.2 Common knowledge

Possession of highly specialized knowledge is the basis of the economic success of all professions – we choose to go to a doctor because we believe they are best able to understand and treat our ailments. Of course, all sorts of medical practitioners have always claimed to have some form of special understanding or skill. However, until the late eighteenth century, medicine was divided between different groups of practitioners who possessed special sets of skills: surgeons knew about wounds and skin lesions, physicians understood internal disease, and apothecaries were skilled in the preparation of drugs. In the nineteenth century, practitioners began to share a common body of knowledge, which was acquired through a similar training.

Until the eighteenth century, surgeons had received a practical training through apprenticeship to an established practitioner, while physicians learned medicine through books and lectures in universities. But, as you have read in earlier chapters, from the eighteenth century, trainee surgeons were taught alongside physicians in universities, hospitals and in the new medical schools. In continental Europe, medical schools were set up by the state. In 1794, the French government founded medical schools in Paris, Montpellier and Strasbourg. In the German states, between 1716 and 1808, schools were set up in Munich, Innsbruck, Berlin, Hanover, Dresden, Salzburg and Bamberg (Bonner, 1995, pp.53–5). In Belgium, new medical courses were established in 1806. As well as these state institutions, established practitioners founded private medical schools, especially in London, Paris and Edinburgh. Many were associated with large hospitals. Teaching in these schools was a commercial venture: practitioners hired rooms, advertised their courses and pocketed the students' fees. In both universities and medical schools, lectures were the main form of teaching; practical training was gained through anatomical demonstrations and dissections. In the hospitals, opportunities were provided for students to observe patients and their treatment, either as part of a large class or as the privileged pupil of a member of the hospital staff (Lawrence, 1996, pp.162–211).

From the late eighteenth century, physicians and surgeons not only went through the same form of training, but also began to study the same subjects. At first, the courses offered by medical schools were those traditionally studied by physicians – anatomy, botany, chemistry, the theory and practice of medicine and ***materia medica***. But their curriculum soon expanded to include classes in surgery and midwifery. By the early nineteenth century, the curriculum included courses in specialized subjects such as the diseases of women and children and ophthalmology. This medical training excluded pharmacy and dentistry (previously practised by apothecaries and surgeons, respectively), both of which became occupations in their own right.

Just as medical training was reorganized, so were the divisions of medical practice. Training at a medical school did not provide students with a formal qualification, but prepared them to sit licensing examinations. Traditionally, different guilds and colleges had licensed physicians, surgeons and apothecaries. But in continental Europe, governments took over responsibility for licensing in the late eighteenth and early nineteenth centuries. Practitioners were divided into new categories. Broadly speaking, these were an elite of university-trained practitioners and a large body of general practitioners educated in medical schools. The exact divisions varied from country to country. From 1803, practitioners in France and its territories (which included modern Holland and Belgium) were divided into doctors, who held a degree in either medicine or surgery, and *officiers de santé*, lower-grade practitioners who studied a three-year course at a medical school, completed an apprenticeship or attended a hospital, before sitting a licensing examination. The Prussian government recognized three classes of practitioner: doctors (*approbieter arzt*), who had a degree, first-class surgeons (*wundarzt erster klasse*) and second-class surgeons (*wundarzt zweiter klasse*), who trained in medical schools. After achieving independence from French rule in 1818, the Belgian government licensed no less than eleven classes of practitioner.

Licensing in Britain followed a rather different course to the rest of Europe since the government took no role in licensing practitioners. Students could qualify either by obtaining a degree from the handful of universities that offered medical training, including Edinburgh, Glasgow, Oxford and Cambridge, or by sitting licensing examinations organized by the colleges of physicians and surgeons in England, Scotland and Ireland and the Society of Apothecaries in London. These institutions perpetuated the traditional divisions by offering licences in either medicine or surgery. However, many practitioners chose to take two licences, one in medicine and one in surgery. There was no formal distinction between a degree and a licence: practitioners with either qualification enjoyed the same freedom to practise where and how they chose.

During the course of the century, these licensing regulations were gradually revised, so that by the 1890s, in much of continental Europe, a university degree was the only qualification for medical practice. This change came about when the lower grades of practitioner were abolished, and the medical men who had previously formed the elite took over all medical practice. Medical schools began closing in the 1830s: the Belgian government closed all the country's schools in 1835, the Bavarian schools were shut in 1842 and the Prussian government shut its surgeons' schools in 1852. At the same time, new medical faculties were opened in universities across Europe: Germany had twenty-four medical faculties by the 1830s. Medical courses were offered for the first time in Berlin and Bonn. In Belgium, all practitioners were required to hold university degrees from 1836, and the degree requirements were increased in 1849 (Schepers, 1994, p.248). In France, the government refused to do away with the *officiers de santé* until 1892, but did make the qualifications more rigorous, extending the period of study to three and a half years in medical school (Bonner, 1995, pp.185–8).

Britain, as ever, followed a slightly different course. Licences were not abolished, but the standards of training required for both licences and degrees were gradually increased under the supervision of the General Medical Council (GMC). Established in 1858 by the Medical Registration Act, the GMC ensured that the sixty medical licences offered by nineteen licensing authorities required a similar standard of training. More and more students chose to take a degree and as a result university medical schools flourished. The moribund medical faculty in Cambridge was revitalized and new universities, such as the University of London, began to offer medical training. Some universities amalgamated with established private medical schools. By the early twentieth century, students could acquire a medical degree from schools in seven provincial centres in England and Wales, as well as from Oxford, Cambridge, London and the Scottish universities. The large hospital medical schools, with their good facilities for clinical teaching, also thrived. Small private medical schools struggled to offer the expanding curriculum of medical subjects and went out of business (Bonner, 1995, pp.193–5, 259–64; Digby, 1999, pp.53–9).

We can get a snapshot of the impact of these changes in medical training and licensing by comparing the education of two Glasgow practitioners – Robert Cowan (1796–1841) and his grandson, John Marshall Cowan (1879–1947). The Cowans were a well-off family, and both men received a very good medical education by the standards of their day.

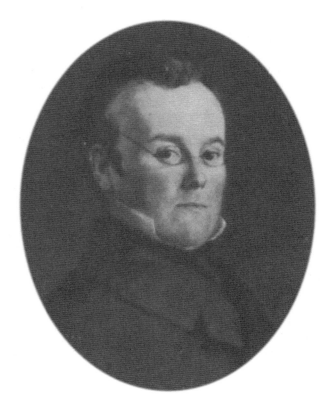

Figure 5.1 Portrait of Robert Cowan. By permission of the Royal College of Physicians and Surgeons of Glasgow

In 1812, aged 16, Robert Cowan (Figure 5.1) began his medical training. At the medical faculty of Glasgow University, he took courses in anatomy, dissection, chemistry, *materia medica*, midwifery, botany and clinical medicine. In 1815, he left Glasgow and spent one winter at Edinburgh, studying in the medical faculty of the university and in private medical schools in the city. There he attended a similar set of courses to those he had already completed in Glasgow, plus a course in the theory and practice of medicine. Robert returned to Glasgow and worked as a resident clerk at the Royal Infirmary to obtain more clinical experience. In 1818, he went to Paris – then the centre for the new study of pathological anatomy – where he attended a course in midwifery and probably went to other classes. In 1819, he returned home and passed the examinations to obtain a licence from the Faculty of Physicians and Surgeons of Glasgow.

Before embarking on his medical training, John Marshall Cowan (Figure 5.2) took an arts degree at Cambridge University. He entered the university medical school in 1891, where he worked through a prescribed curriculum of courses. In his first

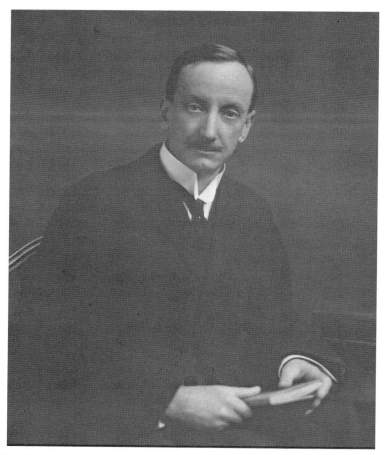

Figure 5.2   Portrait of John Marshall Cowan. By permission of the Royal College of Physicians and Surgeons of Glasgow

year, he studied the basic sciences, including biology and chemistry, then went on to take courses in anatomy, physiology, pathology and pharmacology. His later years of study were devoted to clinical medicine, attending the wards of hospitals, and to more specialist subjects such as hygiene, midwifery and various aspects of surgery. Throughout his studies, he passed a series of rigorous examinations. In 1895, at the end of his course, he passed a final set of examinations and was awarded an MB, ChB degree (bachelor of medicine, bachelor of chirurgery – the old form of the word surgery).

Before embarking on their medical studies, John Cowan and students of his generation were required to undergo some preliminary training – a degree or special courses – or to sit entrance examinations. Compared with students of Robert Cowan's generation, they had less freedom to shape the progress of their studies, and had to train for a fixed period, usually at one institution. They were also subject to rigorous examinations.

What drove these changes in medical education? They were part of a broader context of educational reform. The late nineteenth century saw a rapid expansion of university education, with the creation of more institutions teaching more students. A university degree increasingly was becoming the preparation for a career in many fields, from the civil service to the emerging professions of chemistry, engineering, veterinary medicine and teaching (McClelland, 1991, p.81; Perkin, 1969, pp.252–76).

However, the main force driving change was demand from medical students and practitioners. In the nineteenth century, medical students paid for their education and saw it as an investment, so they wanted training which would equip them for successful practice. In the first part of the century, this meant a broad training in medicine and surgery, which would prepare them for a career in general practice, treating a wide range of ailments and injuries among the expanding middle ranks of society. From the 1830s, a high-quality medical training was at a premium. At this time, practitioners all over Europe complained that the medical profession was overcrowded; there were too many practitioners competing for a finite number of patients' fees. The best possible education at a reputable school or university, studying under well-known teachers, improved the chances of a student succeeding in practice. Higher standards of education also promised to benefit established practitioners by reducing the number of entrants to medicine. And practitioners in Britain, France and Germany all lobbied their governments to increase the standards for licensing.

The changes in medical education also reflected the growing interest of governments in protecting the health of populations through the provision of good quality health care. In continental Europe, states had established medical schools to provide well-trained practitioners for the army and navy and for civilian service, as well as doctors to serve as public practitioners treating the poor and as public health officers. Although we think of state medicine as a feature of the twentieth century, some nineteenth-century governments employed large numbers of medical practitioners. In Prussia, around one-third of all practitioners were employed as military or as public health practitioners in the 1830s and 1840s, while in Russia, virtually all practitioners worked for the state. However, governments were also concerned that the numbers of practitioners be kept within limits – there was no point in producing more doctors than could find work.

While practitioners and governments may have wanted licensing reform, who benefited from the raising of educational standards? Was it the public – who had access to better-trained practitioners – or practitioners themselves? The following exercise asks you to read two contrasting accounts of professional reform: one by Ivan Waddington, the other by Irvine Loudon.

Exercise

Read 'Occupational closure and the 1858 Medical Act' (Source Book 2, Reading 5.1) and 'The Medical Act of 1858' (Source Book 2, Reading 5.2). What sources are used? What does each author see as the force for change? What is the effect of the Act?

Discussion

Waddington's account is based largely on published medical journals, such as the *Lancet*. He is clearly influenced by sociological ideas about professions and his view is that the demand for reform came from the whole medical profession. Waddington portrays practitioners as a clearly defined group, pursuing a clearly identified common interest. According to Waddington, practitioners, rather than the general public, were the main beneficiaries of the 1858 Act, which reduced the numbers of qualified practitioners, marginalized untrained practitioners and increased medical incomes. However, he claims that everyone benefited from the raising of licensing standards.

Rather than institutional records or medical journals, Loudon uses the writings of individuals to capture the views of practitioners on the new legislation. He dismisses Waddington's claim that the 1858 Act came in response to the demands of a unified group pursuing the goal of professionalization. Rather, he sees the Act as a response to earlier changes in education. According to Loudon's account, the Act reinforced the power of the old licensing bodies and ended the hopes of ordinary general practitioners that they might establish their own authority.

5.3 Unity and conflict

In the nineteenth century, licensing reform and developments in medical education brought a new unity to the profession. Like the Bristol students you read about in Chapter 1, students had a similar education, trained in large groups and developed a strong sense of allegiance to their institutions and to their teachers (Figure 5.3). Links formed at medical school were maintained after graduation, with former students keeping in contact, calling on each other for help with operations and consulting each other or their former teachers on difficult cases.

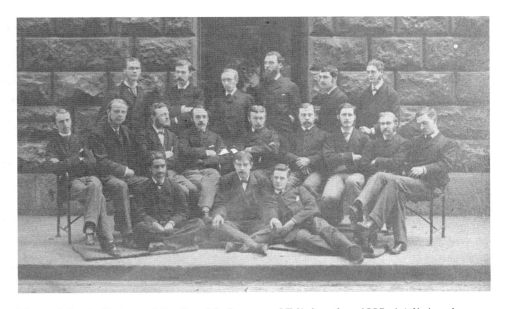

Figure 5.3   A clinique of the Royal Infirmary of Edinburgh, *c*.1895. A 'clinique', or 'firm' as it was known in England, was made up of the students working with the staff of a particular hospital ward. Photographs like this appeared at the end of the century and are a visual representation of the new allegiances of medical students to their classmates, the schools and hospitals where they trained and their teachers. Such pictures were often taken by commercial photographers and sold to students as a memento of their studies. Lothian Health Services Archive/SCRAN

This sense of a collective identity – of belonging to a body of practitioners with similar patterns of work and common interests – was greatly strengthened by the many new medical societies and journals founded in the nineteenth century. Medical journals were most popular in Britain, where more than 400 new titles were launched during this period. One of the first and most successful was the *Lancet*, founded in 1823 by Thomas Wakley (1795–1862), a general practitioner with a real flair for firebrand journalism. The *Lancet* served as a model for many other journals, including the *London Medical Gazette* (1827) and the *Provincial Medical and Surgical Journal* (1849), which became the *British Medical Journal* in 1857 (Bynum *et al.*, 1992) (Plate 7). Medical journals were founded in rather smaller numbers in Europe at the same time – in France, Germany and Belgium, where the *Scalpel* (surely in homage to Wakley's *Lancet*) appeared. Even in Russia, twenty-three new journals were established around the middle of the century.

This period also saw the foundation of large numbers of new medical societies throughout Europe. In Britain, most societies were local affairs, based in a town or region. But the Provincial Medical and Surgical Association, founded in 1832, was a national society and eventually became the British Medical Association (Bartrip, 1996). In France, there were twenty-one associations in Paris and fifty-eight in provincial centres by 1845, and in that year French practitioners came together in a Grand National Congress. The national Association Générale de Médecins was created in 1858. In the German states, a flurry of new societies were founded in the 1840s, and by 1872 there were at least 130. These were brought together in a formal union in 1873. In Russia, twenty-five new societies were founded between 1850 and 1864. The Norwegian Medical Society was formed in 1833, the Dutch Medical Association in 1849 and the Belgian Medical Federation in 1863.

A relatively small number of societies and journals were concerned with specific areas of research or practice. Their activities focused on the exchange of information – reading or publishing research findings and discussing and reviewing books and articles. Most societies and journals had a wider range of functions. They provided practitioners with a forum where they could exchange information and also air their views on professional matters – their status, income and working conditions. The *Lancet*, for example, carried reports of clinical research and reprinted and reviewed research papers. Editorials and letters discussed a wide range of professional issues, including ethics, employment conditions, public health legislation and medical insurance schemes. The journal also carried reports of operations at the London hospitals and the curriculum in medical schools. The letters pages included stories of amazing cures (not just of patients, but even of a practitioner's horse!). Journals and societies also had a social function – practitioners could meet face to face, or follow the fortunes of colleagues through their contributions to journals, reports of their appointments to office and finally through their obituaries.

While education, societies and journals all helped to bring practitioners together, professionally and socially, this did not mean that all members of the profession thought alike, worked in the same way, or enjoyed equal status. You saw in Chapter 4 how some practitioners embraced laboratory science and others rejected it. Such divisions of opinion often reflected divisions between groups of different status within the profession. In the nineteenth century, as in the modern profession, practitioners were divided into two groups – general practitioners, who had received a thorough basic training and provided primary care, and a smaller elite group. The identity and practice of this latter group has changed over time.

As you have seen, in continental Europe, during the first part of the nineteenth century, practitioners were divided by their qualifications. The elite was composed of practitioners who held a degree, while general practitioners, trained in medical schools, held licences. However, this distinction was lost as universities became the main sites for medical training. By 1830, almost half of Belgian practitioners held a degree. In the Netherlands, one-third of practitioners held a degree in the 1830s and by 1860 this figure had risen to 80 per cent. Instead, a new grouping of elite practitioners emerged who were distinguished by their institutional affiliations. They held prestigious but unpaid posts in large general hospitals and belonged to particular associations. In Belgium, for example, the elite belonged to the Académie Royale de Médecine and were appointed by government ministers to the provincial medical boards which examined and licensed new practitioners.

In Britain, where licensing did not create a formal hierarchy among practitioners, the elite were distinguished in a similar way. They held senior posts in hospitals and many were involved in teaching. They were fellows of the Royal Colleges of Physicians or Surgeons, and thus were responsible for examining and licensing new practitioners. Practitioners entered the elite institutions through patronage – senior hospital posts were filled from the more junior ranks – and by recommendations from other elite practitioners. Towards the end of the century, the career ladder to a senior hospital position grew longer and longer. Young practitioners moved from the ranks of clerks and dressers to residents and housemen before becoming assistants and then full physicians or surgeons. This increase in the different ranks of hospital staff reflected the general growth in the numbers of practitioners and nurses as hospitals began to treat acutely sick patients and to undertake more surgery (Peterson, 1978, pp.136–93). These developments are explored in Chapter 2.

These nineteenth-century elite practitioners were not the equivalent of today's consultants, who have gone through a long postgraduate training in some special aspect of medicine and work full-time within that area. In the early part of the century, specialism was associated with quackery, and was viewed with suspicion. Some young practitioners sought to advance their careers by founding specialist hospitals, but they found a place in the professional elite only if they were able to use their specialist skills as a stepping stone to a post in a general hospital. The move towards an elite composed of specialist consultants happened very gradually. At the end of the nineteenth century, medical schools introduced specialist postgraduate courses, and students would further develop their skills by working in a specialist department in a general hospital or in a specialist hospital. In these posts, junior doctors could carry out clinical research, which in turn helped them to rise up the career ladder. But even in the 1930s, the pinnacle of a medical career remained a position as senior physician or surgeon (Figure 5.4).

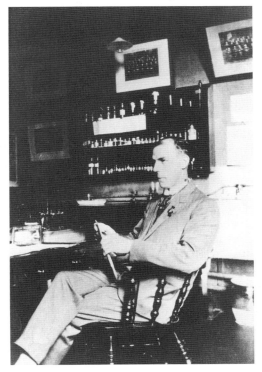

Figure 5.4   David Lyon Murray (1888–1956), professor of clinical medicine, c.1925. Murray was physician, one of the most senior staff, at the Edinburgh Royal Infirmary from 1919 to 1953, and taught at the University Medical School. Murray was involved in the development of specialist care at the hospital, although he did not hold a post in a new specialty. Like many photographs from this period, Murray is shown in his workplace, in this case a biochemistry laboratory. In the background are the bottles of chemicals used in analysing fluids, and group photographs of students. Lothian Health Services Archive/SCRAN

Although hospital posts were vital indicators of membership of the medical elite, paradoxically, elite practitioners spent most of their time working as general practitioners. Only two aspects of their work distinguished them from the rank-and-file GP: the fact that they were called in by general practitioners to consult on difficult cases and the social class of their patients – the elite worked among the upper classes and tended to charge higher fees (Lawrence, 1999). Later, specialists also developed private practices that used their specialist skills and worked as consultants on cases within their area of expertise, but they still spent part of their time working in general practice among the upper classes.

Anne Digby's work on general practice in Britain between the mid-nineteenth and mid-twentieth centuries suggests that we need to think not of GPs and specialists, but of medical careers falling along a continuum between general and consulting practice. Digby (1999, pp.294–8) has identified five career patterns:

- the 'classic' GP, who practised general medicine among a mix of social classes;

- the GP/surgeon who practised general medicine and had a part-time appointment as a surgeon in a small hospital;

- the GP/specialist, who worked as a general practitioner but also did some consulting work in one area of medicine, such as obstetrics or rheumatism;

- GPs who became consultants – men who started their careers in general medicine but switched to full-time consulting;

- 'pure' consultants, who belonged to prestigious medical institutions, held posts in major hospitals and had a private practice.

Conflict and cooperation: elite and general practitioners in nineteenth-century Britain

Elite and general practitioners, then, went through a similar education, held similar qualifications and practised in similar ways. However, the small body of elite practitioners held a disproportionate amount of professional power, especially over licensing. It was therefore not surprising that the two groups engaged in protracted and sometimes violent struggles. In Belgium, the Medical Federation attacked the elite Académie for being unrepresentative and incompetent. In France, the elite attacked the *officiers de santé*, who had an inferior education but competed for patients' fees. However, the fiercest battles seem to have occurred in Britain. The large number of societies and journals – many of which explicitly sought to represent the views of general practitioners – allowed them to air their grievances and campaign for change and sometimes stirred up trouble. From the end of the eighteenth century until the 1840s, general practitioners in England and Wales demanded a new licence which reflected their training in both medicine and surgery and was free of the influence of the old colleges (Loudon, 1986, pp.138–70, 282–96). In the 1820s and 1830s, the *Lancet*, self-appointed champion of the general practitioner, mounted a concerted campaign against the elite medical men of the London Colleges of Surgeons and Physicians and the London hospitals. Wakley attacked the elite for using their influence to advance the careers of their friends and relations, and he had no qualms about using extreme and colourful language. In one editorial, he described the college members as 'crafty, intriguing, corrupt, avaricious, cowardly, plundering, rapacious, soul-betraying, dirty-minded BATS' (*Lancet*, 1831–2, vol.1, p.2). Guy's Hospital was a particular target, perhaps for good reason: in 1840, all five members of the junior surgical staff were former pupils of one of the senior surgeons, Sir Astley Cooper (Plate 8). Three of the junior surgeons were related to Cooper by marriage.

One of the most colourful (and tragic) disputes came in 1828, when a patient of Bransby Cooper (1792–1853) (Figure 5.5), one of Guy's surgeons and a nephew of Astley Cooper, died shortly after an operation to remove a bladder stone. Wakley promptly accused Cooper of incompetence. Look at Figure 5.6, a cartoon that appeared in the *Lancet* in 1828. It is rich in puns and assumes that the audience is familiar with the controversial operation. Cooper is portrayed holding an adze – a heavy woodworking tool used in making barrels (a pun on the name Cooper). But

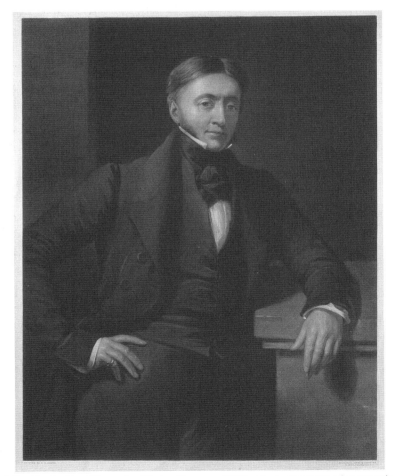

Figure 5.5   Portrait of Bransby Blake Cooper, 1842, photogravure of mezzotint by W.H. Simmons. Wellcome Library, London

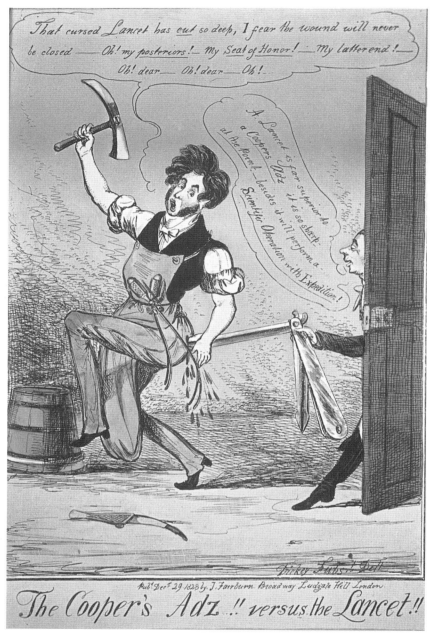

Figure 5.6   *The Cooper's Adz!! Versus the Lancet!!*, 1828. Wellcome Library, London

his actual occupation is made clear by the surgeon's apron and the instruments used for removing bladder stones that are tucked into the belt. Cooper is shown being stabbed in the bottom, not just for comic effect but also as an allusion to the operation to remove a bladder stone. 'Seat of Honor' refers to another cartoon satirizing the nepotism of Guy's Hospital. The lancet carried by the figure that represents Wakley is a pun on the name of his journal. The *Lancet*'s attacks on Cooper and other elite practitioners were extremely pointed and undoubtedly caused pain to their targets. The words attributed to Cooper refer to the exclamations he allegedly made about the difficulty of the case during the operation.

Read 'An operation by Bransby Cooper' (Source Book 2, Reading 5.3). What criticisms does Wakley level at Cooper, at the hospital and at the students? What overall impression is made by such a broad attack?

Wakley criticizes Cooper for being an incompetent surgeon – he took a long time to perform a simple operation, and this lack of skill killed his patient. In the final paragraph, he also implies that Cooper did not behave as a surgeon should – with 'coolness and self possession'. He criticizes the system of appointing surgeons at Guy's Hospital, claiming that Cooper and other surgeons got their posts through connections and patronage, not ability. He dismisses the attempt by students to defend their teacher, arguing that they are caught up in the same network of patronage. They have to stay in their teacher's good books in order to get their certificates, and they have to curry favour with Astley Cooper to ensure they get their licences from the College of Surgeons. The overall impression is that the whole medical hierarchy – hospitals, teachers and licensing institutions – is corrupt.

Elite and general practitioners also clashed over their fees. General practitioners complained that consultants charged the same as they did – in such a situation, patients would always choose to employ a consultant. They also complained that elite practitioners 'poached' patients. When they were called in to assist with a difficult case, the elite practitioner would gradually take over the patient's care and when the patient recovered they would pocket the whole fee. The elite, in turn, complained that general practitioners refused to refer cases on, even if they were unable to offer any effective treatments, fearing that they would lose any part of their fee.

These highly public conflicts gradually died away in the second half of the nineteenth century. The power struggles between consultants and general practitioners were partly resolved by the reform of education and licensing, which somewhat reduced the power of the old institutions. The power of the elite also declined as patronage became less important than research or clinical skills in hospital appointments.

Reports of disputes between individual practitioners over cases also became less frequent – perhaps partly because of their adoption of codes of ethics. (Although in theory the Hippocratic oath established a framework of ethics, in practice it carried little authority.) The first British book on ethics in medical practice was published in 1803 by Thomas Percival (1740–1804), but in the 1830s and 1840s many other books and articles were written on the subject. Unlike modern works on ethics, these were not simply concerned with defining the responsibilities of medical men to their patients, but also dealt with issues of etiquette – defining the roles of different practitioners at the bedside and thus avoiding unseemly conflicts. An extract from one of these works, written by W. Fraser and published in 1847, is given in the next exercise.

Exercise

Read 'Medical ethics' (Source Book 2, Reading 5.4).

I   Would you say that Fraser is more concerned about disputes between practitioners (etiquette) or the practitioner's responsibility towards his patient (modern ethics)?

2   How would you summarize Fraser's ideas on how doctors should behave towards each other?

Discussion

I   Fraser is clearly concerned with both etiquette and ethics. A number of his questions directly address what should happen when two practitioners are involved in treating the same patient and the rules they should follow in dealing with one another. But he also addresses ethical questions about a practitioner's responsibilities towards his patient. Some of his questions relate to particular situations – such as when a patient requests that his life should not be prolonged (still an ethical problem today); but there is also a broader ideal – that the patient's wishes and welfare must always come first.

2   Fraser assumes that practitioners will act as gentlemen in their dealings with each other. They should avoid conflict and public disputes by respecting each others' opinions, and by not attempting to take over another doctor's patients.

We have to be cautious, however, in claiming that writings on ethics helped to change medical practice because no historian has shown that practitioners changed their behaviour as a result of reading them.

Health insurance schemes are discussed in more detail in Chapters 9 and 13.

In the twentieth century, amicable relations between general practitioners and consultants were helped by the advent of health insurance schemes. These schemes clearly laid out the roles of general practitioner and consultant within a referral system. Patients had automatic access to a general practitioner, but had to be referred to a specialist. GPs who sent patients to a specialist had no fear of losing fees, since they were always paid for their work on the case by the insurance scheme.

5.4   Monopoly of practice

In the eighteenth and early nineteenth centuries, formally trained practitioners worked alongside an even larger body of irregular practitioners, who provided a similar range of medical treatments. These untrained healers offered many services, including diagnosis and treatment of ailments (sometimes by magical means), prescription and sale of medicines and midwifery. Some treated particular conditions, for instance, bonesetters and practitioners who dealt solely with hernias. They came from a range of different backgrounds: the clergy and upper classes gave free advice to the poor; retail chemists and druggists dispensed advice along with their medicines; and ordinary workers combined medical practice with some other trade. A few healers worked full-time. They travelled from town to town, putting on shows to draw a crowd before selling their remedies, much as charlatans or quacks had done in the sixteenth and seventeenth centuries (Ramsey, 1977, pp.562–720). Sequah was one of the healers who practised successfully in Britain in the late 1880s (Plate 11). Alleged to be an American, Sequah dressed as a cowboy and began his show by extracting teeth free of charge (a technique traditionally used by charlatans to gain an audience's attention). He then launched into a lecture on the failures of modern medicine and the virtues of native American remedies – including his 'Prairie Flower' water and oil. These remedies proved so popular that the show was franchised and several 'Sequahs' travelled the country (Schupbach, 1985).

The nineteenth century also saw the emergence of unorthodox practitioners offering new systems of medicine including **herbalism**, homeopathy, **hydropathy** and **hypnotism**. Herbalism was founded in 1822 by Samuel Thomson (1769–1843), who published a complete therapeutic system based on the use of a limited range of plant remedies to treat all conditions. Homeopathy was based on treatment by highly diluted drugs intended to stimulate the body's healing mechanisms. Hydropathy, a system of therapeutics devised by an Austrian farmer, Vincent Priessnitz (1791–1851), used pure water, both internally and externally, to expel poisons and to stimulate the body's natural healing processes. Hypnotists, or 'mesmerists', put their patients into a trance to diagnose and treat disease. (For a fuller account of these systems, see Porter, 1999, pp.389–96.) These unorthodox practitioners claimed that their remedies were in some way 'natural' (and, by implication, harmless) and worked in harmony with the patient's body. In contrast, the therapies used by orthodox practitioners (often called allopathic remedies) consisted of 'unnatural' chemicals and minerals and were declared to be 'poisons'. Unorthodox medicine flourished in Europe in the mid-nineteenth century, and in 1854 it was reported that there were at least 6,000 unorthodox practitioners working in Britain. They treated patients from all social classes. Herbalism was popular in working-class industrial areas, while homeopathy was adopted by all classes, from the gentry to the poor. Unorthodox medicine was allied with other unorthodox movements, such as non-conformist religion, vegetarianism, anti-vivisection and temperance (Jutte *et al.*, 2001).

Until the 1830s, the work of irregular practitioners was largely tolerated by trained, orthodox medical men, although some of the more flamboyant and successful quacks were attacked in an effort to discredit their work. However, the rising popularity of unorthodox systems of medicine posed a threat to the incomes of orthodox practitioners, especially as it occurred just when they were investing increasing amounts of time and money in their medical training. Unorthodox medicine also challenged the claims of orthodox medicine to possess a unique insight into health and disease. As general practitioners bonded into a strong occupational group, they realized it was in the interests of all orthodox medical men to drive both irregular and unorthodox healers out of the medical marketplace. Thus they could establish a monopoly of practice for qualified, orthodox practitioners.

Historians have often assumed that orthodox practitioners established a monopoly by using the new licensing regulations passed by governments and the legal system to prosecute unqualified healers. As we have seen, throughout Europe governments and medical institutions required practitioners to pass examinations and hold a licence before they could practice. These laws explicitly banned all unqualified healers from practising medicine. However, when orthodox practitioners attempted to apply the law, they met with mixed success. In the Netherlands, the courts were sympathetic to the orthodox practitioners' cause and routinely prosecuted irregular practitioners. In France, the law proved less effective. Under the 1803 regulations, a few irregular healers were licensed. The law allowed for any practitioner, regardless of their level of training, to be appointed as an *officier de santé* if they had testimonials from the local mayor and two notable citizens proving that they had practised successfully. A number of irregular practitioners, including bonesetters and patent medicine sellers, were duly appointed as *officiers*. When licensed practitioners attempted to prosecute irregular practitioners they met with little success. Local administrators were often reluctant to pursue cases against well-established irregular practitioners who treated the poor for a very small fee or even free of charge. If brought to court, defendants were often acquitted on the grounds that their treatments were as effective as those of regular practitioners. Any irregulars sent to jail simply resumed their practice once they were released (Ramsey, 1977, pp.575–9). In other countries, there was no law against unqualified practice. In Britain, after 1858, irregular and unorthodox practitioners could be prosecuted only for claiming to have qualifications that they did not possess. If they made no such claims, they could practise freely. A few were taken to court by licensed practitioners on charges of manslaughter when patients died under their care. In Germany, after 1871, irregular practice was tolerated. Under *Kurierfreiheit* ('freedom of cure') any sort of practitioner could work freely.

Orthodox medical men also sought to distance their practices from those of irregular and unorthodox practitioners. Although they are often portrayed by historians as being clearly differentiated, there was a considerable overlap between them. (The fact that this overlap is often obscured is testament to the efforts of nineteenth-century medical men.) Irregular healers treated the same conditions as orthodox practitioners using similar therapies. Unorthodox practitioners of homeopathy and hydropathy, for instance, used an orthodox understanding of the body and disease but applied different therapies. And although many medical men were sceptical of the value of traditional medicines, claims that these systems stimulated the body's natural healing processes were attractive to a small but significant number of regular practitioners. These men offered unorthodox medicine instead of or alongside their orthodox practice (Bradley and Dupree, 2001, pp.419–21).

Orthodox practitioners set out to discredit their irregular and unorthodox competitors and to discourage the public from using their services. As the historian Matthew Ramsey has shown in his studies of French healers, orthodox medical men drew sharp and unflattering comparisons between their behaviour and that of irregular practitioners. They portrayed irregular healers, most of whom were drawn from the ranks of the working classes, as people who had taken up medicine as an easy option to avoid the hard work appropriate to their proper station in life. They knew their treatments were useless or dangerous, yet these unscrupulous 'swindlers' continued to sell them to a gullible public (Ramsey, 1977, pp.571–4). Unorthodox medical treatments were subjected to similar attacks. In the next reading, Alison Winter discusses the professional conflicts which accompanied efforts to introduce mesmeric anaesthesia (a form of hypnosis) to surgical practice, at a time when, as you saw in Chapter 2, surgery was seen to be a particularly innovative and successful area of medicine.

Exercise

Read 'Mesmerism vs ether: a professional battle' (Source Book 2, Reading 5.5).

1   Why was mesmerism not supported in conventional medical circles?

2   What did the supporters of mesmeric anaesthesia do to make their unorthodox practice acceptable to all practitioners?

3   How did orthodox medical men attempt to discredit mesmeric anaesthesia?

Discussion

1   Mesmerism did not fit with the image and status of medicine as a respectable, scientific pursuit as the practice was associated with discredited revolutionary politics and did not fit with established knowledge of how the body functioned.

2   Supporters of mesmerism tried to prove its clinical value through experiments, which were described in the conventional way through medical journals. They also emphasized that mesmeric anaesthesia gave the surgeon control over pain, and over the anaesthetized patient – a desirable result for the surgeon (although, as you have seen, a source of concern to patients).

3   Orthodox medical practitioners tried to discredit the results of experiments with mesmeric anaesthesia, claiming that patients only pretended to feel no pain. However, according to Winter, such arguments were not conclusive – the jury was out until the arrival of ether, which was heavily promoted as a respectable and more reliable form of anaesthesia. Ether was not subjected to the same critical scrutiny as mesmerism, despite its disreputable past as a recreational drug. And experimental operations using ether showed that it was not clinically superior to mesmeric anaesthesia. The crucial factor in the success of ether over

mesmerism was the weight of support for it from elite members of the orthodox profession.

There are clear parallels between the practitioners' responses to mesmeric anaesthesia and to the new means of diagnosis and treatment that were later to emerge from the laboratory (which you read about in Chapter 4). In both cases, elite practitioners rejected practices they felt undermined their established knowledge and skills. Orthodox practitioners who took up unorthodox forms of medicine were the subjects of particularly vituperative attack. Qualified unorthodox practitioners could not be prosecuted, but orthodox practitioners could (and did) ruin their careers by denying them access to professional institutions and to practice. The editors of medical journals refused to publish articles on unorthodox medicine. Thus, it appeared that the new ideas had no merit and unorthodox practitioners were denied the kudos of publishing original research. Unorthodox practice was not taught in medical schools, ensuring that students did not learn about such therapies. Medical societies threw out any member who worked with unorthodox practitioners. Such strategies were also used against other groups seen as inappropriate members of the profession – including female and Jewish practitioners.

Unorthodox practitioners fought back, seeking to give their practice a new respectability by adopting the trappings of the orthodox profession. They too established strict standards of education and systems of licensing. They founded their own journals and societies. British herbal practitioners, for example, could join the National Association of Medical Herbalists or the Society of United Medical Herbalists. As they were pushed out of posts in hospitals, unorthodox practitioners created their own hospitals and dispensaries. The London Homeopathic Hospital provided free treatment to the deserving poor and trained students in homeopathic practice. Many countries had homeopathic schools of medicine, with a curriculum similar to that taught in regular schools, except, of course, when it came to therapeutics (Saks, 2003, pp.65–77).

Efforts by orthodox practitioners to establish a monopoly of practice ultimately failed, and both irregular and unorthodox healers continued to flourish into the twentieth century. A parliamentary report produced in Britain in 1910, for example, found herbalists, faith healers, bonesetters and a multitude of other types of practitioner still working all around the country. Patent medicine sellers also plied their trade well into the twentieth century. Practitioners seemed to become resigned to their continuing presence. At the end of a campaign against secret remedies in 1912, the British Medical Association was forced to admit that such medicines might even do some good, since 'for the most part they are made of materials in common use in medical practice' (quoted in Digby, 1994, p.65).

5.5   Autonomy and the right to self-regulation

Licensing and self-regulation

Sociologists have identified the right to self-regulation – to set standards of education, qualification and behaviour – as one of the key features of modern professions. They claim that this autonomy was acknowledged by governments in recognition of a profession's possession of a body of highly specialized, esoteric knowledge and their high level of internal organization. However, some historians of medicine have argued that this is a false impression, based on studies of professions in Britain and America. As you have already seen in this chapter, in many European countries it was governments rather than medical practitioners that were responsible for licensing. Ramsey has laid down a further challenge to the sociologists' arguments, claiming that the right to self-regulation was not won by professions, but was gifted by governments. The acquisition of the right to control licensing had little to do with the organization of the medical profession, but was dependent on wider political circumstances. Broadly speaking, governments which exerted stricter regulation over all aspects of social and commercial life were more likely to regulate the medical profession. Laissez-faire governments, which took a more relaxed attitude to regulation, were more likely to grant the medical profession the right to self-regulation. In Europe, Ramsey has identified several types of regulation including:

- corporate monopoly – where licensing is controlled by medical guilds and colleges;

- bureaucratic regulation – where the state identifies qualified individuals;

- a 'modified free field' – where licensed practitioners have no legal monopoly but have additional rights.

In nineteenth-century France (and also in Prussia until the 1860s), corporate monopoly was replaced by bureaucratic regulation. Under regulations passed in 1803, the state dictated the education of different grades of practitioner, and banned any unqualified healer from practising medicine (although, as you have seen, the law was not always strictly applied). These regulations also specified where the lower grades of practitioner, the *officiers de santé*, could work, and what treatments they could provide. *Officiers* were not supposed to perform major surgical operations, as attempted so disastrously by Charles Bovary in Gustave Flaubert's novel *Madame Bovary* (1857). This organization reflected the strength of French central government under Napoleon. The medical profession had no objection to such state regulation.

In keeping with its minimal regulation of trade and industry, the British government exerted very little control over the medical profession. Until 1858, all licensing was a corporate monopoly, and while in theory all practitioners required a college licence or university degree, in practice those without a formal qualification were unlikely to be prosecuted. In 1858, a modified free field was created by the Medical Act. The law restricted medical practice to those men whose names appeared on the Medical Register, while the General Medical Council (representatives of the profession) set the standards for entry to the register. However, the penalties against unqualified practice were not rigorously enforced. Qualified practitioners did not have a monopoly of practice, but they enjoyed a privileged status. They alone could hold certain public posts, as Poor Law medical officers, for example. Such privileges were increasingly important. Under the 1911 National Health Insurance Act and the National Health Service, only orthodox practice was provided, thus unorthodox and irregular practitioners were finally marginalized.

While the British government's minimal control over medical licensing was in keeping with its laissez-faire doctrines, the story of licensing in Germany appears to run counter to the image of increasing government regulation. Until 1868, throughout the German states, medicine was subject to bureaucratic regulation. In 1868, however, the Prussian government abolished all these controls on medical practice – a move copied by other states and retained after unification in 1871. This created a 'free field' in which any practitioner could work without restraint. This move has often been seen as a peculiar backwards step in the formation of the German medical profession. However, it was taken as part of a wider move to do away with a number of regulations on a range of trades and professions, and was supported by members of the medical elite. They welcomed the freedom from restrictions on the work of different grades of practitioner and on where they could practise. Perhaps because they had lucrative practices among the upper classes, the elite were not concerned with competition from irregular and unorthodox practitioners. Such competition would have concerned general practitioners, but they failed to organize their opposition to *Kurierfreiheit*. Although the government allowed all types of practitioners to work freely, Ramsey's model of a 'modified free field' can be applied to the German situation. Members of the orthodox medical profession still enjoyed certain privileges: only they could be employed as medical practitioners by the government, practise midwifery or run an asylum (Ramsey, 1984).

Working for the state

Ramsey's argument focuses on the autonomy held by medical practitioners over licensing. However, as Rita Schepers, a Dutch historian of the medical profession, points out, there are different forms of autonomy:

> economic autonomy, the right of doctors to determine their remuneration; political autonomy, the right of doctors to make policy decisions as the legitimate experts on health matters; and clinical or technical autonomy, the right of the profession to set its own standards and control clinical performance.
>
> (Schepers, 1994, p.237)

Not all these rights are determined by licensing regulations. In the newly unified Germany, the regulation of clinical matters was in the hands of the Ärztekammer (literally: a chamber of physicians), a body of practitioners responsible for maintaining professional discipline. All medical men were required to join their local Ärztekammer who could fine incompetent practitioners (McClelland, 1991, pp.83–4).

The right to political autonomy was a particularly contentious issue. The impact of government employment varied widely, as we can see in the differing experiences of British and Russian practitioners. In Russia, working for local government increased the political autonomy of practitioners. There, more than in any other European country, doctors were state employees. All practitioners trained in state medical schools and had to pay for their education by working in government posts. It was virtually impossible for doctors to make a living through private practice. Practitioners were of low status in the strict social hierarchy and were poorly paid. However, from 1864, doctors found new appointments as *zvemsto* ('local government') practitioners. By the 1870s, successful initiatives on public health and welfare, and in particular their campaign to control the 1892–3 **cholera** epidemic, brought doctors a new prestige. As a result, the state began to acknowledge doctors as experts and to seek their advice on public health policy (Frieden, 1975).

Other public health initiatives are discussed in Chapter 7.

In Britain, working for the Poor Law authorities – the government bodies responsible for looking after the poor and sick – appeared to threaten the clinical and political autonomy of doctors. (The work of the Poor Law authorities is described in Chapter 2.) My research into public vaccination against smallpox provides a good case study of this type of conflict. In 1840, as part of a wider movement to tackle epidemic disease, parliament passed an Act requiring the Poor Law authorities in England and Wales to offer free vaccination. Boards of guardians, the administrators who distributed poor relief, were required to appoint, supervise and pay public vaccinators. While practitioners approved in principle the provision of free vaccination, they had serious objections to the proposed system of provision. First, there was the issue of control. Practitioners argued that professional men, with their specialist skills and knowledge, should not have to work under the supervision of the lay guardians, who understood nothing of the medical issues involved. Second, there was the issue of pay. While guardians were concerned to keep costs down, and thus pay as little as possible for vaccination (1s 6d per case was the recommended fee, but some boards paid less), medical men argued that they should receive a larger fee, similar to that paid by private patients, which reflected the skills required to conduct the operation. Finally, practitioners protested that forcing parents to have their children vaccinated by a designated public vaccinator denied them the right to choose their own doctor. In 1840 and 1841, across England, practitioners went on strike, refusing to vaccinate for less than 2s 6d per case. They did not see such behaviour as incompatible with professional status (as we might do now), but portrayed it as heroic mutual support. A *Lancet* editorial described the action of one group of practitioners as a demonstration of '*esprit de corps*, a liberal feeling, a freemasonry of sentiment'. Such actions rarely succeeded – usually the Poor Law authorities could find a practitioner willing to defy his colleagues and take on the work.

Conflicts such as this happened occasionally all over Europe. In Germany, from the 1890s, practitioners working for insurance schemes made similar protests that the administrators provided low rates of pay and denied patients a free choice of practitioner. By 1903, more than 10,000 doctors had joined the Hartmann League to fight for better pay, and conducted local strikes. The insurance companies could not find enough medical men to maintain the schemes, and were forced to give in to the strikers' demands (McClelland, 1991, pp.140–1). Similar actions in Holland were unsuccessful. Perhaps the longest dispute was conducted by Norwegian practitioners who refused to take up military posts from 1854 to 1861 as a protest against the low level of pay. (Disputes between practitioners and governments continue to this day, whenever the state tries to change doctors' contracts.)

5.6 The status of medical men

Sociologists have described professionalization as a process of 'collective social mobility' whereby members of an occupational group improve their social standing. You have read in Chapter 3 that surgeons improved their professional standing in the late eighteenth and early nineteenth centuries. But what about other practitioners? Did they achieve high social status in the nineteenth century? Status is very difficult to measure so here I look at it from the viewpoints of contemporary practitioners and the public and through the work of historians who have explored the experience of British practitioners.

Did medical men themselves think that the status of their profession improved during the nineteenth century? In the 1840s and 1850s, many British practitioners complained that the public held them in low esteem. The public did not value their services but were happy to employ the practitioner who charged the lowest fees. The public conflicts between elite and general practitioners dragged down the reputation of all medical men. And, so long as practitioners made up and sold their own medicines, their work would not be seen as a profession but as a form of trade. Some of these commentators described the ideal practitioner who could command public respect. Interestingly, his status rested not on his superior knowledge (although he had received a good education in both the arts and medicine) but on his behaviour. The ideal medical man was skilful, polite and considerate, remaining calm and firm even in a crisis. He respected the opinions of his colleagues and treated the poor free of charge, as part of the social obligation shared by the upper classes.

It seems unlikely that all practitioners could have lived up to such an ideal. However, medical men did their best to drill the next generation of practitioners in good behaviour. From the 1830s, medical courses opened with lectures on appropriate behaviour and the need for students to work hard during their studies. Medical schools began to provide living accommodation, where students were required to keep regular hours, and respectable outlets for students' energy, such as cricket and rugby clubs (Figure 5.7). Students indulging in riotous behaviour were expelled. This had some effect. The early nineteenth-century stereotype of the callous, loud-mouthed and ignorant medical student who drank, skipped lectures, cheated in exams and stole body parts from dissecting rooms for macabre pranks was replaced by an image of a diligent and serious student. Drinking and practical jokes were not eradicated, but these were seen as occasional aberrations and accepted as necessary for 'letting off steam' after long hours in the classroom (Waddington, 2002).

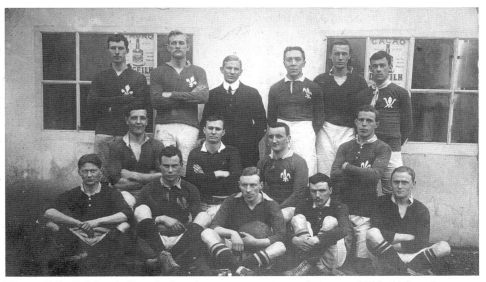

Figure 5.7   St Mary's Hospital rugby team, on a tour of France, 1908. Although originally introduced as an outlet for students' energy, sport became a very important aspect of life at medical school and an expression of the camaraderie among students of a particular institution. At Edinburgh, the students associated with different wards at the Royal Infirmary played for their clinique in a competition. Some schools argued against the admission of women on the grounds that it would reduce the number of students available for the sports teams. Wellcome Library, London

Grumbles about the low status of medicine died away in the second half of the nineteenth century. Peter Eade (1825–1915), an elite physician, who became mayor of Norwich, wrote in his autobiography:

> Looking back at the state of the medical profession ... one can only thankfully observe the great changes which have taken place in its tone and morale. In 1840–1850, the rivalry between neighbouring country practitioners was often intense ... Not only were small appointments often made into heated personal competitions, but in any complaint against a medical attendant, the matter would be followed up by the Guardians [of the poor] ... in a quite partisan manner ... Party spirit ... ran high ... and in public matters doctors were almost afraid to vote, because of offense liable to be taken by patients of opposite views.

(Long, 1916, p.35)

By the late nineteenth century, according to Eade, practitioners no longer had to toady to their patients and employers but enjoyed a certain respect.

Ultimately, social status lies in the eye of the beholder. Did the general public regard medical men with greater respect by the end of the nineteenth century than they had at the beginning? Various popular images and descriptions in fiction suggest that at least the middle classes – who were the main employers of doctors – did so. As you read in Chapter 4, the nineteenth century saw huge social upheavals, with the breakdown of an old social order based on rank and privilege. All over Europe, there emerged a more meritocratic society, where entry to the universities, to the professions and ultimately to the powerful ruling elite was based on ability rather than patronage. Medical practitioners exemplified the new middle-class values of hard work, self-advancement, respectability and public service.

At the beginning of the century, cartoons relentlessly poked fun at fat, greedy, incompetent doctors. However, by the middle of the century, the hard-working general practitioner was presented in a much more sympathetic light, as in the following reading, an extract from Anthony Trollope's *Dr Thorne* which contains a wonderfully accurate portrayal of a medical dispute.

Exercise

Read 'A squabble between doctors' (Source Book 2, Reading 5.6). How does Trollope portray Dr Thorne and Dr Fillgrave? What qualities do they possess?

Discussion

Trollope's sympathies clearly lie with Dr Thorne, who is well trained (he holds a degree), hard-working and provides the services his patients need (all sound middle-class values). Thorne is not worried about appearing undignified – he is happy to accept a standard fee from his patients. In contrast, Trollope portrays Dr Fillgrave as a pompous, conceited man who has an inflated sense of his own professional dignity and is overly concerned with social niceties, such as whether Dr Thorne should dine with the gentry (a reflection of the old social order, where advancement relied on patronage). Dr Fillgrave condemns Dr Thorne for working like a tradesman. Regardless of the comfort of his patients, he upholds the outdated divisions between different groups of practitioners and refuses to consult with Dr Thorne.

By the last decades of the century, medical practitioners had even become the subject of sentimental high art. Luke Fildes's painting *The Doctor* (1891) (Plate 9), showing a middle-class practitioner treating a poor child out of selfless disinterest, proved enormously popular among a middle-class audience when first exhibited, and reputedly helped to raise the standing of medical men in the eyes of the public. Practitioners hung reproductions of the image in their waiting rooms – perhaps hoping to inculcate a respectful, grateful attitude in their patients. At the same time, cartoonists working for popular magazines (which also had a middle-class readership) began to present a more positive image of the doctor. Late nineteenth-century cartoonists still occasionally poked fun at the profession, but were equally likely to make the patient the butt of the joke. A few cartoons portrayed practitioners as acutely perceptive. Look now at Figures 5.8, 5.9 and 5.10 and read the captions.

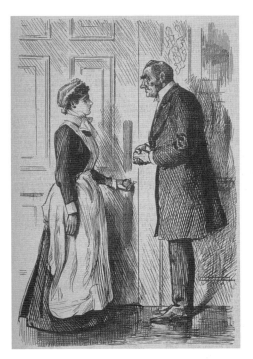

Figure 5.8   The caption to this cartoon, entitled *A Lucid Interval*, reads: 'Doctor: "How is the patient this morning?"; Nurse: "Well – he has been wandering a good deal in his mind. Early this morning I think I heard him say, 'what an old woman that doctor is!' – and I think that was about the last really rational remark he made."' This cartoonist, for one, was still happy to poke fun at doctors – in this case, the sick patient complains that his doctor is fussing too much. Note the doctor's frock coat and stiff collar – this dress became the stereotype of the late Victorian physician, and reflected their improved incomes. From *Punch*, 28 November 1891, p.258. Wellcome Library, London

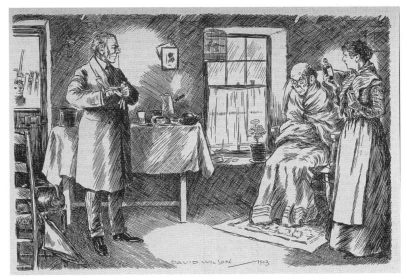

Figure 5.9   The caption to this cartoon reads: 'Doctor: "Well, Mrs O'Brien, I hope your husband has taken his medicine regularly, eh?"; Mrs O'Brien: "Sure, then, Doctor, I've been sorely puzzled. The label says, 'One pill to be taken three times a day', and for the life of me I don't see how it can be taken more than once!"' This is one of a number of cartoons in which working-class patients are the butt of the joke. It is no coincidence that these appear at the time when insurance schemes were giving the working classes greater access to medical practitioners than ever before. From *Punch*, 7 October 1903. Wellcome Library, London

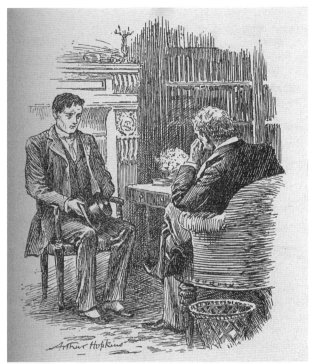

Figure 5.10   The caption to this cartoon, entitled *Diagnosed*, reads: 'Patient: "I'm feeling wretched, Doctor. I take no interest in anything, have no appetite, can't sleep – "; Doctor: "Why don't you marry the girl?"' Here the patient is again the butt of the joke. The perceptive doctor instantly realizes that the source of his symptoms is emotional not physical. From *Punch*, 23 April 1898. Wellcome Library, London

Why did practitioners enjoy greater social standing by the end of the century? Medical men had certainly acquired a new role as experts, and were using their specialist knowledge to deal with new medical and social problems. They applied their expert status in all sorts of situations – as coroners in the law courts judging cause of death and as public health officers and factory inspectors pronouncing on the health of the environment. Even general practitioners began to assess the future health of applicants for health insurance. Doctors also rose to control the running of hospitals. In the past, historians have linked the increased status of nineteenth-century medicine to the development of the medical sciences. However, we cannot draw a simple connection between expert status and the perception that medicine had become 'scientific'. As you saw in Chapter 4, there is no simple link between science and authority. While some doctors embraced the new sciences and actively sought a role as a 'medical expert', elite practitioners chose to stress the need for clinical skills over scientific analysis. These elite practitioners did not lose social standing by rejecting the use of laboratory science. They 'were themselves wealthy and lived in a style not unlike that of the plutocrats they treated. They enjoyed aristocratic leisure activities, such as dining well, gardening and motoring ... [Their practice] depended on face-to-face encounters to maintain and promote social relations and attract clientele' (Lawrence, 1999, p.425).

Exercise

Look back at the portraits reproduced in this chapter (Figures 5.1, 5.2, 5.4 and 5.5) and at Plates 7 and 8. If you did not know these were medical men, would you be able to guess at their occupation? If not, then how are these men portrayed?

Discussion

Figure 5.4, the most modern image, shows a practitioner in a research setting surrounded by laboratory equipment. In the earlier, more formal portraits, there is nothing to suggest that the sitters are doctors. But you may have noticed the books or papers shown in some of the portraits. This visual convention suggests that the sitter is well educated. Overall, these medical men have chosen to be portrayed as gentlemen rather than as doctors.

While the improved status of medical men owed something to their position as experts, it was not linked to the recruitment of new practitioners from the higher social ranks or to increased incomes. Researchers have shown that throughout this period, most practitioners were members of respectable, middle-class families, prepared to work hard for a living (Crowther and Dupree, 1996, pp.396–400; Peterson, 1978, pp.194–214). However, new entrance requirements and the increasing length of medical training meant that, as the century progressed, poorer students would have struggled to qualify. Historians working in the 1970s (including Ivan Waddington, whose work on the 1858 Medical Act you read earlier), assumed that practitioners' incomes rose over the century, as regulation reduced the number of qualified medical men and irregular practitioners were marginalized. But more recent studies have pointed to the complexity of the issue. Across Europe, the effect of new licensing regulation seems to have been at best temporary. There was a slight dip in the numbers of practitioners around the middle of the century, but then numbers climbed again. However, the increasing number of practitioners did not mean that all struggled to earn a living. The nineteenth-century growth in population and the advent of health insurance schemes meant that more people could afford to pay for medical services. Digby has looked in detail at the earnings of British practitioners and concludes that they remained fairly stable throughout the nineteenth century. Between 1800 and 1850, practitioners could expect to earn between £150 and £400 per annum. By 1857, this had risen slightly to around £500. At the end of the century, the average yearly income was around £600 (Digby, 1994, pp.135–48).

5.7 Conclusion

So did the modern medical profession emerge in the nineteenth century? For much of the century, medicine did not look like a modern profession. Practitioners were divided into different grades by licensing regulations which in most countries were set by governments. Different groups of practitioners squabbled over power and over fees. They had relatively low social status, and they engaged in fierce competition with irregular and unorthodox practitioners. Thus, nineteenth-century medicine had a form and character that was unique to its time. By the end of the century, there is a stronger case for seeing medicine as a profession. Practitioners formed a more cohesive group, sharing the same forms of education, qualifications and codes of ethical behaviour. They enjoyed the status of experts, and had greater (though by no means total) control over licensing. However, they still had no monopoly of practice.

Did these changes come about through a process of professionalization or reform? There is no clear answer. On the one hand, nineteenth-century practitioners wanted to be seen as members of a profession, distinguished by gentlemanly codes of behaviour. This may have encouraged the development of medical ethics. On the other hand, change was also driven by economics. The key attribute of modern professions – the possession of a body of specialist knowledge – was also a means by which individual students could ensure that they would succeed in practice. However, as the experience in many European countries shows, governments also had an interest in driving up educational standards in order to ensure that their populations had access to well-trained practitioners. The role of social, cultural, economic and political contexts in shaping the development of the medical profession remains poorly understood. As we have seen in this chapter, professionalization occurred right across Europe – from Russia and Norway to Britain, France, Holland, Belgium and Germany – and in each nation, licensing standards were pushed up, practitioners developed a strong collective identity and they were concerned with their low status. Why this should have happened at the same time under widely differing political regimes and against different cultural backgrounds remains a puzzle for future historians.

References

Bartrip, P. (1996) *Themselves Writ Large: The British Medical Association*, London: British Medical Association.

Bonner, T.N. (1995) *Becoming a Physician: Medical Education in Britain, France, Germany and the United States, 1750–1945*, New York: Oxford University Press.

Bradley, J. and Dupree, M. (2001) 'Opportunity on the edge of orthodoxy: medically qualified hydropathists in the era of reform, 1840–60', *Social History of Medicine*, vol.14, pp.417–37.

Bynum, W.F., Lock, S. and Porter, R. (eds) (1992) *Medical Journals and Medical Knowledge: Historical Essays*, London: Routledge.

Crowther, A. and Dupree, M. (1996) 'The invisible general practitioner: the careers of Scottish medical students in the late nineteenth century', *Bulletin of the History of Medicine*, vol.70, pp.387–413.

Digby, A. (1994) *Making a Medical Living: Doctors and Patients in the English Market for Medicine, 1720–1911*, Cambridge: Cambridge University Press.

Digby, A. (1999) *The Evolution of British General Practice, 1850–1948*, Oxford: Oxford University Press.

Frieden, N. (1975) 'Physicians in pre-revolutionary Russia: professionals or servants of the state?', *Bulletin of the History of Medicine*, vol.49, pp.20–9.

Jutte, R., Eklöf, M. and Nelson, M.C. (eds) (2001) *Historical Aspects of Unconventional Medicine: Approaches, Concepts, Case Studies*, Sheffield: European Association for the History of Medicine and Health Publications.

Lawrence, C. (1999) 'A tale of two sciences: bedside and bench in twentieth-century Britain', *Medical History*, vol.43, pp.421–49.

Lawrence, S.C. (1996) *Charitable Knowledge: Hospital Pupils and Practitioners in Eighteenth-Century London*, Cambridge: Cambridge University Press.

Long, S.H. (ed.) (1916) *The Autobiography of Sir Peter Eade*, London: Jarrold.

Loudon, I. (1986) *Medical Care and the General Practitioner, 1750–1850*, Oxford: Clarendon Press.

McClelland, C.E. (1991) *The German Experience of Professionalisation*, Cambridge: Cambridge University Press.

Parry, N. and Parry, J. (1976) *The Rise of the Medical Profession: A Study of Collective Social Mobility*, London: Croom Helm.

Perkin, H. (1969) *The Origins of Modern English Society, 1780–1880*, London: Routledge & Kegan Paul.

Peterson, M.J. (1978) *The Medical Profession in Mid-Victorian London*, Berkeley: University of California Press.

Porter, R. (1999) *The Greatest Benefit to Mankind: A Medical History of Humanity from Antiquity to the Present*, London: Fontana.

Ramsey, M. (1977) 'Medical power and popular medicine: illegal healers in nineteenth-century France', *Journal of Social History*, vol.10, pp.560–87.

Ramsey, M. (1984) 'The politics of professional monopoly in nineteenth-century medicine: the French model and its rivals' in G. Geison (ed.) *Professions and the French State, 1700–1900*, Philadelphia: University of Pennsylvania Press, pp.225–305.

Saks, M. (2003) *Orthodox and Alternative Medicine: Politics, Professionalisation and Health Care*, London: Continuum Press.

Schepers, R.M.J. (1994) 'Towards unity and autonomy: the Belgian medical profession in the nineteenth century', *Medical History*, vol.38, pp.237–54.

Schupbach, W. (1985) 'Sequah: an English "American medicine" man in 1890', *Medical History*, vol.29, pp.272–317.

Waddington, K. (2002) 'Mayhem and medical students: image, conduct and control in the Victorian and Edwardian London teaching hospital', *Social History of Medicine*, vol.15, pp.45–64.

Source Book readings

I. Waddington, *The Medical Profession in the Industrial Revolution*, Dublin: Gill & Macmillan Humanities Press, 1984, pp.136–43, 147–52 (Reading 5.1).

I. Loudon, *Medical Care and the General Practitioner, 1750–1850*, Oxford: Clarendon Press, 1986, pp.297–301 (Reading 5.2).

Editorial, *Lancet*, 1827–28, vol.2, pp.20–2 (Reading 5.3).

W. Fraser, 'Queries in medical ethics', *London Medical Gazette*, 1849, vol.2, pp.181–7, 227–32 (Reading 5.4).

A. Winter, 'Ethereal epidemic: mesmerism and the introduction of inhalation anaesthesia to early Victorian London', *Social History of Medicine*, 1991, vol.4, pp.6–11, 13–14, 17–23, 25–6 (Reading 5.5).

A. Trollope, *Dr Thorne*, London: Wordsworth Classics, 1996, pp.25–8 (Reading 5.6).

6

Women in Medicine

Doctors and Nurses, 1850–1920

------------------ Maxine Rhodes ------------------

Objectives

When you have completed this chapter you should be able to:

- demonstrate how and why women were restricted in developing a career as a doctor;

- understand why these restrictions applied to the medical profession, but not to nursing;

- explore the forces that brought about change in the nursing profession;

- understand how different historical approaches describe women's place in medicine.

6.1   Introduction

Women have always cared for the sick. They have nursed family members within the home and worked as nurses, healers and midwives within the community. In the eighteenth century, a few women worked as 'doctresses' and 'surgeonesses', having received some form of training similar to male practitioners. However, when formal medical training began to be developed in hospitals and medical schools in the early nineteenth century, women were not admitted. Thus they were excluded from the ranks of the medical profession. It was not until the late nineteenth and early twentieth centuries, after a long and often bitter struggle, that women gained access to formal medical training. But even after this barrier had been crossed, women still encountered difficulties in pursuing a career as a doctor.

In the practice of nursing, there were major changes in the late nineteenth century, with a massive increase in the number of nurses working in hospitals and the development of formal training and qualifications. The role of nurses was subtly redefined, shifting from solely domestic care to a combination of caring with more medical tasks. Nurses, however, remained firmly subordinate to doctors. The physician was in charge of the patient's care, and a nurse was expected to simply follow his instructions. At the beginning of the twentieth century, there was another period of change, when nurses sought to secure professional status for their occupation. Many of the strategies used by male doctors to keep women out of medicine were employed by nurses to ensure only the 'right sort' of woman gained entry to the profession – those with some education and a 'good' moral character.

In this chapter, I examine these changes in the medical and nursing professions and look at the forces that drove them. Given that their way was often blocked, how did women gain a foothold in the medical profession and then further their careers? How effective were nurses in turning a low-status occupation into a profession? I also examine the historiography of the topic, showing how historians have studied women in the medical and nursing professions, moving from biographies of heroic pioneers to accounts which explore the social and professional context in which these women worked.

6.2 Gender, medicine and society

To understand the reaction to attempts by women to both enter the medical profession and raise the status of nursing, you need to look at some contemporary views about women's capabilities and their role in society. The view that prevailed among most upper- and middle-class commentators was one developed by doctors, that women's abilities were defined principally by their physiology.

This commonly held belief about women is reflected in contemporary writings, including the *Manual of Midwifery*, which was written by Dr Michael Ryan for a medical audience. First published in 1828, it was reprinted into the 1840s.

Exercise

Read 'The biological destiny of women' (Source Book 2, Reading 6.1).

1   According to Ryan, how does female physiology determine women's role in society?

2   Does he allow for any exceptions to this rule?

Discussion

1   Ryan claims that every aspect of the female character – mind, emotions, behaviour, health and strength – is ultimately related to women's reproductive role. Women are biologically preprogrammed for a life within the home, caring for husbands and children. Although Ryan does not state this, it is implicit in his argument that women are therefore not capable of having professional careers.

2   There is no possible exception to this rule – however intelligent they may be, women will 'naturally' desire a domestic role.

These ideas about physiology underpinned the notion of **separate spheres** for men and women. Women belonged in the private sphere of the home, providing a caring environment for husband and children. Men were equally determined by their physiology. Physically strong, rational and not ruled by their emotions, they were fitted for a role in the public sphere, dealing with the rough and tumble of the world of work.

These views were widely held throughout Europe and remained dominant into the twentieth century. In France, in the late eighteenth century, writer and philosopher Jean-Jacques Rousseau (1712–78) glorified the female domestic role and praised the values of selfless and devoted motherhood. 'Virtuous' women who remained within their 'natural' sphere of home and family were extolled. 'European women were continually told that motherhood was women's special role and that mothering was what they should devote themselves to' (Anderson and Zinsser, 1988, p.151). The implications for women of such ideas were enormous. They were used to justify the existing organization of society and to place limitations on middle-class women's access to education and work. (Ironically, at the same time, thousands of working-class women were engaged in paid employment outside the home, without any apparent damage to their health.)

Exercise

Read 'Women as doctors and women as nurses' (Source Book 2, Reading 6.2).

1   How does the relationship between doctors and nurses portrayed in this editorial relate to the roles of men and women in the home?

2   What does the author believe will be the result of women entering the medical profession? Can you see any contradictions within the argument?

Discussion

1   The author accepts the argument that women have natural capabilities as wives and mothers. By nature they are helpful, sympathetic and caring. These are the key characteristics required of a nurse, and thus women are equipped for this role by their physiology. Women are naturally subordinate to men, in all aspects of life. Wives defer to their husbands and daughters to their fathers. This hierarchy is replicated in the medical setting. Nurses are happy to assist doctors in caring for patients. Men are natural leaders and the cooperation of nurses and doctors is presented as a form of natural harmony. Each complements the other and this reflects the domestic hierarchy. The author suggests that men would make excellent nurses, but would find it difficult to adopt a subordinate role. In contrast, women are entirely unfit to be doctors because by their nature they are not suited to a dominant role.

2   If women do succeed in becoming doctors, they will lose their natural female capacities for caring and nurturing. Worse, the whole social order will be put at risk. Neither female nurses nor male patients will happily follow orders given by women (an odd idea in a world of female servants supervised by female housekeepers and householders). As a result, nurses will become dissatisfied with their role and the quality of the care they offer will deteriorate. Nurses will increasingly demand medical training, and will abandon their traditional role to become doctors. Such a challenge to the natural order in the sickroom threatens to be the first step in a much wider set of changes, in which women break away

from their traditional domestic role. While the author paints a picture of social chaos, he also argues that the natural order of things will prevail. An absence of good nurses will result in women doctors nursing their own patients and thereby realizing that nursing is in fact their true vocation. This contradicts the earlier claim that nurses will become dissatisfied with their role. Given the chance, women will turn to men for guidance on all matters, including medical treatment.

Opposition to women doctors was not confined to medical journals, but was also expressed in popular novels, which showed the folly of a young woman's desire for a medical career. While the narratives in these novels differed, the outcomes were remarkably similar. 'In each, the young woman repents, abandons her medical studies and finds true fulfilment by marrying the hero, usually a doctor himself' (Anderson and Zinsser, 1988, p.54).

These ideas about the social role of women did not go totally undisputed. In the late nineteenth and early twentieth centuries, feminist campaigners increasingly challenged this pervasive ideology (Bland, 1995; Vertinsky, 1990). While nine-teenth-century feminism in Britain has come to be associated in the public imagination primarily with the demand for the vote, it was not a single-issue campaign. Rather, it encompassed a number of issues which ultimately sought to challenge the established idea of women's role in society. Middle-class women fought for the right to go to universities and to enter the professions. Other campaigns focused on the rights of working-class women. While their views had some influence, the idea that women were the 'weaker sex' and needed protection persisted well into the inter-war period, acting as an obstacle to equality (Dyhouse, 1995).

6.3   Gaining admission: access for women to a medical education

Despite the arguments against female doctors, a small number of European women (many of whom were involved in or sympathetic to the feminist movement) sought to enter the medical profession in the second half of the nineteenth century. As you read in Chapter 5, the medical profession was less strictly regulated in the eighteenth century, and there were various routes into a career in medicine. Trainee practitioners could undertake apprenticeships, attend lectures and courses in medical schools and gain clinical experience in hospitals. In Britain, a few women continued to gain entrance to the profession in this way until the middle of the nineteenth century. In 1858, Elizabeth Blackwell (1821–1910), a British-born woman living in America, was accepted onto the Medical Register in Britain by virtue of her foreign degree. As a consequence of her actions, the British Medical Association promptly barred admission to holders of foreign qualifica-tions. In 1865, Elizabeth Garrett (1836–1917) (Figure 6.1) also gained a medical qualification, through a long and difficult route. She attended clinical classes in London hospitals, and after threatening legal action against the authorities who refused to let her sit the examination she acquired a licence from the Society of Apothecaries, the rules of which did not specifically exclude women. The society

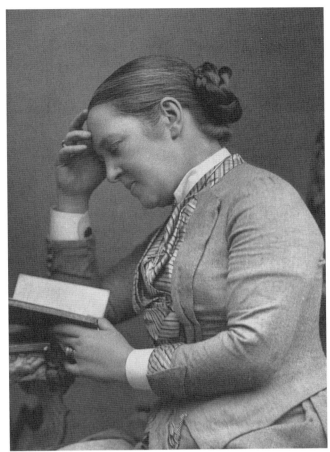

Figure 6.1   Portrait of Elizabeth Garrett Anderson, after her marriage to J.G.S. Anderson, a businessman. Garrett Anderson is shown reading intently, which is unusual in a portrait and emphasizes the high level of education she attained. Like many women doctors, she continued to practise after her marriage and had a very successful medical career, mainly in general practice. Her daughter Louisa also became a doctor. Wellcome Library, London

promptly closed this route to other women by refusing to examine any candidate who had not studied at a recognized medical school.

In the past, historians tended to see women's entrance to medical education simply in terms of the life stories of such pioneering individuals. However, these accounts give a very partial view.

Exercise

Read 'Elizabeth Blackwell, a medical pioneer' (Source Book 2, Reading 6.3).

1   How is Blackwell portrayed? Think about the incidents described here.

2   Is anything missing from this account?

1   This biographical account stresses the heroic efforts Blackwell made to acquire her medical training, and the disastrous loss of her sight in one eye. It portrays Blackwell in a very positive light, attributing to her such virtues as high intellectual ability, perseverance, adaptability and 'superhuman courage'. A lighter side to Blackwell's character is suggested in her liking for champagne.

2   The author describes how Blackwell constantly has to struggle to achieve her goals, but gives no reason as to why she is denied access to medical training. Initially, the author is negative about the training route open to Blackwell at La Maternité hospital, but later admits that Blackwell herself found it extremely useful. Throughout, the author describes a life of tremendous suffering in the face of great opposition. There is little consideration of the context of the times or of what motivated Blackwell to continue her training. As a result, the account offers a rather one-dimensional picture of Blackwell's career, which appears to have developed in an arbitrary way and was dependent on the support of specific individuals.

This account is typical of the rather old-fashioned biographies of Victorian pioneering women, which elevate individuals to heroic status without fully exploring the social context from which they emerged. However, since the 1980s, historians of medicine have developed alternative, more contextualized interpretations of women's access to medicine. These studies have re-examined the careers of the first medical women, and have looked at the experiences of later generations of female doctors. Instead of simply showing that women had to fight to gain entry to medicine, these studies have explored the reasons why and how women were excluded from medical education and practice. They have set these reasons into a social context, examining the background of those women who chose to defy contemporary opinion. They have also put women's entry to medicine into the context of the professional changes described in Chapter 5 – the reform of medical education and practitioners' efforts to secure higher social status. Feminist historians, in particular, have explored the ways in which the medical profession became dominated by men, and how male practitioners used arguments about women's intellectual and physical capabilities to prevent women gaining ground within the profession at a time when they were trying to raise the status of their occupation.

Look back to Chapter 5 if you need to refresh your memory about educational reforms and efforts to raise medicine to professional status.

These later studies have also shown that women coming after Blackwell and Garrett Anderson faced even greater problems in entering medicine because the education received by girls did not usually prepare them for an academic career. In the late nineteenth century, as medical training began to shift to universities, there was an expectation that students would have received a good school education or even completed a degree prior to medical study. This inequality in education was again justified by physiology. Women's bodies were thought to be particularly at risk of damage during and just after puberty. Energy expended at this time on education would cause menstrual disorders and ultimately sterility, leaving women 'unsexed' and therefore unfit for marriage and domestic life. Even women trying to enter higher education worried about the effects of intense study. One American student recalled: 'We did not know when we began whether women's health could stand the strain of education. We were haunted in those days by the clanging chains of that gloomy little specter [sic] Dr Edward H. Clarke's *Sex in Education* [a book that warned of the dire effects of study on women's health]' (quoted in Blake, 1990, p.165). Such concerns were shared by European women. There were few opportunities for women to enter university. In France, for example, where public secondary education for girls lacked an academic focus, there were only 4,254 women attending universities in 1913, as opposed to 37,783 men (Anderson and Zinsser, 1988, p.188).

Even when they were admitted to university, women were not always allowed to study medicine. In Russia, women were admitted into the university system from 1876 (only to be barred again between 1881 and 1905), but they could not attend classes that taught medicine. Across Europe, medical education was opened to women only very slowly. Switzerland had a reputation for being a liberal society, especially on issues of women's education, and Zurich, in particular, was regarded as being intellectually open. In the 1860s, Zurich University opened its doors to female medical students, and by 1870, seven women (from Russia, England, America and Switzerland) had matriculated. Women also began to study in Paris in 1868, and by 1874 more than 150 women were enrolled on medical courses in France and Switzerland. In Sweden, women could enter medical schools from 1870, but it was not until 1888 that the first Swedish woman completed her studies. In Denmark, two women overcame faculty opposition and enrolled in medicine in 1877. In Belgium, Norway, Spain and Portugal women were admitted to university medical schools in the 1880s (Bonner, 1992, pp.31–80).

Once enrolled in medical schools, women then faced fierce opposition from staff and fellow students:

> almost everywhere it was opposition from faculty in the medical schools, and their links with senior staff and managers of local hospitals and infirmaries, that delayed the universities' formal provision for the full acceptance of women students to classes and examinations.
>
> (Dyhouse, 1995, p.13)

Male students and practitioners complained that if faced with a mixed class, lecturers would have to modify the content of their teaching, so as not to shock or offend their female listeners.

In Britain, the campaign for access to the medical profession began at Edinburgh University in 1869, and was led by Sophia Jex-Blake (1840–1913). Influenced by the feminist movement of the time, Jex-Blake had a wide-ranging education and was keen to earn an independent living. She fought a relentless battle with the Edinburgh University authorities. Initially, the university refused to admit a lone female student, so Jex-Blake recruited a small group of women. Once admitted, the women were denied access to the university's medical classes so they made their own arrangements for learning these subjects, organizing separate classes with professors sympathetic to their cause and attending courses taught outside the university. They were then denied access to clinical training at Edinburgh's Royal

Infirmary, and were only admitted after a long battle with the hospital authorities. Finally, they were denied the right to graduate. Jex-Blake eventually qualified in Bern, Switzerland, and received her licence through the Irish College of Physicians (Blake, 1990, pp.97–155).

Female medical students also faced physical violence. Despite medical students' growing reputation for studiousness, Jex-Blake and her fellow female students were roughly handled by the male students. During a 'riot' in Edinburgh, Jex-Blake and her companions were jeered at and had the gates of the medical school slammed in their faces. Later, a live sheep was pushed into their classroom, and on leaving the lecture the women had mud thrown at them and were pushed and jostled (Blake, 1990, pp.125–8). Across Europe, similar resistance was shown to women who wanted to study medicine. In Spain, a group of female medical students passed their examinations but were refused a full degree. And one Spanish student, Pilar Tauregui, was attacked by her male classmates when she attended medical school in 1881 (Anderson and Zinsser, 1988, p.189).

Why were medical men so violently opposed to women becoming practitioners?

Exercise

Read 'The impact of women doctors' (Source Book 2, Reading 6.5).

1   Why is the author of this editorial so worried about the prospect of women qualifying as doctors? How does it reflect the concerns of mid-nineteenth-century practitioners explored in Chapter 5?

2   What arguments are used to oppose the entry of women to the profession?

Discussion

1   The author is deeply concerned about the effect that women will have on the medical profession. As he boldly states towards the end of the extract: 'the profession is overstocked'. Such claims were used to justify raising the requirements for medical licensing in order to reduce the number of male practitioners. Competition from women doctors will mean that the income of each will further decline, and fewer men of ability will be attracted to the profession. The presence of female doctors also threatens the status of the profession. At this time, medical men were trying to raise the status of their occupation by emphasizing the need for practitioners to possess highly specialized knowledge. If women, who were thought to have very limited intellectual capacities, could qualify, then this devalued medical knowledge.

2   The editorial reiterates the argument that women are not physiologically suited to a career in medicine. They lack the physical stamina, they would be overcome with emotion at the sight of a patient in pain and they cannot be trusted to respect patient confidentiality. (The author here assumes a biological tendency to 'gossip'.) If women do complete a medical training, they run the risk of losing their natural female qualities of compassion and kindness. The author also introduced some new arguments. While denying that women patients are

demanding female physicians (the author suggests that a 'thoughtful' woman regards the idea of a female medical attendant as repulsive), he seems to assume that female doctors will concentrate on midwifery. Such specialism is equated to quackery and poor standards of practice, and is seen as a backward step. Doctors have only recently saved obstetrics from the practice of untrained **wise-women**. The author claims that female practitioners who work only in obstetrics will not acquire, and are not capable of acquiring, a full medical education – another sign of the quack doctor. This will further devalue all medical training, resulting in a reduction in the quality of service, and will threaten the status of the whole profession.

The idea that women could not become competent practitioners was not confined to the medical press. It was also the subject for cartoons in the popular press (Figure 6.2).

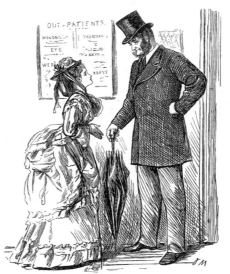

Figure 6.2   The caption to this cartoon, entitled *The Coming Race*, reads: 'Doctor Evangeline: "By the bye, Mr Sawyer, are you engaged tomorrow afternoon? I have rather a ticklish operation to perform – an amputation, you know." Mr Sawyer: "I shall be very happy to do it for you." Doctor Evangeline: "O, no, not *that!* But will you kindly come and administer the chloroform for me?"' The humour rests on the way the cartoon turns on its head the stereotype of the helpless woman and strong man. It portrays a 'comic' situation – where a fashionably dressed, small female doctor claims greater surgical competence than a man. At the same time, it accurately captures the way doctors did ask each other for help in administering anaesthetics. The cartoonist reflects the ambiguous views held of women doctors. In the 1870s, when only a few women were training as practitioners, they were depicted as small, elaborately dressed feminine figures. By 1900, when a small number of women were practising successfully, a more 'mannish' stereotype emerged, wearing a plain skirt and masculine jacket. She was often the butt of the joke. From *Punch*, 14 September 1872, p.113

Why in the face of such resistance did women wish to become doctors at all? Until recently, many authors have argued that women pursued a medical career as a form of service and for altruistic reasons. Women doctors claimed to be serving the public (one of the features of a profession) by preserving the modesty of women patients and ending their suffering at the hands of male doctors who did not understand the female body. This idea of women being called to serve for the betterment of others is a common feature of many autobiographies written by pioneer women doctors and contemporary biographies. However, recent scholarship suggests that women may have constructed narratives of their lives in ways that would be acceptable to society.

> Given the obstacles that had to be faced, the fact that women doctors often told their stories in terms of having received a calling, or having been possessed by a mission is scarcely surprising. To have felt possessed by forces outside one's own control was probably easier than owning up to one's own driving ambition.

(Dyhouse, 1998, p.324)

Exercise

Read 'Motives for medical training' (Source Book 2, Reading 6.4). According to this account, what motivated Mary Murdoch to qualify as a doctor?

Discussion

This account suggests that Mary Murdoch (1864–1916) (Figure 6.3) was bored by the life of a 'lady of leisure' and did not want to waste her years in the 'small activities' of a country town. As the only daughter left at home, she cared for her mother until her death and was then left with the problem of how to support herself. With a small legacy and no husband she had to find a career. The family physician clearly had some influence. Thus her career choice might have resulted from changes in her family life and from a desire for freedom.

In the second passage, Murdoch is shown as offering herself to medicine in a way similar to that of a noviciate offering herself to God. Murdoch was a deeply religious woman, and her Catholicism seeps through the piece as she justifies her choice of career. Her medical career is presented as a life of self-sacrifice. While loving her chosen profession, Murdoch presents it as a life of service and devotion to the detriment of other pleasures, as medicine has taken away her liberty.

Murdoch's biography hints at the role played by male supporters in encouraging women in their chosen path. While women did face fierce opposition, mainly from elite practitioners who made up the staff of the largest medical schools and teaching hospitals, they also received help and advice from individual men. At Edinburgh, for example, Jex-Blake had invaluable support from two men. Alexander Russel was editor of the *Scotsman* newspaper and did much to publicize the unfair treatment meted out to the female medical students. David

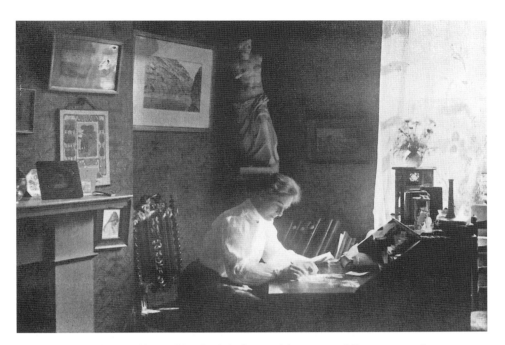

Figure 6.3   Portrait of Mary Murdoch in her writing room. Like many male contemporaries, Murdoch is portrayed without any sign of her occupation, but is shown as a woman of culture – note the paintings, statue and books. By permission of the British Library, shelfmark: 010855.cc.8

Masson was professor of English at Edinburgh University, and a strong supporter of education for women.

Having been denied access to established medical schools, some British women were determined to found their own training courses. This was quite possible in Britain where, as you read in the previous chapter, there were many private medical schools set up by practitioners. Opinion was divided on the matter among medical women. Garrett Anderson and Blackwell opposed the idea of a separate education for women, fearing that it would be regarded as inferior to that received by men. After she failed to graduate from Edinburgh, Jex-Blake moved to London in 1874 and began to plan a women's medical school. The London School of Medicine for Women (LSMW) was opened in October 1874 and received the support of some men, including the Earl of Shaftesbury, and some intellectual radicals, including lawyers (for example, William Shaen, who acted as solicitor to the school) and politicians (for example, James Stansfeld, who supported women's suffrage). The LSMW did not provide a way into medicine for all women: the founders limited admission to the very brightest and charged high fees of £200 per annum. Lectures were given by male and female doctors already in hospital posts and, from 1877, the female students were able to gain clinical experience at the Royal Free Hospital (Blake, 1990, p.186). While the LSMW offered opportunities for education to women when other routes to medicine were blocked, it did not provide the same springboard to a medical career as a 'male' education could do. Its staff did not belong to the medical elite and could not offer their graduates entry to junior posts in prestigious hospitals. Without support from distinguished hospital staff when seeking posts, many of the LSMW's students worked in lowly positions within the medical hierarchy – as medical missionaries for instance.

Until 1914, the number of women attending medical schools grew slowly (Figure 6.4). In Britain, even after the 1876 Enabling Act allowed medical examining boards to grant licences to women, universities could still legally exclude women from their medical schools. By 1881, there were only twenty-five women doctors in England and Wales – a total of 0.17 per cent of the profession. By 1911, there were 495 women on the register, comprising just under 2 per cent of the profession (Harrison, 1981, p.51). In Germany, there were only a total of 138 women physicians in the entire Reich by 1913. It was in Russia that female medical students were the most numerous. By the First World War more than 1,600 had qualified and were practising – more than the combined number of qualified women throughout the rest of Europe (Bonner, 1992, p.78).

The assumption that the First World War opened up medicine to new ideas and practices is explored in Chapter 12.

The First World War is often portrayed as a watershed for women, opening up many new employment opportunities. The war certainly gave medical schools an incentive to open their doors to women, as the number of male applicants fell and the call up of male doctors offered increased opportunities for women to practise on the home front. Some women were able to work close to the battlefield itself, in the Scottish Women's Hospitals (SWH). Funded through charitable donations, the SWH saw service under French command (the British Army refused the services of the women) on the western front and in Serbia. However, the idea that the war irrevocably improved the situation for women wishing to pursue a career in medicine is overstated.

Many medical schools persisted in their opposition to women, and, at the end of the war, limits were once again put in place.

> One by one the London teaching hospitals again closed their doors to female students. University and King's College Hospitals retained limited places, but otherwise the Royal Free was the only London hospital offering them clinical induction.
>
> (Leneman, 1994, p.176)

At St Mary's Hospital Medical School in London (which had supported the admission of women from 1916), male students and staff started to complain about the female students. The arguments reached a crisis point in April 1924, when ninety-six male students signed a petition for the removal of the female students (Garner, 1998, p.83). The hospital discussed the matter and decided that from 1925 no more women would be admitted. Although St Mary's chose to exclude women, in other medical schools the backlash against female students was dying away. The number of women studying in British medical schools increased during the late 1920s and 1930s. By 1931, there were 3,331 qualified women, accounting for about 10 per cent of the medical profession (Cherry, 1996, p.33). This was not the case throughout Europe, however. In Germany, for instance, the proportion of women in medical schools actually fell by 17 per cent between 1923 and 1928 (Bonner, 1992, pp.162–5).

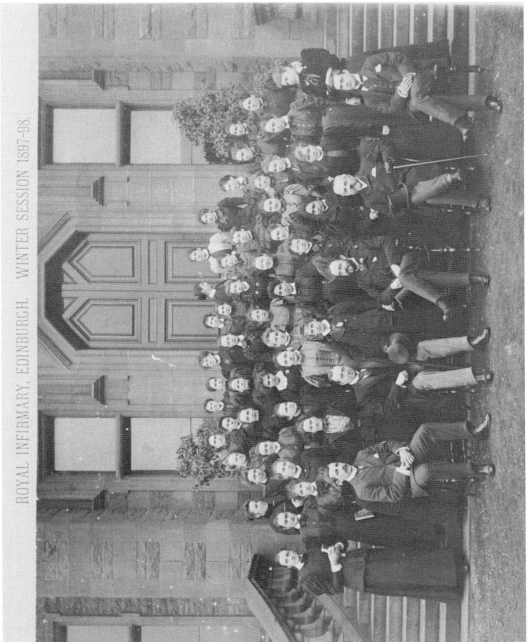

ROYAL INFIRMARY, EDINBURGH.   WINTER SESSION 1897-98.

Figure 6.4   Women medical students, Royal Infirmary, Edinburgh, 1897–8. Women students were finally admitted to Edinburgh University in 1892, but they were taught separately from the men. This group photograph was taken in front of the main door, exactly where the male classes were photographed. Note the all-male teaching staff seated in the front row. Lothian Health Services Archive/SCRAN

The inter-war period was also characterized by gains and setbacks in the career paths of individual women. Male practitioners were still able to push women into the margins of the profession – just as they had marginalized practitioners who practised unorthodox forms of medicine – by denying them access to research opportunities and prestigious posts. For some, such as Mary Walker (1888–1974), barriers remained to their career progression. Walker spent much of her career working in London Poor Law hospitals (regarded by most practitioners as a low-status post) despite a clear aptitude for research. Her doctoral thesis won the Edinburgh Gold Medal in 1937, but she did not take up the offered post at the Elizabeth Garrett Anderson Hospital to pursue research in neurology. Whether this was a consequence of male opposition, lack of desire or the impact of marriage and a family is unclear. Others, such as Letitia Fairfield (1885–1978), were able to have careers which mirrored those of their male colleagues. From an intellectual family (her sister was the novelist Rebecca West), Fairfield took a post with the London County Council in 1911, and eventually became its first female senior medical officer. She served in a medical capacity in both world wars and had interests in maternal, child and geriatric medicine (Hall, 1994, pp.194–5).

Women's access to the medical profession was thus fraught with difficulties, which even by the 1920s were not completely removed. As Porter has noted, women faced two obstacles to entry into the medical profession: first, medicine was a 'chummy male monopoly' (1999, p.356) and second, it required a university education which was largely denied to women. Biological arguments about women's suitability for medical work were utilized in specific ways to maintain and protect existing professional structures and to prevent equal access and progression for women well into the inter-war years.

6.4   Caring not curing: the role of the nurse and nursing reform

In the middle of the nineteenth century, the situation for nurses was very different from the experience of women doctors. Large numbers of women were engaged in nursing, but the personnel, their organization and even their place of work were a far cry from the highly trained, professionally regulated and hospital-based nurse of today. Nursing was carried out by women from a wide range of social backgrounds, from those caring for their own children, to inmates of the workhouse system nursing fellow paupers, to elite 'sisters' in charge of wards in large hospitals. While the latter group were distinguished by their experience, most nurses had little training.

Exercise

Read 'Nurses and servants' (Source Book 2, Reading 6.6). How can we distinguish between nurses and servants in the early nineteenth century?

In the early nineteenth century, it was very difficult to distinguish nurses from other serving occupations. Although some women specialized in nursing work, as private nurses or in hospitals, many drifted into nursing by chance. Others, such as the pauper nurses, were forced into nursing by circumstances. No specialist training or knowledge was required as nursing consisted of basic care – cleaning the sickroom or ward and looking after the comfort of patients. Judging by advertisements, nurses in hospitals were distinguished by their good character, and private nurses by an acute sense of their ambivalent social position, somewhere above ordinary servants, but firmly subservient to their employers' families.

This association of nursing with domestic work and the lack of formal education required of nurses gave the occupation a poor and gendered image. Nurses were not regarded as specialists in medicine but rather as a workforce engaged in caring, under the direction of an employer, doctor or the administrator of some institution.

How then did nursing develop into a profession? It is not a straightforward story, and has at least three distinct phases. First, nursing was split off from domestic care and became a respectable occupation for middle-class and poorer women. Second, and occurring at about the same time, nurses began to develop a recognized body of skills, taught in nursing schools. In the final phase, a system of registration was created which established common standards of training for all qualified nurses.

Florence Nightingale and nursing reform

Nursing reform is firmly associated with the work of Florence Nightingale (Figure 6.5). She has become an icon of British history and is one of the few women who has been celebrated on a banknote. The following extract is typical of past writing on Nightingale's legacy:

> It was not until the great Florence Nightingale returned in glory from the Crimean War, in the year 1855, that steps were taken to train nurses systematically for a period of years, after which they could work independently as professional nurses. Money publicly subscribed to Florence Nightingale for her wonderful work in the Crimean War was used by her to found the Nightingale School for Nurses at St Thomas's Hospital. These Nightingale nurses went to the ends of the earth founding nurse-training schools, after the pattern of their alma mater in London.
>
> (Hardy, 1955, p.18)

Just as the heroic accounts of pioneering women doctors have been revised by historians, Nightingale's work has also come under critical scrutiny in the last two decades. Whereas once she was revered for single-handedly bringing down mortality rates in the army hospitals in the Crimea and for reforming nurse training, her work is now seen as more significant in that it made nursing a

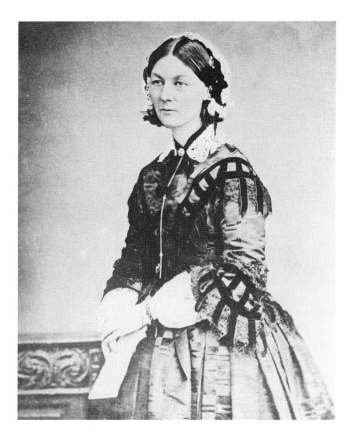

Figure 6.5   Portrait of Florence Nightingale, 1856. Nightingale is shown here in a highly conventional pose, not smiling or looking at the camera, against a rather neutral background. The paper in her hand hints at her intellectual abilities – and she was a prolific letter-writer. Compare this conventional picture with the heroic image of Nightingale in Plate 13. Wellcome Library, London

respectable occupation – a crucial element in making the occupation into a profession. The work was opened up to upper-middle-class women, whose middle-class morals and norms of behaviour were then imposed on working-class nurses and patients. Drinking, swearing, gambling and 'wandering about' were not acceptable on the strictly regulated Nightingale ward. This reinforced earlier efforts to control the behaviour of hospital patients through strict rules – which you read about in Chapter 2.

Nightingale's influence in reforming training for nurses has also been questioned. Until the 1980s, she was regarded by historians as the architect of modern nursing. Through the foundation of the Nightingale School for Nurses at St Thomas's Hospital, she was said to have created a body of institutionally trained, regimented and competent carers who brought new ideas of sanitation and health to the care of the sick. Nightingale argued that nursing had to be learnt and carefully mastered and could not be left to the untrained and ignorant. Nursing knowledge did not arrive 'by inspiration to the lady disappointed in love, nor to the poor workhouse drudge hard up for a livelihood' (Nightingale, [1860] 1969, p.134). Unlike earlier nurses, who picked up their skills informally, nurses at St Thomas's went through a structured programme of training, spending time as a trainee before qualifying as a nurse.

However, a close study of the training at St Thomas's shows that its reputation for novelty represented a triumph of public relations, rather than a root and branch reform of nurse education. That said, there were some novel and important elements in the St Thomas's training. First, nurses learned an unquestioning obedience to a hierarchy: trainee nurses (called probationers) answered to ordinary nurses who answered to sisters and matrons who held authority over the work on the wards (Figure 6.6). Second, nurses were responsible for high levels of hygiene on the ward and were taught that cleanliness was crucial to the recovery of the sick. In part, this was achieved by hospital design (discussed in Chapter 2) as well as the work of nurses. However, while this new emphasis on hygiene in theory separated nursing from the work of domestic servants, in reality the content of work for rank-and-file nurses changed little.

Despite Nightingale's stated dislike of nurses 'picking up' skills in the ward or sickroom, the method of acquiring nursing skills at St Thomas's was little different from earlier times. The diaries of trainee nurses illustrate the continued reliance

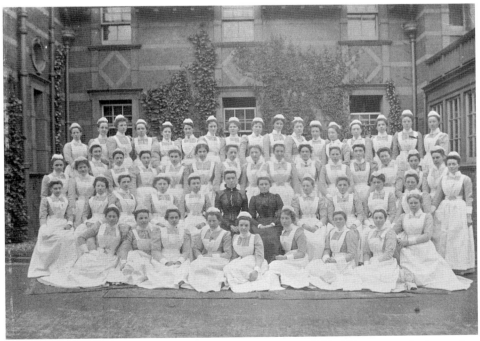

Figure 6.6   Night nurses, Royal Infirmary, Edinburgh, 1900. This group photograph exemplifies the order and discipline of nursing. All the staff are dressed in exactly the same uniform, apron and cap, except for the matrons (or superintendents, as they were known at this time). They wear darker dresses and no apron, because they were administrators and did not work on the wards. Lothian Health Services Archive/SCRAN

on practical experience over academic teaching. At St Thomas's, the duties of student nurses included preparing food, making beds and attending to the comfort of patients. They also performed some medical tasks but these were designed to train nurses to assist doctors, not to be independent of them. It appears that during their period of training, nurses primarily were expected to work on the ward, without instruction, and to pick up the traditional elements of nursing work from others. Rebecca Strong (1843–1920), who trained at St Thomas's in 1867, recalled:

> Very little was expected from us, as progress was slow in regard to organised teaching. Kindness, watchfulness, cleanliness, and guarding against bed sores were well ingrained. A few stray lectures were given ... There was a dummy on which to practise bandaging, and some lessons were given, also a skeleton, and some ancient medical books, one, fortunately, on Anatomy for those who attempted self-education.
>
> (quoted in Summers, 1988, p.93)

Initially, Nightingale nurses received little formal medical teaching, given Florence Nightingale's strong disapproval of such training for nurses.

Read 'Florence Nightingale on nurse training' (Source Book 2, Reading 6.7).

1   Why did Florence Nightingale disapprove of medical training for nurses? Did other nurse trainers share her views?

2   What effect do you think that Nightingale's insistence that nurses did not need to be trained in medicine have on the status of the occupation?

1   Nightingale saw cleanliness – not medical treatment – as the most important means of recovering health. It was the nurses' responsibility to control the environment of the ward or sickroom. Medical knowledge – such as the role of bacteria in spreading disease – was simply irrelevant to the nurses' work. Educated women involved in training nurses at the time appeared to be more receptive to the idea of a 'medical model' and were more willing to introduce lectures on medicine into nursing training.

2   Nightingale's insistence that cleanliness was a crucial aspect of nursing and that practical skills and a good character were the essential qualifications for a nurse reinforced the traditional connection between nursing and domestic work. It supported the idea that nursing was not an intellectual occupation that required technical knowledge.

However, limited medical teaching did become a standard part of the training of Nightingale nurses. The quality of this teaching differed between schools and over time. At St Thomas's, lectures were given by visiting medical practitioners and by matrons. However, they were not strictly timetabled: the busy matron had little time to give lectures and the probationer had little time to attend them. It also proved difficult to teach groups of women with varying abilities and from different educational backgrounds. Overall, Nightingale training reinforced the idea that caring was more important than specialist knowledge, and that nursing skills could be learnt by good example and experience. Student nurses were offered a practical training in return for their labour. Not surprisingly, the scheme proved very beneficial to hospitals. At a time when hospitals were increasingly involved in caring for the acutely ill, often through surgical treatment, senior staff began to press for the numbers of probationers to be increased.

But did this training improve standards of nursing? The following entry in the diary of Mrs Deeble, a qualified Nightingale nurse, is evidence that training at St Thomas's was no guarantee of a nurse's competence.

> Sister L was asked to take the temperature of a patient and she replied that she did not know how ... Sister Clarke made a sad mistake in the application of leeches to the eye of a patient. She applied one so close to the inside of the eye as to cause haemorrhage [sic] ... The Ward Orderly remarked to Sister Lennox next morning that if Sister C. had used the Eye-glass such a thing could not have happened. The glasses are always used here but Sister C. had never seen them.
>
> (quoted in Summers, 1988, p.93)

It seems that despite St Thomas's reputation for training nurses to a high standard, the busy hospital environment and the mixed abilities of the probationers meant that this did not always happen. However, Nightingale nurses did become skilled in controlling the moral and physical environment of the wards and in organizing the work of the nursing staff.

This emphasis on practical skills rather than medical knowledge at St Thomas's, reflected Nightingale's vision of a strict division of labour between doctors and nurses. She did not wish for nurses to be of equal status with doctors; indeed, she was clear that their roles should not overlap. Her model nurse was a competent assistant to the doctor. She had a specific and important role in carefully observing the condition of the patients, caring for their needs and controlling the environment of the ward or sickroom. But nurses did not challenge a doctor's authority or usurp their role in determining treatment: 'to cultivate ... observation and experience in women ... is just the way to do away with amateur physicking, and if the doctors but know it, to make the nurses obedient to them' (Nightingale, 1969, p.132).

Unlike those women who wished to become doctors, there appeared to be nothing here to worry the medical profession. Nightingale's vision for the role of the nurse closely matched contemporary notions of the nurturing qualities inherent to women. But in fact there was some opposition to the introduction of Nightingale nurses into voluntary hospitals. Doctors regarded this new internal hierarchy of matrons and nurses as a threat to their own status. At Guy's Hospital, for example, the medical staff was opposed to the matron controlling nurse rotas and work schedules, and a bitter dispute raged through 1879 and 1880 (Waddington, 1995, pp.211–30). However, in broad terms, matrons appear to have been successful in establishing for themselves an important role in the hospital hierarchy – as support for medical staff and as disciplinarians of nursing staff.

Historians have also reassessed Nightingale's contribution to raising the status of nursing as a profession, and have concluded that she was less forward-thinking than historians had previously believed. She argued for improvements in the status of nursing, but was careful to highlight the nurse's caring role rather than her medical expertise. This image persisted in photographs of nurses into the twentieth century (Figure 6.7). For Nightingale, nursing was firmly linked to vocation and service. She was not a feminist campaigner. Nightingale did not see why a woman should be limited in her role, but did not support the idea of equality. Instead, she argued that women should rise above the contemporary discussions about women's access to a medical education and equal citizenship to 'bring the best she has, whatever that is, to the work of God's world' (Nightingale, 1969, p.135).

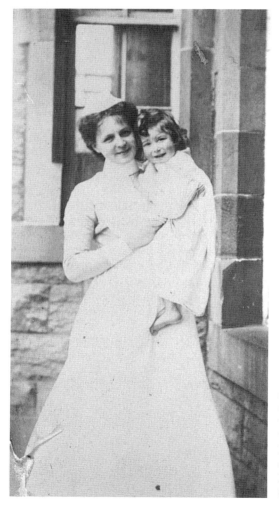

Figure 6.7   Nurse Playfair and patient outside Corstorphine Convalescent Home, Edinburgh, c.1900. Photographs like this one – of nurses with babies or small children – are common in the late nineteenth and early twentieth centuries, showing the continuing importance of caring and nurturing as characteristics of the ideal nurse. Such images are far more common than those that show nurses actually treating patients (except during the First World War, when nurses acquired a new heroic status). Lothian Health Services Archive/ SCRAN

Nor did the Nightingale School for Nurses at St Thomas's help to create a homogenous occupational group. Rather than encouraging professional unity, the hierarchy of matron, sister and probationer reinforced social differences between groups of nurses. Middle-class girls, who entered as 'lady probationers', were groomed to be future matrons, while it was hard for the working-class recruit to rise through the ranks. 'Those who entered as special probationers at voluntary hospitals, especially in London, had the greatest advantage, with the Poor Law trained nurse achieving the least advantage' (Brooks, 2001, p.20). Campaigners such as Nightingale were convinced that exclusionary tactics – where nursing work was portrayed as suitable for a particular type of woman – would improve its status. Others of a more feminist persuasion also campaigned for nursing reform, viewing the work as one way for the educated, middle-class young woman to earn a respectable living. The result was that opportunities were available to a range of women, from those with limited education, but of good character and not afraid of hard work, to middle-class women looking for a career. These ideas helped to ensure that nursing remained a predominantly female occupation to the present day. In 1901, there were 64,209 female nurses which represented 93 per cent of the workforce. In 1921, women still accounted for 90 per cent of nurses (Cherry, 1996, p.35).

Just as historians of medicine have sought to explore the wider social context of early women doctors, historians of nursing have looked beyond Nightingale to find other influences on the development of the occupation. Recent scholarship has revealed how religion shaped the role and status of nurses in a similar way to Nightingale's reforms. In Catholic countries, such as Italy and France, nursing had always been provided through religious orders. And in Protestant countries, the evangelical movement of the late nineteenth century led to the creation of new orders of nursing sisters, who worked in hospitals and in the homes of the poor and lent a new meaning to the work of nurses. Like Nightingale, these nursing orders saw the nurse's role as including the exertion of a moral influence over her patients. Similarly, the philanthropists who employed nurses to care for the poor expected them to deal not only with the physical condition of their sick patients, but also with their moral and spiritual well-being. Nurse-visiting schemes, which were often associated with a religious mission, would only employ women of suitable moral character and Christian tendency (Summers, 1979).

This emphasis on the moral nature of the work and its capacity to reform individuals lifted the nurse from domestic drudge to Christian reformer. Thus, nursing became a more attractive career for women from a wider section of society. As Martha Vicinus has commented:

> A life of hard work under difficult conditions was transformed ideologically into fighting for spiritual regeneration among the poor patients and respect for the educated working women among the doctors and the general public. Power, self-fulfilment, and moral duty could all be satisfied by serving the sick.

(Vicinus, 1985, p.87)

Such lofty aspirations fitted neatly with the ideal of womanhood. Many women involved in home visiting 'were ardent Christians who espoused deeply conservative political principles; and many were, indeed, explicitly anti-feminist' (Summers, 1979, p.59).

The rise of the hospital-trained nurse

In Chapter 2, the changing function of hospitals in the nineteenth century is discussed in detail.

Nightingale nurses were closely allied to hospitals. The school at St Thomas's provided a model, and soon every large hospital had its own nurse training school. The hospitals benefited from the free labour of trainee nurses. The greater numbers of trained nurses, working within a strict hierarchy, was intimately linked to the changing function of hospitals – from places of care for the sick poor to centres of high-tech, specialized medical care. The closer association of nurses with hospitals not only brought about changes in the way nurses carried out their jobs, but also fostered the idea that nurses possessed specialist skills and knowledge. This idea was a crucial step towards the claiming of professional status for nursing (you have already seen how a similar process occurred in the development of surgery as a prestigious area of medicine). Doctors gradually came to accept that by carefully observing patients and monitoring their symptoms, nurses could assist practitioners without interfering with their control over the patient's treatment. This was, of course, more easily organized in the institutional setting of the hospital than in the home, where nurses had greater autonomy over the care of their patients. Nurses in the late Victorian period did not see their job as medical, but they had created their own sphere of influence – the sickroom or ward – and had, by the 1880s, clearly established their authority therein (Figure 6.8). By the end of the nineteenth century, nurse education began to incorporate more theoretical and medical training. And the syllabus increasingly was influenced by doctors. In Britain, for example, doctors were often involved in the design of courses, which varied between institutions. In this way, doctors were 'inculcating nurses with the rationalist ethos and values of scientific medicine, thus facilitating compliance with medical orders' (Rafferty, 1996, p.12).

At the same time, the status of nursing was also changing. The inroads made by middle-class women into nursing during the nineteenth century had transformed nursing from working-class domestic service to a respectable occupation. With its religious and moral overtones, and with training now located in the civilized environment of the hospital, nursing could be presented as suitable work for a wider constituency of women. The low pay and closed community of the nurses' home (regarded as a morally protected environment by virtue of its being strictly regulated and women only) made it possible to argue that nursing was a respectable vocation rather than simply a job, with opportunities for career development through the nursing hierarchy.

The First World War, nurse registration and professionalization

A profession is often defined as a skilled occupation that requires specialist training and the application of specialist knowledge usually in the service of others. If we use this definition, then nursing had developed a degree of professionalism prior to the First World War. Standards of nurse training were

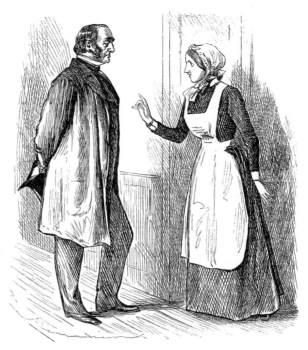

Figure 6.8   The caption to this cartoon, entitled *Laborare Est Orare* [To Work is to Pray], reads: 'Senior Surgeon: "I wish particularly to see Case No. 36 in your ward before I leave. I fear the symptoms are not so favourable—"; Nurse: "You cannot enter now, Sir George. We are just going to have *Evensong!*"' While poking fun at the nurse's excessive solicitousness for her authority, this cartoon neatly captures the way nurses had acquired control over wards, especially with regard to their routines and organization. It also accurately portrays the moral influence of the nursing staff – on many wards the day did end with the singing of a hymn. From *Punch*, 18 December 1880, p.228

rising, with some medical knowledge required in addition to practical skills (Figure 6.9). Access to that training was regulated by the entry requirements for nurse training schools. The status of nursing was also rising, and nurses were developing their own specialist knowledge of patient care. While their knowledge was regarded as inferior to that of medical practitioners, nurses were establishing for themselves an area of expertise as carers, moral guardians and experts in the order of the sickroom (Dingwall *et al.*, 1988; Maggs, 1980; Vicinus, 1985, pp.101–20).

For many historians, it was the experience of nurses in the First World War that raised the status of their occupation into that of a profession. In Britain, for example, traditional accounts of the development of the modern profession have tended to argue that the First World War gave new impetus to a campaign for professionalization which had begun in the 1880s. As the demand for trained nurses grew, and public admiration for their work increased, more and more nurses pressed for their occupation to be acknowledged as a profession. In this interpretation, nurse registration, which was introduced in Britain in 1919, was, like the vote, offered in recognition of women's wartime role.

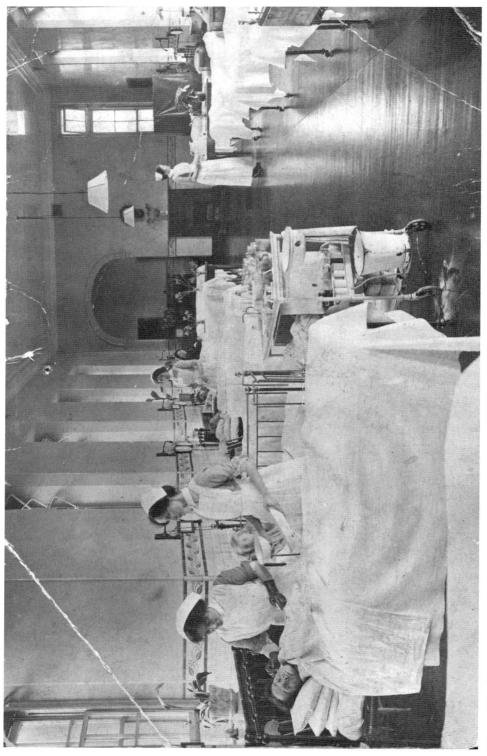

Figure 6.9 Nurses on a ward, Leith Hospital, Edinburgh, 1917. This image encapsulates the order and cleanliness of the hospital ward, with its rows of beds and polished floor. This picture is unusual in that it does not show the medical staff, only the nurses, some of whom are tending to a patient. The trolley of dressings and bottles is visual evidence of how the role of nurses had expanded from providing care to undertaking medical treatment. By courtesy of the Trustees of the National Museums of Scotland/SCRAN

While there is no doubt that nursing on the battlefield and on the home front was dangerous and arduous, historians have questioned whether women's wartime activities really resulted in long-term changes to their position in society. Indeed, in her study of British military nurses, Anne Summers has concluded that nurses were not powerful nor was their leadership radical. She concludes that: 'the war had shown how easily the state could override the nurses' criteria of professionalism, by "diluting" hospital staffs with barely trained **VADs** [Voluntary Aid Detachment nurses]' (Summers, 1988, pp.253–70).

After 1918, a boundary of expertise was drawn around nursing by the introduction of nurse registration. It defined a particular body of knowledge as essential to the qualified nurse and identified those nurses who had been trained in that knowledge. During the 1880s, nurses began to see registration as the best way to regulate the nursing profession. Nurse leaders argued that nurses themselves should organize a system of registration which, like medical licences, would guarantee a common minimum standard of nursing knowledge and practice throughout the country. However, the association of nursing with 'women's work' and the nineteenth-century restructuring of nursing made this process neither straightforward nor inevitable.

The campaign for nurse registration in Britain began in 1888 with the foundation of the British Nurses Association, which was created specifically to lobby for the legal status of profession for nursing. The campaign ended with the passing of the Nurses Registration Act in 1919, which offered a legislative framework for registration and regulation. This episode has tended to dominate in nursing history, being seen as the key moment in time when nursing became a profession (Abel-Smith, 1979, pp.81–113). However, the campaign for registration also demonstrates the limits to the power of nurses as an occupational group. Demands for registration were interpreted as a challenge by nurses to the power of the hospitals. In Britain, hospitals were important not only in selecting and training recruits, but in finding employment for nurses. Essentially they acted as agencies for nursing labour, offering positions in domiciliary settings as well as being large employers in their own right. Hospital administrators resisted registration fearing that the longer training period suggested by reformers would exacerbate an existing shortage of trained nurses. And, more importantly, they also feared such measures would undermine the power of hospitals as employers by placing some control of nursing labour in the hands of nurses themselves. The hospitals were a powerful lobby group and effectively halted legislation until 1919. Many doctors, while accepting that nurses had some specialist sphere of influence, saw nurse registration as a challenge to their own authority and practice. However, the medical profession is a complex entity and not all practitioners thought alike on this matter, as on many others. Specialists in the royal colleges felt less ambivalent to the proposed reforms than GPs. It is possible that GPs may have regarded better-trained nurses as competitors in the medical marketplace. The interests of the state also influenced the timing of the Nurses Registration Act. The Act fitted into the wider agenda of the post-war Liberal government, which sought to expand health and welfare services as part of the post-war reconstruction (Rafferty, 1996, p.95). Additional trained nurses were needed to staff these new services.

A superficial examination of the campaign for registration would see it as a lengthy but ultimately successful process. In 1919, the Nurses Registration Act was passed and the General Nursing Council (GNC) was established to oversee the registration process and to regulate nursing, just as the GMC controlled doctors. Dominated by nurses, the GNC was apparently the institution which finally transformed nursing into a fully fledged, self-governing profession. However, more detailed scrutiny reveals that the Act itself was a piece of political compromise. It served the needs of hospitals and doctors by leaving the issues of pay, conditions and content of nurse training in their hands with final power resting with the state (Witz, 1995, p.166). The GNC was responsible for the registration of nurses, the approval of training schools and devising a model training syllabus, but its powers were severely limited by internal strife, administrative difficulties and political weakness. Criteria for admission to the Register (which was opened in 1921) were low – one year's formal training, or three years' practice prior to 1919, but, even so, many nurses were reluctant to put themselves forward for admission, which cost a guinea. The council's syllabus of training was not compulsory and it was not until 1925 that the first nurses taking state examinations were admitted to the Register. As Dingwall *et al.* have noted, the GNC was, ultimately, weak and thus its influence in raising the status of nursing as a profession was limited. Its rulings could be (and were) overturned by the newly created Ministry of Health (Dingwall *et al.*, 1988, p.88).

In the final analysis, the campaign for registration did little to enhance the position of nurses within the hierarchy of medical health-care professionals. Instead, registration provides an illustration of just how powerless nurses were against the requirements of the state, the hospitals and GPs. The campaign offers a way to understand how nursing retained its low status within the hierarchy of medical health-care professions. Despite the efforts of personalities, it was the wider context of politics, reform and professional self-interest which shaped nursing into the twentieth century.

> The passage of the Nurses Registration Act in 1919 did not represent a victory for pro-registrationist nurses. The nursing profession had not come to power. Instead nurses were henceforth to be tightly constrained within a state–profession relation within which they were the weaker partner, as well as within the employment relation between hospitals and nurses and the inter-professional relation between doctors and nurses.
> (Witz, 1995, p.165)

6.5   Conclusion

In this chapter, I argue that women found it easier to make a career in nursing than in medical practice because of the way in which these occupations (and the role of women) were constructed in the nineteenth century. Essentially, medical practice, with its emphasis on intervention and cure, was considered a male occupation, and unsuitable for women. It was argued that women were not capable of the intellectual effort required to qualify as medical practitioners. Reasons for excluding women were not simply based on physiological arguments; serious, virulent and sometimes violent professional objections were also raised. This period was one of great change for the medical profession and different groupings of medical men were keen to establish and protect their range of influence. Women's entry to the profession was regarded as unnecessary competition as well as immoral and inherently wrong. In some respects, little had changed by the end of the First World War. While more women had gained a medical degree, barriers to their career remained in place. However, women were not passive victims of patriarchy and the power of the medical profession. Indeed, feminist campaigns met with some success, and some middle-class, unmarried women began to be viewed as capable of an intellectual working life. In the inter-war years, more women qualified to practise medicine, but their numbers remained small in comparison with men and their career paths were often different from those of their male counterparts.

Throughout the period, the fundamental notion that nursing was women's work was not in dispute. Women found it easier to establish a career in nursing because it looked to their supposed natural abilities and talents rather than to the intellectualism required for a medical training. This meant that women were able to establish the occupation as their own. The consequence of this, however, was that nursing continued to be regarded as inferior to medical practice. In Britain, nurses did achieve their goal of professionalization, and improved their status in society. But the process did not necessarily improve their position in relation to the medical profession or to the state, which ultimately remained more powerful in reshaping their profession.

References

Abel-Smith, B. (1979) *A History of the Nursing Profession*, London: Heinemann.

Anderson, B.S. and Zinsser, J.P. (1988) *A History of their Own: Women in Europe from Prehistory to the Present*, vol.2, London: Penguin.

Blake, C. (1990) *The Charge of the Parasols: Women's Entry to the Medical Profession*, London: The Women's Press.

Bland, L. (1995) *Banishing the Beast: English Feminism and Sexual Morality, 1885–1914*, London: Penguin.

Bonner, T.N. (1992) *To the Ends of the Earth: Women's Search for Education in Medicine*, Cambridge, Mass.: Harvard University Press.

Brooks, J. (2001) 'Structured by class, bounded by gender: nursing and special probationer schemes, 1860–1939', *International History of Nursing Journal*, vol.6, no.2, pp.13–21.

Cherry, S. (1996) *Medical Services and the Hospitals in Britain, 1860–1939*, Cambridge: Cambridge University Press.

Dingwall, R., Rafferty, A.M. and Webster, C. (1988) *An Introduction to the Social History of Nursing*, London: Routledge.

Dyhouse, C. (1995) *No Distinction of Sex? Women in British Universities, 1870–1939*, London: UCL Press.

Dyhouse, C. (1998) 'Driving ambitions: women in pursuit of a medical education, 1890–1939', *Women's History Review*, vol.7, no.3, pp.321–44.

Garner, J.S. (1998) 'The great experiment: the admission of women students to St Mary's Hospital medical school, 1916–1925', *Medical History*, vol.42, pp.68–88.

Hall, L.A. (1994) 'Chloe, Olivia, Isabel, Letitia, Harriette, Honor and many more: women in medicine and biomedical science, 1914–1945' in S. Oldfield (ed.) *This Working Day World: Women's Lives and Culture(s) in Britain, 1914–1945*, London: Taylor & Francis, pp.192–202.

Hardy, G.M. (1955) *Nursing as a Career and Livelihood*, London: Edward O. Beck.

Harrison, B. (1981) 'Women's health and the women's movement in Britain, 1840–1940' in C. Webster (ed.) *Biology, Medicine and Society, 1840–1940*, Cambridge: Cambridge University Press, pp.15–72.

Leneman, L. (1994) 'Medical women at war, 1914–1918', *Medical History*, vol.38, pp.160–77.

Maggs, C. (1980) 'Nurse recruitment in four provincial hospitals, 1881–1921' in C. Davies (ed.) *Rewriting Nursing History*, London: Croom Helm, pp.18–40.

Nightingale, F. [1860] (1969) *Notes on Nursing: What It Is, and What It Is Not*, New York: Dover Publications.

Porter, R. (1999) *The Greatest Benefit to Mankind: A Medical History of Humanity from Antiquity to the Present*, London: Fontana.

Rafferty, A.M. (1996) *The Politics of Nursing Knowledge*, London: Routledge.

Summers, A. (1979) 'A home from home – women's philanthropic work in the nineteenth century' in S. Burman (ed.) *Fit Work for Women*, London: Croom Helm, pp.33–63.

Summers, A. (1988) *Angels and Citizens: British Women as Military Nurses, 1854–1914*, London: Routledge & Kegan Paul.

Vertinsky, P. (1990) *The Eternally Wounded Woman*, Manchester: Manchester University Press.

Vicinus, M. (1985) *Independent Women: Work and Community for Single Women, 1850–1920*, London: Virago.

Waddington, K. (1995) 'The nursing dispute at Guy's Hospital, 1879–1880', *Social History of Medicine*, vol.8, pp.211–30.

Witz, A. (1995) *Professions and Patriarchy*, London: Routledge.

Source Book readings

M. Ryan [1841] *A Manual of Midwifery* in P. Jalland and J. Hooper (eds) *Women from Birth to Death: The Female Life Cycle in Britain, 1830–1914*, Atlantic Highlands: Humanities Press International, 1986, pp.20–1 (Reading 6.1).

Editorial, *Lancet*, 17 August 1878, vol.2, pp.226–7 (Reading 6.2).

M. Forster, *Significant Sisters: The Grassroots of Active Feminism, 1839–1939*, London: Penguin, 1984, pp.70–4 (Reading 6.3).

H. Malleson, *A Woman Doctor: Mary Murdoch of Hull*, London: Sidgwick & Jackson, 1919, pp.16–17, 36–7 (Reading 6.4).

Editorial, *Lancet*, 1873, vol.2, pp.159–60 (Reading 6.5).

R. Dingwall, A.M. Rafferty and C. Webster, *An Introduction to the Social History of Nursing*, London: Routledge, 1998, pp.9–18 (Reading 6.6).

M.E. Baly, *Florence Nightingale and the Nursing Legacy*, London: Croom Helm, 1986, pp.23–5 (Reading 6.7).

7

Dealing with Disease in Populations
Public Health, 1830–1880

—————————— *Deborah Brunton* ——————————

Objectives

When you have completed this chapter you should be able to:

- understand how social, geographical and economic factors shaped nineteenth-century public health practice;

- explain how interpretations of the history of public health have shifted over time;

- interpret simple tables of mortality.

7.1   Introduction

The late nineteenth century is usually seen as the great age of public health. Populations were frequently attacked by epidemics of fevers, smallpox and cholera, especially in the new and rapidly growing cities. Tuberculosis and childhood diseases, such as measles, scarlet fever and diphtheria, were rife. In Britain, death rates were around twenty-two per thousand people per year. Life expectancy (the average lifespan) was just 40 years for men and 42 years for women, but substantially less in cities like Manchester. The average lifespan was reduced by high infant mortality – 16 per cent of infants did not survive until their first birthday. By 1900, life chances had improved substantially. While infants and children continued to suffer from high **mortality rates**, deaths from smallpox and fevers had been checked and cholera eradicated from western Europe. Life expectancy had risen – to 44 years for men and 47 years for women (Smith, 1979, pp.195–7; Wohl, 1983, p.329). With the important exception of **vaccination** against smallpox, this success was not based on any new techniques to prevent disease. Rather, it was achieved through massive programmes of sanitary reform, by the isolation of infected persons and the disinfection of goods and property.

It is not surprising, then, that successive generations of historians of medicine have studied the history of public health in the nineteenth century. But our understanding of this aspect of medical history has changed radically during the last fifty years. From the 1950s, historians portrayed public health reform as a response to the 'intolerable' levels of disease that resulted from rapid urbanization and industrialization. Much of their work focused on Britain, the first industrial nation, whose public health reforms were assumed to have set the pattern for countries in mainland Europe. Public health history was fitted into a broader story of medical progress – from inadequate to 'modern' ideas of disease causation and from dirt and disease to cleanliness and health. Historians analysed the work of the government administrators responsible for drawing up legislation (thus giving public health history a reputation for being dull), and of the medical men who developed the germ theory, the idea that diseases were caused by specific bacteria.

From the late 1980s, historians of medicine began to challenge many aspects of this account. They showed that governments had been concerned with public health well before the nineteenth century, and that the policies and practices adopted then had a long history. Far from being a simple story of progress, public health practices were controversial and were hindered by a wide range of problems. International comparisons of public health across Europe have shown how reforms in each country were shaped by unique combinations of factors. And detailed research has identified local not central government as the key player in implementing health reform. Recent research has also revealed new facets of public health history. The public, once seen as a monolithic and silent recipient of 'public health', are now known to have held widely differing views on sanitary reform. And historians have shown that sanitary reform did not just consist of huge government-funded infrastructure projects, but also of educational programmes, targeted at the domestic environment and delivered by voluntary agencies.

This new approach owes much to the input of a range of scholars from different academic disciplines. Historians of medicine sometimes boast of the openness of their field to methods and approaches associated with other disciplines, and public health history has proved to be a fertile area for the exchange of ideas. Historical demographers have brought their specialist skills and techniques to bear on nineteenth-century disease statistics, rigorously examining the impact of public health reform. Historians have alerted medical historians to the class dimension of public health and to the importance of local studies in understanding the variation in public health practices.

This chapter presents a history of European public health. But rather than trace its chronological development, I look in turn at the four main aspects of public health: understandings of mortality; theories of disease causation; public health practices; and debates on the impact of public health reform. I also explore the historiography of the subject, showing how historians' understanding of public health in the nineteenth century has changed during the last forty years. We begin by looking at an early account of nineteenth-century public health by historian of medicine Erwin Ackerknecht. This account provides a reference against which we can compare later research.

Exercise

Read 'An early account of public health history' (Source Book 2, Reading 7.1).

1   Which aspects of public health history does Ackerknecht deal with in detail?

2   Are some aspects of public health history neglected in his account?

1   Ackerknecht deals in some detail with the understanding of mortality and with theories of disease causation. He outlines the diseases that caused high levels of mortality in Europe in the early nineteenth century. His work emphasizes the role of 'great men' and of political ideas in shaping public health policy. He identifies some of the men responsible for analysing mortality, such as Edwin Chadwick (1801–90) and William Farr (1807–83). He discusses developments in theories of disease causation, from the 'erroneous filth theory', which claimed that epidemic disease arose from **miasmas**, to an understanding that certain diseases were carried in water and, finally, to the 'correct' theory that bacteria caused disease.

2   Ackerknecht pays relatively little attention to public health practice. He lists the targets of reform and claims that public health measures were effective in combating disease without producing any evidence to prove his point. He also pays a lot of attention to public health in England and says little about public health practices elsewhere in Europe.

7.2   Understanding patterns of mortality

Ackerknecht claims that it was in part the high levels of mortality, revealed by government investigators such as Chadwick and Farr, that prompted action on public health in the nineteenth century. Industrialization and urbanization were certainly associated with increasing rates of mortality and declining life expectancy. Death rates were particularly high in Britain, where industrial development was very rapid. However, more recent work by historians of medicine and social historians has shown that the analysis of disease and mortality has a much longer history and was motivated by developments in political economy and social science.

Data on deaths had been regularly collected from the late sixteenth century. City authorities published bills of mortality recording the number of deaths from different causes within their community (Figure 7.1). From the seventeenth century, these bills were analysed by political economists. In 1662, for example, John Graunt (1620–74) published *Natural and Political Observations ... made upon the Bills of Mortality*, which compared the death rates of different age groups and the deaths from different types of diseases in London. The eighteenth century saw an outpouring of such analyses of mortality in particular communities. Writers in Britain, Holland, Spain, France and the Italian and German states tried to explain variations in mortality by correlating deaths to environmental factors, such as rainfall, wind velocity, temperature and atmospheric pressure. However, as study after study failed to uncover the crucial factor linking disease and the environment, interest in the project began to wane (D. Porter, 1999, pp.49–51).

In the nineteenth century, data on disease and death were collected much more systematically. From the end of the eighteenth century, governments began to collect data on their populations in order to better understand how to regulate and

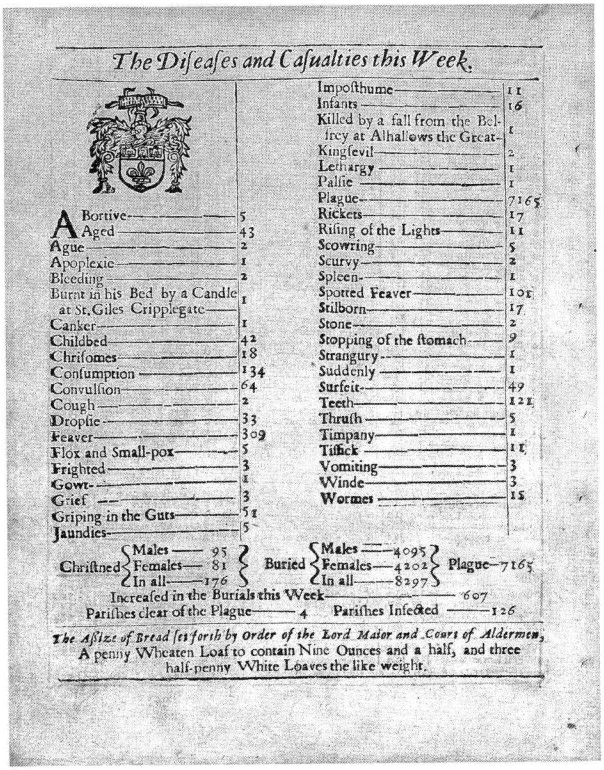

The Diſeaſes and Caſualties this Week.

Abortive	5	Impoſthume	11
Aged	43	Infants	16
Ague	2	Killed by a fall from the Belfrey at Alhallows the Great	1
Apoplexie	1	Kingſevil	2
Bleeding	2	Lethargy	1
Burnt in his Bed by a Candle at St. Giles Cripplegate	1	Palſie	1
Canker	1	Plague	7165
Childbed	42	Rickets	17
Chriſomes	18	Riſing of the Lights	11
Conſumption	134	Scowring	5
Convulſion	64	Scurvy	2
Cough	2	Spleen	1
Dropſie	33	Spotted Feaver	101
Feaver	309	Stilborn	17
Flox and Small-pox	5	Stone	2
Frighted	3	Stopping of the ſtomach	9
Gowt	1	Strangury	1
Grief	3	Suddenly	1
Griping in the Guts	51	Surfeit	49
Jaundies	5	Teeth	121
		Thruſh	5
		Timpany	1
		Tiſſick	11
		Vomiting	3
		Winde	3
		Wormes	15

Chriſtned { Males — 95, Females — 81, In all — 176 } Buried { Males — 4095, Females — 4202, In all — 8297 } Plague — 7165

Increaſed in the Burials this Week — 607

Pariſhes clear of the Plague — 4 Pariſhes Infected — 126

The Aſſize of Bread ſet forth by Order of the Lord Maior and Court of Aldermen, A penny Wheaten Loaf to contain Nine Ounces and a half, and three half-penny White Loaves the like weight.

Figure 7.1 Bill of mortality, London, 12–19 September 1665, from *London's Dreadful Visitation: or a Collection of all the Bills of Mortality for this Present Year*, 1665. Bills of mortality, like this seventeenth-century example, simply listed the number of deaths from various causes. There was no attempt to analyse the data in any way. The records of two specific fatal accidents were reported in exactly the same way as the huge death toll from plague. Note that apart from plague (which disappeared from Britain in the eighteenth century), the biggest killers in 1665 were fevers and consumption (tuberculosis), diseases which continued to kill many people in the nineteeth century. Wellcome Library, London

legislate for their people. In the 1830s, the break up of old patterns of life and work through urbanization and industrialization and the fear of popular unrest prompted a new body of researchers to analyse social data. By doing so, they hoped to uncover the rules by which society operated and thus advise governments on how to promote its harmonious working. Some data were acquired through existing institutions: the Swedish government used the clergy to record information on births, deaths, disease and literacy (the ministers worked so assiduously that their data now provide an unparalleled source of information for historical demographers). New methods of data collection were also devised: censuses (the first British census was conducted in 1801), special studies (France established a bureau of statistics in 1800) and the compulsory registration of births, deaths and marriages. Individual researchers, including medical men, amassed their own statistics on education, crime, housing and disease among the urban working class.

Armed with this data, researchers began to discover the links between social conditions and mortality. In the 1830s, the use of statistics in medical studies thrived, particularly in France among a group of investigators known as the hygienists. Louis René Villermé (1782–1863), an ex-army doctor, used data on death rates and rental values of property in Paris to prove that mortality was not linked to environmental factors – the traditional explanation for the relative healthiness of different areas – but to social conditions (Table 7.1). Villermé found a clear correlation between the proportion of poor families living in a district and death rates: mortality was highest in the poorest districts of Paris and lowest in the wealthiest. This disproved the long-held belief that the luxurious lifestyle of the wealthy classes caused them to die earlier than their poorer counterparts (Coleman, 1982; La Berge, 1992).

Table 7.1   Social conditions and mortality in Paris

Arrondissement (district)	Percentage of poor families	Mortality
2nd	7	1/62
3rd	11	1/60
1st	11	1/58
4th	15	1/58
11th	19	1/51
6th	21	1/54
5th	22	1/53
7th	22	1/52
10th	23	1/50
9th	31	1/44
8th	32	1/43
12th	38	1/43

(La Berge, 1992, p.62)

The analysis of mortality was taken even further by later generations of observers, including William Farr, a British medical practitioner. Farr spent part of his medical education in Paris with Pierre Louis (1787–1872), a pioneer in the use of medical statistics. He was later appointed as the first compiler of abstracts at the Registrar-General's Office, where he had access to data on births and deaths for the whole of England and Wales collected under the 1836 Registration Act. This huge pool of information allowed Farr to produce elaborate statistical tables, comparing the number of deaths caused by different diseases, the death rates among different age groups and in different areas and the changes in mortality over time (Eyler, 1979). We can use Farr's statistics to get a detailed picture of mortality in England and Wales in the mid-nineteenth century.

Mortality in England and Wales, 1848–55

Look at Table 7.2, which lists the main causes of death in England and Wales in the mid-nineteenth century. You may be surprised by some of the causes listed. Nowadays 'age' is not seen as a direct cause of death, and 'convulsions' or 'atrophy' (a gradual wasting away) would be seen as symptoms of some underlying condition. In the 1850s, doctors had few means of diagnosis beyond their powers of observation, so diseases and deaths were categorized by these visible signs.

Table 7.2   Main causes of death arranged in order of mortality, 1848–55

Cause of death	Number of deaths
Consumption (tuberculosis)	354,542
Age	186,457
Convulsions	168,026
Pneumonia	154,402
Premature birth	127,590
Typhus	124,910
Scarletina (scarlet fever)	113,743
Diarrhoea	106,955
Atrophy	86,080
Cholera	83,097
Heart disease	77,197

(Registrar-General's Office, 1857, p.176)

Compared with modern populations, people in England and Wales in the middle of the nineteenth century suffered far more from infectious diseases – tuberculosis, pneumonia, typhus, scarlet fever and cholera – which now cause very few deaths. However, Victorian Britons suffered much less from heart disease – a common cause of death in the twenty-first century.

Public health reforms were not targeted against the diseases that caused the greatest number of deaths. Instead, they focused on just two of the diseases which appear in Table 7.2, typhus and cholera. By 1848, there was also a Europe-wide campaign to control smallpox through vaccination – the practice of infecting children with cowpox, a mild disease which provided immunity against smallpox. The technique was developed in 1796 by Edward Jenner (1749–1823) and it spread rapidly across Europe. By the middle of the century, many countries had schemes of free vaccination for the poor, and some had even made the practice compulsory for all infants. As a result, death rates from the disease declined significantly.

Why did reformers target typhus and cholera and not other diseases which caused many more deaths? There are several reasons. The first was simply practical – there was no means of reducing the number of deaths from 'age' or convulsions. And until the bacteria responsible for tuberculosis was discovered in 1882, medical men believed that tuberculosis was a hereditary condition, which could be treated but not prevented.

Public health strategies were also shaped by perceptions of disease. Look now at Table 7.3. It is always tempting to see numbers as presenting an accurate and objective record of mortality, but even Farr's data were not complete. The number of deaths from specified causes is always smaller than the total number of deaths. We also need to be cautious in assuming that nineteenth-century categories of disease are identical to modern categories. Where a Victorian doctor would diagnose typhus fever, a modern practitioner would see cases of typhus and typhoid fever. The two diseases were not differentiated in the Registrar-General's figures until 1869.

Table 7.3   Number of deaths from selected infectious diseases in England and Wales, 1848–55

Cause of death	1848	1849	1850	1851	1852	1853	1854	1855
Smallpox	6,903	4,644	4,665	6,997	7,320	3,151	2,808	2,525
Measles	6,867	5,458	7,082	9,370	5,846	4,895	9,277	7,354
Scarletina (scarlet fever)	20,501	13,123	13,371	13,634	18,887	15,699	18,528	17,314
Whooping cough	6,862	9,622	7,770	7,905	8,022	11,200	9,770	10,185
Croup (diphtheria)	3,777	4,038	4,322	4,180	4,058	3,660	3,998	4,419
Diarrhoea	11,067	17,831	11,468	14,728	17,617	14,192	20,052	12,770
Dysentery	2,629	3,050	2,036	2,185	2,756	1,891	1,943	1,437
Cholera	1,908	53,273	887	1,132	1,381	4,419	20,097	837
Influenza	7,963	1,618	1,380	2,152	1,359	1,789	1,061	3,568
Typhus	21,406	17,896	14,294	17,122	17,845	18,015	18,332	16,032
Consumption (tuberculosis)	51,663	50,299	46,618	49,166	50,594	54,918	51,284	52,290
Bronchitis	14,472	14,826	14,611	17,294	17,073	22,391	20,062	27,182
Pneumonia	21,862	21,194	20,303	22,001	21,421	24,098	23,523	26,052
Age	26,188	26,750	25,567	25,980	26,376	29,130	26,466	29,714
All causes	398,531	440,839	368,995	395,396	407,135	421,097	437,905	425,703
Specified causes	387,416	432,710	361,536	388,675	400,439	414,197	432,242	419,798

(Registrar-General's Office, 1857, pp.180–1)

Study Table 7.3 carefully and note how the number of deaths from each disease varies over time. Can you see any patterns?

The mortality of every disease varies, but some vary more dramatically than others. Consumption and croup, for instance, show relatively little change. The highest annual total is only around one-fifth greater than the lowest. But cholera shows a very different pattern, with huge death tolls in 1849 and 1854 and relatively few deaths attributed to the disease in other years. Smallpox, too, shows quite a wide variation, with deaths in 1852 more than double the number in 1853.

Consumption and croup were **endemic** – they were present at all times and caused a fairly consistent number of deaths each year. Diseases such as cholera and smallpox occurred in **epidemics** – they flared up at intervals and caused many deaths over a short period. In the case of cholera, this epidemic pattern was particularly extreme. Cholera was unknown in Europe until the 1830s, when it spread out from the Near East, creeping across the continent of Europe and reaching Britain in 1831. It died out in 1832, but further waves of the disease reached across Europe in 1848–9, 1854 and 1866. Its novelty and the high death toll made cholera particularly frightening. The unpleasant symptoms of cholera added to the fear of the disease. One report described the symptoms:

> from a state of apparent good health ... an individual sustains as rapid a loss of bodily power as if he were suddenly struck down or poisoned; the countenance assuming a death-like appearance, the skin becoming cold ... The pulse is either feeble, intermittent, fluttering, or lost ... vomiting soon succeeds ... spasms, beginning at the toes and fingers, soon follow ... the next severe symptoms are an intolerable sense of weight, and constriction felt upon the chest ... a leaden or bluish appearance of the countenance ... at length a calm succeeds and death ... The powers of the constitution often yield to such an attack at the end of four hours, and seldom sustain longer than eight.

(quoted in Mort, 1987, p.11)

Not surprisingly, governments made great efforts to deal with this terrifying killer. By contrast, endemic diseases and those epidemic diseases that appeared fairly regularly were far less frightening and prompted less action.

But why did governments act against typhus – an endemic disease?

Table 7.4   Causes of death by age group, 1848–55

Cause of death	Under 1	Under 5[1]	5–	10–	15–	25–	35–	45–	55–	65–	75–
Smallpox	9,219	24,961	4,748	1,224	2,661	1,626	691	359	126	65	25
Measles	8,875	44,003	3,857	516	229	109	50	18	6	2	3
Scarlet fever	7,540	72,056	31,066	6,543	2,369	772	497	218	117	63	29
Whooping cough	24,824	58,254	2,664	153	37	9	5	12	6	1	3
Croup	4,381	24,037	3,689	202	36	23	20	9	6	5	5
Diarrhoea	53,072	76,660	1,896	774	1,633	2,046	2,152	2,695	4,337	6,947	7,801
Dysentery	3,162	6,452	655	289	709	1,076	1,040	1,351	1,666	1,958	1,287
Cholera	3,326	14,029	7,216	3,688	7,712	11,896	11,778	10,183	8,428	5,571	2,545
Influenza	2,737	4,552	400	233	450	492	674	1,006	1,988	3,706	3,819
Typhus	2,130	19,605	15,234	11,641	24,460	14,777	11,223	9,620	8,419	6,839	3,074
Consumption	11,465	27,270	10,199	15,462	87,379	83,878	59,507	37,664	22,163	9,262	1,687
Bronchitis	22,345	40,506	1,756	605	1,981	3,150	5,586	10,105	16,797	22,477	17,752
Pneumonia	57,956	107,831	5,096	1,684	4,622	4,968	5,596	6,244	7,169	6,842	4,327

[1] Note that the total of deaths under 5 years includes the deaths in the first year of life
(Registrar-General's Office, 1857, pp.150–1)

Exercise

Study Table 7.4, which shows deaths from specific diseases by age group. You will see that children under the age of 5 were especially vulnerable to infectious disease. But which were the main diseases to kill adults of working age (between 15 and 55 years)?

Discussion

Cholera, typhus and consumption all caused very high mortality among adults of working age, although a large number of infants also died of these diseases.

By killing adults of working age, typhus and cholera posed a serious economic problem – they removed productive workers and left behind orphaned children who had to be supported by charity or the state. Typhus was associated with poverty, and epidemics tended to occur in periods of economic downturn (Figure 7.2). As workers lost their jobs, they crowded together in poorer housing to save money. In these conditions, the body lice which spread the disease flourished. Local authorities took action against typhus for humanitarian reasons, in an effort to prevent social unrest and protect the lives of workers.

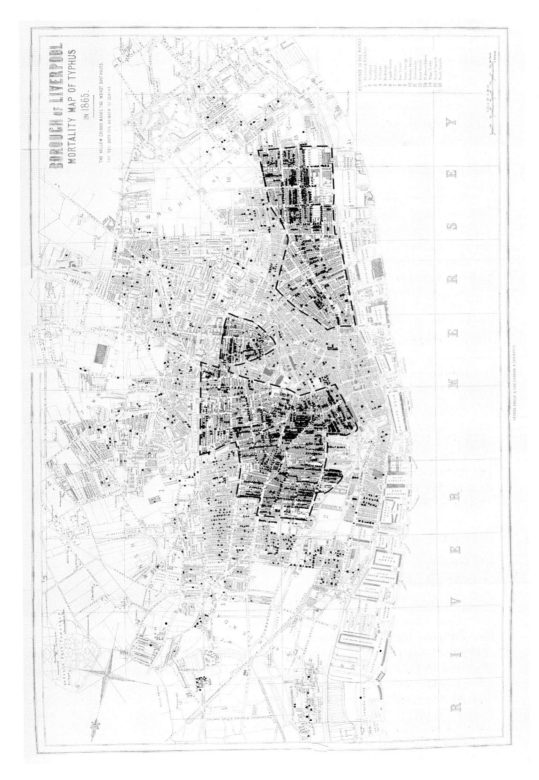

Figure 7.2   Mortality map of typhus in Liverpool, *c.*1865. This map represents an alternative way of analysing disease, showing where typhus occurred rather than when it appeared. Such 'fever maps' graphically illustrated the correlation between disease and poor living conditions. In this example, the cartographer has highlighted a few areas – although typhus was common across Liverpool. He may have wished to make a point about slum areas inhabited by the poorest people. Wellcome Library, London

7.3   Understanding the causes of disease

As you saw in the extract by Ackerknecht, the early historians of public health treated developments in the understanding of disease causation (or **aetiology**) as one of the most important aspects of public health history. They described how at the beginning of the nineteenth century practitioners thought that most diseases were caused by a combination of environment and lifestyle. Epidemic diseases were assumed to be transmitted from person to person through some agent or material. By the 1840s, ideas of disease causation were dominated by the miasma theory. This was the idea that the vapours given off by decomposing organic matter in the environment were the direct cause of disease. Ackerknecht refers to this as the 'erroneous filth theory'. This theory was gradually overturned by researchers who returned to the old idea that diseases were spread by some unknown agents. As early as 1849, John Snow (1813–58) suggested that cholera was spread through water contaminated with rotting matter or excrement. In 1856, William Budd (1811–80) showed that typhoid was spread by contact with the faeces of people suffering from the disease. In the 1880s, these unknown agents were identified as bacteria. In 1882, Robert Koch identified the bacterium which caused tuberculosis. In 1883, he identified the cholera bacillus, and thereafter researchers gradually uncovered more and more disease-causing bacteria (Porter, 1999, pp.429–42).

The discovery of the role of bacteria in disease causation was explored in Chapter 4.

However, more recent research has shown that we need to be cautious when interpreting writings about disease causation and that there was no smooth shift from a consensus over miasma theories to a general acceptance of the germ theory.

Exercise

Read extracts (i)–(iv) of 'Unhealthy environments' (Source Book 2, Reading 7.2). Take careful note of the author of each account, the date of publication, the type of publication in which it appeared and the diseases each author discusses.

I   What conclusions would you draw from these sources about theories of disease causation in the mid-nineteenth century?

2   Do they fit with the interpretation given by early historians of public health?

Discussion

I   These sources suggest that both doctors and laymen firmly believe that diseases arise from environmental conditions. General ill health, fevers and cholera are seen to be products of a range of environmental factors: dirt, poor drainage, polluted water courses and damp and dilapidated housing, which occur in both great cities and villages. Mayhew puts a particular emphasis on the unpleasant smells that pervade these places.

2   Three of the extracts fit well with the understanding of theories of disease causation put forward by Ackerknecht and his contemporaries. The extract from

The Times does not – according to the interpretation of early historians, doctors had abandoned miasma theories by 1865.

Recent studies of the medical literature have shown that in the mid-nineteenth century, there was no consensus that all epidemics arose from the environment. Most doctors believed that some diseases were caused by miasmas and some by specific, contagious agents. It was generally believed that smallpox spread from person to person through a specific agent. Doctors had exploited this phenomenon in inoculation – the practice of deliberately infecting children with smallpox using the liquid which formed in the characteristic spots. (This practice was dangerous as some children died as a result of being inoculated. It was quickly abandoned after the development of vaccination.) Many practitioners accepted that other diseases – such as typhus and fevers – did arise from miasmas. But there were differing views. Florence Nightingale, for example, declared that all diseases, even smallpox, arose from dirt, a view that reinforced the need for hospitals to employ trained nurses to ensure high standards of hygiene. The aetiology of certain diseases provoked prolonged and heated debates. Between the 1830s and 1870s, doctors were divided as to whether cholera was spread by miasmas or by some unknown agent in the water supply. As new evidence for the contagious nature of cholera and typhoid built up, practitioners began to change their minds and abandon miasmatic explanations for these diseases. Even in the 1870s, though, some practitioners continued to claim that cholera was caused entirely by environmental factors or that cholera germs played only a small part in spreading the disease.

Recent research has also demonstrated that doctors did not simply see contagion and the environment as completely different and mutually exclusive sources of disease. Michael Worboys (2000) has shown that from the 1850s (well before bacteria had been identified), medical men debated the nature of the agents which caused disease. They hypothesized that diseases were spread by 'zymes', which might be chemicals, fungi, 'germs', parasites or cells originating in the body of disease victims. Some suggested that zymes themselves could arise not only from infected individuals but also from the environment. And even if disease agents did not arise from the environment, they were certainly spread within it through contaminated water and dirt. From 1855, Max von Pettenkofer (1818–1901), the first German professor of public health, developed a theory that cholera was spread by 'germs' which had been 'activated' by contact with damp soil.

Practitioners developed extraordinarily sophisticated (or complicated) ideas about the role of bad air and bad smells in causing disease. For example, in 1862, W.T. Gairdner, later medical officer of health in Glasgow, warned his students:

> How far are 'stinks' ... to be regarded as sources of disease and death? It has, on the one hand, been argued that bad smells are truly the very seeds of disease; and, on the other hand, it has been maintained that they are wholly innocuous ... I think you will see your way through these confusing labyrinths of discussion, if you will only look at the matter in this point of view: – neither a bad smell, as such, nor sulphuretted hydrogen, as such,

nor carbonic acid [these chemicals were associated with rotting matter and the air of overcrowded rooms], as such, contains the special poisons which we have to fear particularly as the sources of epidemic disease. But all of these are, to a certain extent, indications, beneficent, providential warnings, plainly given to us ... to bring before our senses the circumstances in which dangerous poisons may perchance be present.

(Gairdner, [1862] (2001), pp.70–1)

Throughout the nineteenth century, environmental factors were thought to predispose individuals to catch diseases. This idea explained why some people fell ill and died during epidemics, while others remained healthy or recovered. People living in overcrowded and damp accommodation, eating a poor diet, suffering from excessive work or stress and indulging in immoral behaviour – especially drinking – would always be the first victims of epidemic disease. Some middle-class doctors and clergymen reported with satisfaction that drunkards and prostitutes were the first to die during cholera epidemics as a result of their immoral lives, not their poverty. These ideas persisted even after practitioners accepted that bacteria caused disease. Practitioners spoke of the bacteria as 'seeds' which would only produce disease if they landed in fertile 'soil' – the bodies of those individuals predisposed to illness by their environment and lifestyle. Equally, building up the body through fresh air, exercise and good food would ensure that any invading germs would not produce illness (Hamlin, 1992; Worboys, 2000, pp.161–4).

By now, you should have realized that when we read nineteenth-century accounts which link disease with the environment, this does not necessarily mean that the author sees a simple or direct link between bad air and ill health. If you refer back to Source Book 2, Reading 7.2, extracts (ii) and (iv), you can see that Henry Mayhew might be arguing that the environment predisposed slum-dwellers to infection. And while *The Times* editorial on the inquest into deaths from typhoid explicitly states that the disease arises from dirty conditions, Dr Letheby might believe that typhoid was caused by contact with faeces. He describes the poor drainage of the homes where the deaths occurred and it is clear that he thinks the whole atmosphere of the poor dwellings contributed to the fatal cases of typhoid.

7.4 Public health practices

The role of central government

As you saw in the Ackerknecht extract, early historians of public health showed little interest in describing the implementation of public health reform. They were far more interested in the work of central government. Early researchers focused on the work of government administrators (particularly Chadwick) in passing legislation which they assumed were the main means by which diseases were brought under control (Finer, 1952). These historians saw public health reform as fitting into wider programmes of government action. In Britain, a liberal and laissez-faire regime tackled a range of social problems caused by rapid industrialization, applying policies which imposed minimal interference with industry and the liberty of individual citizens. From the 1830s, successive British governments regulated working hours and workplace conditions, provided welfare for the poor and unemployed and improved police and prison services (MacDonagh, 1977). Government action to control disease can also be seen as part of a trend to take action on health issues – including funding for hospitals, research institutes and (in some countries) regulating the medical profession.

Since 1980, historians of medicine have challenged this view in a number of ways. They have argued that sanitary reform and disease control measures were not nineteenth-century innovations but were a continuation of eighteenth-century policies. The political theory known as mercantilism or cameralism equated the strength of a nation with the size of its population (from which was drawn its army and workforce). Governments should therefore seek to prevent disease through the provision of drainage, clean water and street cleaning. They should provide medical care to the sick poor through hospitals and state doctors, and guarantee a supply of healthy children by allowing only healthy people to marry. These policies (known as **medical police**) were put into practice by the authorities in a number of German states. Early researchers portrayed medical police as a system of surveillance and control, and assumed that it was adopted only in authoritarian states. However, further work has shown that medical police policies were embraced most enthusiastically in Sweden, which was perhaps the most democratic regime in late eighteenth-century Europe. There, in an effort to boost the population, the government established more than twenty general hospitals and required local authorities to appoint medical practitioners and midwives to care for the poor. It also introduced compulsory vaccination against smallpox in 1816 – the first European country to do so. Medical police also found a foothold in Britain. In the late eighteenth and early nineteenth centuries, Scottish cities acquired police acts – legislation which allowed them to pave, drain, clean and light streets as well as control crime. English towns and cities acquired similar powers under improvement acts (Carroll, 2002; Rosen, 1974).

Historians have questioned the assumption that central government was the key player in public health reform. They pointed out that although England and Wales had government offices dedicated to health matters, these agencies were small and had little political power (indeed, the General Board of Health, the first government office to deal specifically with public health issues, was so unpopular, it survived only from 1848 until 1854, when the agency was disbanded). While foreign governments expressed their admiration for English public health reform, few created a similar administration until the very end of the century. In Scotland, the Board of Supervision for the Relief of the Poor was responsible for public health, but it employed only one doctor on an ad hoc basis to investigate specific problems. The French government created a High Council of Health in 1822 to deal with quarantine against yellow fever, but it was not until 1886 that a central Bureau of Public Health and Hygiene with substantial authority was established. In Germany, too, central government fought shy of intervening in the lives of its citizens in the late nineteenth century. An Imperial Health Office was finally established in 1873, but it was mostly concerned with collecting data on health and disease (Porter, 1994, pp.53–86, 121–5).

Finally, new research has questioned whether there is a clear link between the political character of a government and its public health policies. In a groundbreaking article in 1948, Ackerknecht had firmly linked public health reforms to the political character of governments. He argued that in the late 1840s, governments were faced with a choice of policies. If they believed that epidemic disease arose from the environment, then they would adopt sanitary reforms (a theory which Ackerknecht called anticontagionism). If disease spread through contagion, it would be controlled through quarantines. Ackerknecht suggested that at this time there was equally convincing evidence for both arguments. In such a situation, 'economic outlook and political loyalty will determine the decision. These, being liberal and bourgeois in the majority of the physicians of the time, brought about the victory of anticontagionism' (Ackerknecht, 1948, p.589). Sanitary reforms designed to clean up the environment were therefore favoured by liberal regimes, while absolutist governments imposed quarantines that restricted trade.

In a detailed analysis of responses to cholera, smallpox and venereal disease in different European countries, the historian Peter Baldwin has shown that government policies on public health do not fall neatly into the model offered by Ackerknecht. Just as few practitioners believed that all disease arose from one source alone, miasma or contagion, governments did not opt solely for either contagionist or anticontagionist theory in dealing with public health. Instead, they tended to adopt a mix of quarantine and sanitary measures. Their exact choice of policies depended on a wide range of factors: earlier experiences of disease prevention, economics, geography and their understanding of disease transmission (Baldwin, 1999). For example, during the first cholera epidemic that swept across Europe from the Near East between 1831 and 1832, the autocratic regimes of eastern Europe – Russia, Austria and Prussia – tried to keep the disease out by imposing quarantines. This technique had been used since medieval times against plague and other epidemics. Ships were held offshore for a period of days or weeks to ensure that none of the passengers was infected. Travellers were inspected and anyone suspected of having cholera was isolated in special hospitals. However, such measures proved ineffectual. Cholera continued to travel westwards, arriving next in south Germany, France and Britain. Armed with the knowledge that quarantines had not worked elsewhere, these governments introduced much less rigorous quarantine policies. The only exceptions were busy port cities, like Marseille and Hamburg, where quarantines were retained to reassure trading partners that action was being taken against the disease. In Britain, the authorities supplemented quarantines with environmental measures. Town authorities organized general cleansings of the streets and the homes of the poor. 'Nuisances' – accumulations of dirt thought to present a particular danger to health – were removed. The experience of this first cholera epidemic shaped policy and practice during the second outbreak in the late 1840s. Thus, despite the failure of quarantines to keep cholera at bay, Prussia continued to favour this practice, while Bavaria, France and Britain emphasized sanitary measures.

The problems of drawing a direct link between the political character of a government and its policy on public health are made clear by the history of Sweden's responses to cholera. According to Ackerknecht's model, democratic Sweden should have rejected the use of quarantine. In fact, Sweden was an enthusiastic supporter of the practice right through the nineteenth century.

Baldwin argues that the Swedish state was predisposed to use quarantines by its geographical position in the far north of Europe. There, its inhabitants could watch the slow march of cholera across the continent. And closing the routes of entry to the approaching disease was the most obvious method of prevention. Quarantine was also a practical option in Sweden, where there were relatively few ports and the country was not dependent on international trade. Finally, quarantine was popular with the people. Far from seeing quarantine as a repressive interference with liberty, local authorities set up their own quarantines, refusing travellers the right to stay in town. The inhabitants of Örebro even blocked all the roads leading into their town to prevent infection.

Although Baldwin identifies many factors shaping public health policies – geography, trade, experience of disease – the work of Christopher Hamlin suggests that economics and politics should be added to the list. Hamlin has re-examined the creation of the *Report on the Sanitary Condition of the Labouring Population* (1842), which was drawn up by Edwin Chadwick, secretary to the Poor Law Commissioners. The *Sanitary Report* is often portrayed as an objective account of the dreadful living conditions of much of the British population, which inspired parliament to pass the 1848 Public Health Act. However, Hamlin argues that the *Sanitary Report* should not be seen as an objective survey.

Exercise

Read 'Reassessing Chadwick's *Sanitary Report*' (Source Book 2, Reading 7.3).

1   According to Hamlin, did Chadwick emphasize the need for sanitary reform to tackle ill health on medical or political grounds?

2   How does Hamlin's argument relate to Ackerknecht's ideas about politics shaping public health?

Discussion

1   Hamlin suggests that Chadwick's ideas of disease causation were shaped by a desire to limit welfare services and were supported, rather than directed, by medical practitioners. The New Poor Law was proving expensive, partly, Chadwick believed, because Poor Law medical officers prescribed food – 'mutton medicine' – for their patients. The object of the *Sanitary Report* was to provide conclusive proof that environmental conditions, not social factors such as diet and poverty, were the principle causes of disease. It would thus justify the wider principle of providing minimal levels of support to the poor in an effort to force them to work.

2   Hamlin's study suggests that Ackerknecht is right to point to the role of politics in shaping public health practice. But it is not the overall character of the government which dictates policy, but rather how an individual public health policy fits with other government programmes.

Hamlin's work shows that Chadwick was able to set the government agenda on public health matters while consulting with only a few practitioners, the views of whom were not typical of medical opinion. There has been little systematic work on how governments devised their health policies. Although it is tempting to assume that public health was one area where practitioners brought their expert knowledge to bear, in fact, very few medical men were directly involved in public health. Within government, a handful of practitioners exerted disproportionate amounts of influence. John Simon (1816–1904), medical officer to the Privy Council, was the most powerful medical practitioner working for the British government in the 1860s. He quickly accepted the idea that cholera could be spread by germs, and under his guidance the British authorities devised more focused quarantine procedures against the disease. However, Simon was also a pragmatist and maintained the existing sanitary measures, which he saw would help to prevent the spread of germs. He stated:

> empirically we know that ... the pestilence [cholera] rages only where there are definite sanitary evils. This knowledge remains unchanged; and unchanged remain also our practical means of applying it ... Excrement-sodden earth, excrement-reeking air, excrement-tainted water, these are for us the causes of cholera.
>
> (quoted in Worboys, 2000, p.115)

At the same time in the German states, governments shaped their policies around von Pettenkofer's theory that cholera germs were released in the excreta of victims and activated by contact with contaminated soil. The German authorities, therefore, focused their preventative strategies on disinfecting lavatories and sewage.

The role of local government

Since the 1980s, historians of medicine have shown that across Europe local, not central, government was largely responsible for the reforms in public health. Town, district and regional authorities, assisted by temporary boards and voluntary associations, implemented legislation as part of a wider civic effort to create civilized, progressive communities which were pleasant to live in. Local authorities were responsible for measures to control epidemics. They set up hospitals where the victims of disease could be isolated and treated and arranged for the fumigation of homes. They were also responsible for sanitary reforms that aimed to reduce overall mortality by making the whole urban environment a healthier place. The goal of the sanitary reform movement was: 'a sewer in every street of every town and every village; a drain for every house, a constant and unlimited supply of good water to every family; pure air at any cost' (*Fraser's Magazine*, 1847, vol.36, p.517).

Such policies were not new. From medieval times and right through the eighteenth century, city authorities had sought to improve the health of their populations by cleaning streets and draining standing water (Riley, 1987). Long before the nineteenth century, authorities in large cities dealt with the problem of refuse by paving streets, laying gutters and organizing gangs of men with brooms to sweep the streets and cart away the dirt. However, from the mid-nineteenth century, the scale of sanitary reform increased. In large cities, the streets were swept and refuse collected daily. Street cleaning was introduced in smaller towns and villages. Local authorities had an economic incentive to institute cleaning as street refuse was sold as agricultural fertilizer. The authorities in Scottish fishing villages turned a healthy profit on the heady mixture of horse manure and the refuse from gutting fish that was collected from the streets. Hamburg, Edinburgh and other large cities actually sold the right to clean the streets to the highest bidder, in the expectation that whoever won the right would make a profit by selling the refuse. In the 1850s, many cities helped the cleansing operations by building new drains to carry off rainwater. This required building on a heroic scale. In London, between 1856 and 1859, 842 kilometres of main sewers and 20,921 kilometres of drains were built (Figure 7.3). The project used 13 million bricks and required workmen to dig by hand 2.8 million cubic metres of earth. And London was not unique. Between 1855 and 1865, 18 kilometres of main sewer and 90 kilometres of pipes were installed in Liverpool. Paris boasted 1,113 kilometres of sewers by 1900. These drains were designed to deal with stormwater, so in 1880, when large numbers of householders began to connect flushing lavatories to the drains, larger sewer systems had to be built to carry away the excrement which had previously been collected in privies and cesspools.

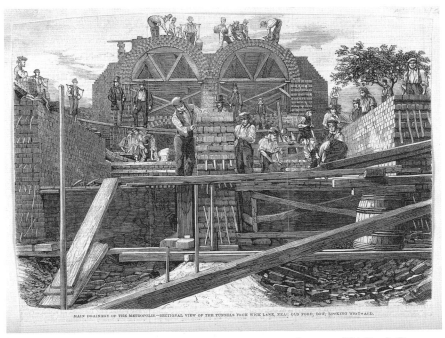

MAIN DRAINAGE OF THE METROPOLIS.—SECTIONAL VIEW OF THE TUNNELS FROM WICK LANE, NEAR OLD FORD, BOW, LOOKING WESTWARD.

Figure 7.3   The construction of the great sewage tunnels, near Old Ford, Bow, London, c.1856–9. This image presents sanitary reform on a heroic scale – the huge tunnels dwarf the workers. At the same time, the chaos of planks and bricks in the foreground and the large number of workers shown reminds us that these engineering projects were almost entirely constructed by hand. Wellcome Library, London

In the late nineteenth century, many local governments also took on responsibility for providing their communities with a clean and plentiful supply of water (Figure 7.4). Until the nineteenth century, all communities relied on natural water courses and wells located within or near the built-up area, or on supplies provided by private water companies. However, with the growth of urban populations and the fact that many rivers and streams were also used to dispose of refuse and industrial waste, water supplies became increasingly inadequate and polluted. The provision of new water supplies was a massive undertaking. Suitable sources of water had to be found and these were often at a great distance. The surrounding land then had to be bought and the right to lay pipes negotiated. Facilities to store, filter and finally distribute the water had to be built. In the 1860s, Baron Haussmann (1809–91) oversaw the building of a system, which included a massive aqueduct, for carrying water more than 160 kilometres to Paris. The combined efforts of local governments and private water companies to increase supplies of water were rewarded within a generation. Throughout Europe, the inhabitants of many towns and cities no longer had to live with an intermittent, polluted communal water supply but could enjoy a constant supply of clean water piped into their homes. By 1890, every house in Hamburg and 95 per cent of houses in Berlin had water on tap.

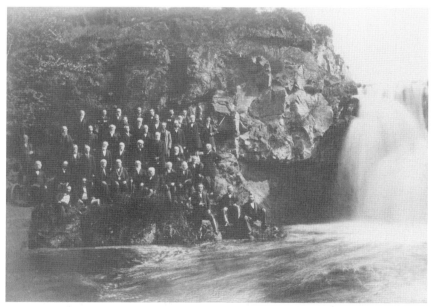

Figure 7.4   The romance of sanitary reform: Glasgow Water Commissioners at the Loch Katrine waterworks, *c*.1880. These reservoirs outside Glasgow were originally built by a private company, the Gorbals Gravitation Water Company. In 1856, they were purchased by the Glasgow Police Commissioners, the body responsible for paving, lighting, draining and cleaning the city, as one part of a major new scheme to supply water. Every year, the Water Commissioners (a subcommittee of the Police Commissioners) travelled out to inspect the reservoirs. Although the backdrop to this photograph has been chosen for its romantic grandeur, the image gives a sense of the scale of the reservoir, and of the Commissioners' pride in their achievement. SCRAN/Glasgow City Archives

The most novel element of late nineteenth-century sanitary reform was the desire to provide urban residents with clean air. Disease had long been associated with bad air and bad smells. During epidemics in the sixteenth and seventeenth centuries, city authorities had tried to drive out bad air by lighting bonfires and burning tar and other substances to make pungent smells. In the nineteenth century, local governments sought to ensure clean air – fresh and free from the smells of rotting substances – as part of the strategy to provide a healthy environment. They tried to ensure that individual homes were well ventilated by passing regulations to limit the numbers of people sleeping in lodging-houses and to stop landlords renting out cellars as dwellings. On a larger scale, whole areas of slum housing were demolished to bring light and air into densely crowded parts of cities (Figure 7.5). The city governments were assisted in this project by the mid-century railway boom, when companies demolished slums to make room for their new lines and stations. Since the displaced residents were not usually provided with alternative accommodation, they squeezed into poor-quality housing in other areas. This tended to shift the problem rather than solve it. The authorities also took action against factory owners, prosecuting them for causing smoke pollution and encouraging the installation of devices to consume smoke. However, such measures had little effect and 'pea-souper' fogs, so beloved of Victorian detective fiction, continued to blight city life into the mid-twentieth century.

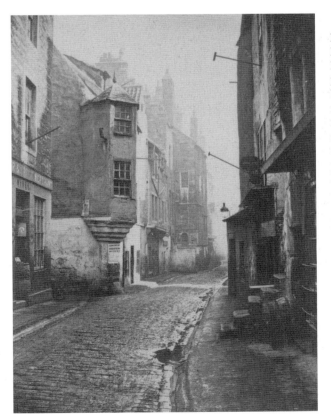

Figure 7.5   Cardinal Beaton's house, Cowgate, Edinburgh, 1868. This once palatial house, originally built in 1509, had by the mid-nineteenth century fallen into serious disrepair and would have been inhabited by very poor people. It was demolished as part of Edinburgh's slum-clearance programme shortly after this photograph was taken. The photograph reveals the ambiguous attitude of the better-off classes towards such ancient buildings – they were 'picturesque' and it was understood that they had a place in history, but they were also the homes of the poorest and unhealthiest people and were therefore places to be avoided. SCRAN/Edinburgh City Libraries

It is very difficult to draw an overall picture of the progress of public health reform across Europe. The authorities in individual areas or towns took up public health with varying degrees of enthusiasm, and implemented policies according to perceived local needs. The rapidly growing cities faced the biggest problems of pollution, environmental degradation and high mortality, and they took the lead in initiating reform. The *département* of the Seine, which included Paris, set the pace of public health reform in France, and its policies were copied by smaller towns and cities. City governments copied successful measures from other countries. Hamburg set up its first public bathhouse in emulation of Liverpool, while supporters of planned improvements to Paris's water supply cited the success of such schemes in British cities (Evans, 1987). The compliment was returned when British municipal authorities copied the design of Paris's public urinals. While public health reforms were aimed at reducing mortality, they also improved unpleasant, dirty and crowded conditions and promised to help maintain good public order. The Paris authorities demolished old buildings and opened up new streets partly to let in light and air but also to give access to the police and army should there be an uprising among the politically volatile underclass. Finally, pragmatism and opportunity played a role in shaping public health practice. Linlithgow enjoyed a reputation as the dirtiest burgh in Scotland because its citizens could dump their rubbish in a local loch belonging to the crown without fear of prosecution. Hamburg used a devastating fire, which destroyed large sections of the old city, as an opportunity to install a major new drainage system.

Recent research has also shown how local authorities faced formidable obstacles when implementing sanitary reforms. In the past, penny-pinching ratepayers were blamed for hampering efforts at improvement. Historians cited contemporary commentators such as Charles Dickens, who caricatured such opposition in the periodical *Household Words* (1853):

> Ratepayers, Cess-cum-Poolton! Rally round your vested interests. Health is enormously expensive. Introduce the Public Health Act [of 1848] and you will be pauperised! Be filthy and fat. Cess-pools and Constitutional government! Gases and Glory!

> (quoted in Finer, 1952, p.435)

More recent studies have shown that ratepayers in some towns did oppose reform. The Hamburg Property Owners Association held up improvements to water quality for thirteen years. In most cases, however, their opposition was short-lived. New research reveals that local authorities did not only have problems with ratepayers. There were also the sheer logistical difficulties of finding new sources of water and building new drainage systems. Local authorities, too, had to balance the conflicting interests of private citizens and the general public. In Edinburgh and Glasgow, residents went to court to stop the local police commissioners from installing public lavatories close to their homes. Such facilities might serve the community, but they were smelly and less than respectable (Hamlin, 1988; Kearns, 1988). Some of the other problems faced by local authorities have been described by Gerry Kearns and Anthony Wohl.

Exercise

Read 'The problems of sanitary reform in Islington' and 'The problems of sewering Farnham' (Source Book 2, Readings 7.4 and 7.5).

1   What was the view of these local authorities on public health reform?

2   What was their relationship to central government?

Discussion

1   The local authorities portrayed here seem keen in principle to introduce sanitary reform. In practice, however, they feel beleaguered by their responsibilities and afraid of taking the wrong action, which might prove costly. In Wohl's account, efforts by the Farnham authorities to build a sewage system are severely hampered by conflicting advice on the technical points of different schemes. Kearns, by contrast, paints a picture of a local authority struggling to work with other institutions – the vestry (which held the purse strings), private companies (who demanded payment beyond Islington's means) and the legal system (which defended the rights of the individual over the public).

2   Both authorities seem rather detached from central government – there is no sense that they are trying to follow a particular agenda that is set down in legislation. Rather, government is a distant resource. The Islington authorities hope that parliament will pass legislation (which will save them money) and Farnham finally approaches central government for advice.

Class and public health

Class differences were not confined to public health but were a feature of all medical provision. This is discussed in Chapter 13.

Recent research has also revealed an important class dimension to reform and shows that 'public' health affected different sections of the public in very different ways. It seems ironic but the upper and middle classes were perhaps the main beneficiaries of sanitary reform. They used their vote in local elections to demand improved drainage and sewage in the areas where they lived. If required, they could contribute to the cost. Upper- and middle-class residents were able to create a healthy environment within their own homes. They could afford to live in the airy suburbs, in houses with good sanitary arrangements. They had bathrooms and laundries, servants, water supplies, drains, sinks, baths, soap and disinfectants to keep themselves and their clothes clean (Figure 7.6). As a result, life expectancy in better areas of town could be ten years greater than in the worst slums. However, even the wealthiest families were not immune to disease. In 1861, Prince Albert died of typhoid contracted from the defective drains of Windsor Castle. Nor did sanitary improvements bring peace of mind: new drainage systems brought the fear of 'sewer gases' seeping into houses to poison the inhabitants (Tomes, 1998).

Middle-class reformers constantly held up the homes of the poor as proof of the need for sanitary improvements. (You have read some examples of this extensive literature in Source Book 2, Reading 7.2.) Their houses were described as being small, dirty, ill-lit, poorly ventilated and insanitary. Many had no water supply,

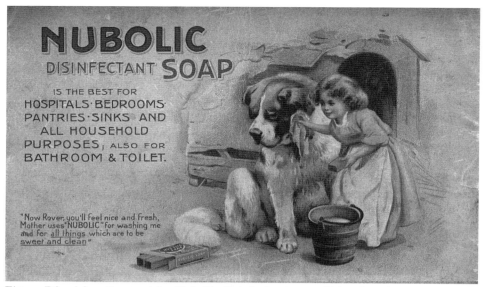

Figure 7.6   Advertisement for Nubolic disinfectant soap. This advertisement shows how women were expected to take responsibility for health and cleanliness within the private space of the home (compare this image with the photograph of the all-male Glasgow water authority). The little girl washing the dog offers sentimental parallels to the mother keeping her home and family 'sweet and clean' and healthy. Wellcome Library, London

shared privies with other households and were in a dilapidated condition. Such houses were criticized for being 'overcrowded', but many families could only afford to rent a single room. (Reformers often overlooked the fact that the poor spent a lot of time away from their homes at work or at leisure in the streets and in public houses.) In the minds of reformers, such housing conditions bred immorality as well as disease. Having unmarried adults of both sexes sleeping in the same room was assumed to lead to incest and illegitimate births. Miners who attempted to keep clean were condemned for bathing in front of other family members. Ironically, while the homes of the poor were acknowledged to be most in need of improvement, sanitary reforms were not targeted at poor areas. Slums and slum-dwellers were thought to be beyond sanitary redemption (they could not be taught to use sinks and lavatories properly) and they could not contribute towards the cost of new drains.

However, there is evidence that poor people were well aware of their unhealthy living conditions and wanted improvements, as this remarkable letter from *The Times* newspaper shows:

> We are Sur, as it may be, livin in a Wilderniss, so far as the rest of London knows anything of us, or as the rich and great people care about. We live in muck and filth. We aint got no priviz [privies], no dust bins, no drains, no water-splies [supplies], and no drain or suer in the hole place. The Suer Company in Greek St., Soho Square, all great, rich and powerfool men, take no notice watsomedever of our complaints. The Stench of a Gully-hole is disgustin. We all of us suffer, and numbers are ill, and if the Cholera comes Lord help us.

Some gentlemans come yesterday ... they was complaining of the noosance and stenche our lanes and corts [courts] was to them in New Oxforde Street. They was much surprised to see the seller [cellar] ... in our lane, where a child was dyin from fever, and would not believe that Sixty persons sleep in it every night ... we hope you will let us have these complaints put into your hinfluenshall paper, and make these landlords of our houses ... make our houses decent for Christians to live in.

(*The Times*, 5 July 1849, p.5, col.f, original spelling retained throughout)

Many working-class women spent huge amounts of time and effort trying to keep their homes clean – a Herculean task without adequate water and in smoke-polluted air. And in northern England, working men founded associations to campaign for sanitary reform (Sigsworth and Worboys, 1994).

Voluntary associations complemented the work of government. Where the state tackled disease through measures directed at public spaces, charities encouraged the poor to follow the example of middle-class households by keeping their homes as clean as possible. The London-based Ladies Sanitary Association tried to educate the poor in hygienic habits through lectures, pamphlets and home visits.

Exercise

Read 'Popular health education' (Source Book 2, Reading 7.6).

1   How is the text of this pamphlet written to reach out to a working-class audience?

2   Does it link hygienic living with any other benefits?

Discussion

1   The pamphlet tries to appeal to a working-class audience by conveying its message through a dialogue between working men. The text also uses simple language. The messages about how to live a healthy life are geared to an audience of poor people – the hints about health are few, simple and cheap. The message being put across is that fresh air and washing go a long way towards preventing disease.

2   The text carries many other messages. It suggests that working-class education is useful: it is through lectures and 'little books' that the participants have learned how to be healthy. Healthy living is closely linked to domestic contentment, happy children and a well-ordered home. Healthy living is also linked to a moral life – the family goes to church, and a peaceful demeanour is rooted in a belief in God.

While sanitary reforms may have passed them by, poor people were the primary target of measures to control epidemic diseases. The better off, who were less likely to suffer during epidemics of fever or cholera, were expected to behave in a socially responsible manner by isolating cases of infectious disease within their own homes and were quietly exempted from public regulations. In 1849, when a zealous Edinburgh medical officer knocked on doors in a respectable street demanding to know if there were any cases of cholera within the houses, he was reprimanded by his local authority employers. The poor were subjected to far more rigorous scrutiny. Local authorities sent medical men to inspect the homes of the poor, identify any cases of illness and arrange for the removal of the sick to isolation hospitals. Fumigation squads would then arrive to disinfect homes with strong chemicals (these often damaged or destroyed clothing and fabrics) and whitewash the walls. Such actions cast doubt on Ackerknecht's assumption that sanitary reform interfered less with the rights of the individual than quarantines.

The poor did not always passively accept such efforts to control disease among them, and cholera, that strange and frightening disease, provoked violent responses. In the 1830s, from Russia to France, the poorer classes saw that they suffered disproportionately from the disease. They concluded that governments and the medical profession were conspiring to kill them, either in cholera hospitals or by poisoning water supplies. Regulations requiring the disinfection and rapid burial of the bodies of cholera victims in special, sometimes unconsecrated, graveyards also caused disquiet. Such measures went against traditional practices of holding wakes and large public funerals, and raised fears of premature burial (especially as the corpses of cholera victims could exhibit muscle spasms hours after death). There were riots in many cities, where doctors, cholera hospitals, police stations and local magistrates were attacked. In Britain, the poor believed that doctors used cholera as an excuse to obtain bodies for anatomical studies. Riots broke out in Manchester and Paisley when evidence was uncovered of bodies and body parts being removed for dissection (Ackermann, 1983; Durey, 1979, pp.155–200; Frieden, 1977). Just as the poor had their own understanding of the causes of cholera, they also had their own methods of prevention. In 1849, the residents of a suburb of Leeds refused to clean their homes, but stood outside a local chemical works for hours on end. They knew that none of the workers in the factory had suffered from cholera in the earlier epidemic, and believed that the strong smells produced by the factory had disinfected the air (Sigsworth and Worboys, 1994, p.244). Religious or magical charms were also used against cholera. In Zurich, Switzerland, in 1867, children wore amulets against 'Madam Cholera' whom they pictured as an evil black woman who strangled her victims.

The only disease prevention strategy under which rich and poor were treated equally was smallpox vaccination. During the first half of the nineteenth century, many European countries passed legislation making vaccination compulsory for all infants – rich and poor alike. However, some parents from all classes doubted that the practice was safe. They feared that their children might become infected with other diseases through the vaccine (it was shown around 1870 that syphilis might be transmitted in this way), or that they would be harmed by the 'unnatural' process of infecting children with a disease of cows. In England, Switzerland and France in the 1860s, a small proportion of parents refused to comply with the law. Efforts in England to quash the opposition by fining or sending parents to jail seemed to increase resistance, and eventually the government was forced to pass a 'conscientious objection' Act allowing parents to opt out of vaccination.

7.5   The impact of public health reform

How effective were all these efforts – installing drains, scrubbing streets, hospitalizing reluctant cholera victims – in reducing the death toll from diseases in the middle and late nineteenth century?

Table 7.5 is very complex, not least because the categories of causes of death change over time. Study it carefully and answer the following questions.

1   When was there an overall decline in the death rate? Which diseases caused fewer deaths?

2   Did the mortality from any diseases increase?

3   Between 1871 and 1900, which diseases show the greatest decline in mortality?

Table 7.5   Average mortality per year per million from various causes in England and Wales[1]

Cause of death	1851–60	1861–70	1871–80	1881–90	1891–1900
Smallpox	221 (1.0%)	163 (0.7%)	236 (1.1%)	45 (0.2%)	13 (0.07%)
Measles	412 (1.8%)	440 (2.0%)	378 (1.7%)	440 (2.3%)	414 (2.3%)
Scarlet fever	876 (3.9%)	972 (4.3%)	716 (3.3%)	334 (1.8%)	158 (0.9%)
Diphtheria	109 (0.5%)	185 (0.8%)	121 (0.6%)	163 (0.8%)	263 (1.4%)
Whooping cough	503 (2.3%)	527 (2.3%)	512 (2.4%)	450 (2.4%)	377 (2.1%)
Fevers	908 (4.1%)[2]	885 (3.9%)[2]	484 (2.3%)[2]	235 (1.2%)[3]	182 (1.0%)[3]
Diarrhoeal diseases	1,080 (4.8)	1,070 (4.7)	935 (4.4%)	659 (3.4%)[4]	713 (3.9%)[4]
Cholera	———[5]	———[5]	———[5]	15 (0.08%)	25 (0.1%)
Tuberculosis	2,679 (12.1%)	2,475 (11.0%)	2,116 (9.9%)	1,724 (9.0%)	1,391 (7.6%)
Respiratory diseases	3,021 (13.6%)	3,364 (15.0%)	3,760 (17.7%)	3,729 (19.5%)	3,409 (18.7%)
Cancer	317 (1.4%)	387 (1.7%)	473 (2.2%)	589 (3.1%)	758 (4.2%)
Circulatory diseases	1,247 (5.6%)[6]	1,349 (6.0%)[6]	1,477 (6.9%)[6]	1,576 (8.2%)[7]	1,657 (9.1%)[7]
Deaths from all causes	22,165	22,416	21,272	19,080	18,194

[1] Note that the data in this table are not directly comparable with the data in earlier tables in this chapter: this table gives the number of deaths per million people living, not the number of deaths in the whole population
[2] Typhus, typhoid and continued fevers [3] Typhus and enteric fever [4] Diarrhoea and dysentery only
[5] Not separately recorded [6] Circulatory diseases and dropsy – which is often caused by circulatory problems
[7] Circulatory diseases
(Registrar-General's Office, 1884–5, p.cxii; Registrar-General's Office, 1895, p.c; Registrar-General's Office, 1905, p.clxxxii)

1   The overall decline in deaths began in 1870 and continued until 1900. However, the pattern of mortality for each disease between 1851 and 1900 did not follow this overall trend. Only two diseases definitely declined throughout the whole period – tuberculosis and fevers. (The decline in fevers was slightly boosted by removing continued fevers from this total after 1881.) There was a trend towards fewer deaths from scarlet fever, diarrhoeal diseases and smallpox, although this mortality increased in some decades.

2   Mortality from three disease categories definitely increased – cancer, circulatory diseases and respiratory diseases. Diphtheria mortality showed an upward trend, but did not rise consistently.

3   The mortality from scarlet fever (which declined from 3.3 per cent of deaths to 0.9 per cent), fevers (2.3 per cent to 1.0 per cent) and tuberculosis (9.9 per cent to 7.6 per cent) fell most substantially. Mortality from smallpox also fell rapidly from 1.1 per cent to 0.07 per cent after 1871, but this decline was exaggerated by the increased deaths in earlier years.

This table shows the beginning of a major shift in patterns of mortality. Between the middle of the nineteenth century and the early twentieth century, the mortality from infectious diseases declined across Europe. More people died from degenerative diseases – cancer and heart and circulatory diseases (such as strokes); a pattern of mortality that we still experience today. This shift is called the 'epidemiological transition'.

But was public health reform responsible for the declining death rates from infectious disease? As with much public health history, the data for England and Wales have been subject to the closest scrutiny. Early historians simply assumed that public health legislation had reduced mortality, but, as we have seen, these historians gathered little concrete evidence on the implementation of reforms, never mind their impact. In 1976, this assumption was challenged by Thomas MacKeown in his book *The Modern Rise of Population*. MacKeown was not a historian, but professor of social medicine at Birmingham University. At the time he was writing, sanitary reform as a policy was in decline, and social reforms – improvements to diet, living and working conditions – were seen as the key to improving public health. MacKeown, then, was open to the idea that factors other than sanitary reform might explain the observed decline in mortality. In his book, he considered a number of possible reasons. MacKeown dismissed late nineteenth-century medical treatment as a means of saving lives, arguing that there was little effective therapy for diseases, and that hospitals were more likely to kill than to cure their patients. (This was a common view at the time, before historians had conducted extensive research into nineteenth-century hospital records.) He argued that while sanitary reforms would have prevented water- and food-borne infections, such as cholera and typhoid, these were not the main contributors to the overall decline in mortality. The reduction in deaths was mainly due to a saving of lives from airborne infections, particularly bronchitis and tuberculosis. Such a

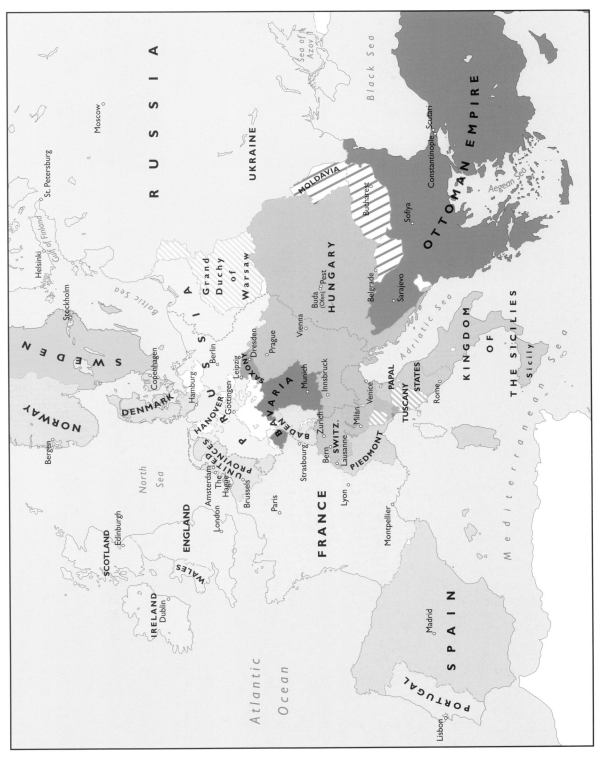

Plate 1   Europe, *c*.1800

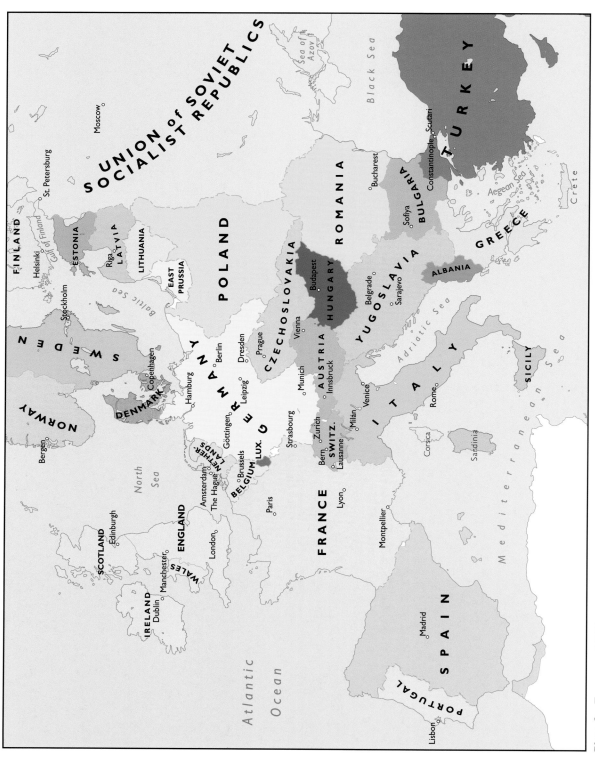

Plate 2 Europe, c.1930

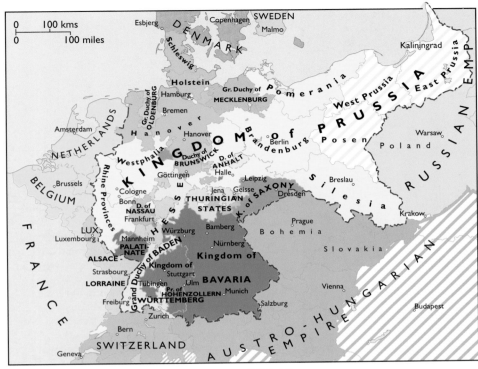

Plate 3   Formation of the German empire, 1864–71

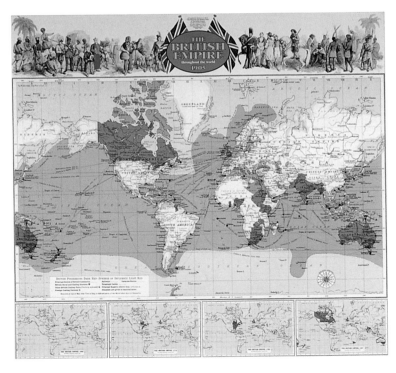

Plate 4   As well as providing geographical information, maps can make political statements. This world map of 1905 celebrates the British empire, emphasizing not only the extent of territory under British control, but also the historical growth of the empire and the array of indigenous people under colonial rule. By permission of Old House Books

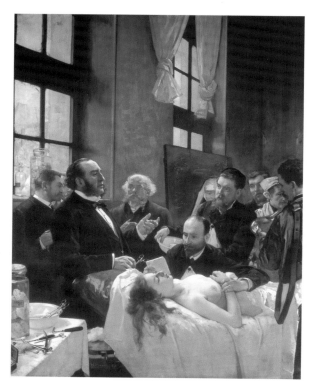

Plate 5   Henri Gervex, *Before the Operation, or Dr Pean Teaching at St Louis Hospital*, 1887, oil on canvas, 242 × 188 cm. In the late nineteenth century, surgeons, more than any other practitioners, seemed to have the knowledge and skills that could save lives, and they were often represented in this heroic manner. Here, Dr Pean is about to operate on a female patient. The patient's nakedness, her hair flowing over the pillow and her passivity under anaesthesia heighten the power relationship between patient and practitioner. The surgeon controls the situation; the patient is powerless and silent.
Bridgeman Art Library/Peter Willi

Plate 6   Thomas Eakins Cowperthwait, *The Gross Clinic*, 1875, oil on canvas, 244 × 198 cm. Knowledge brought power and prestige within the profession. In this portrait, Samuel Gross (1805–84), professor of surgery at Jefferson Medical College in Philadelphia, stands, literally, head and shoulders above his assistants, and turns to address the rows of students who observe his surgical skills within the operating theatre. Although surgery was held in high regard, the public wanted a sanitized view of the field: thus, the patient is almost invisible and depersonalized. However, the depiction of blood, on the scalpel in Gross's hand, caused great controversy.
Bridgeman Art Library, London

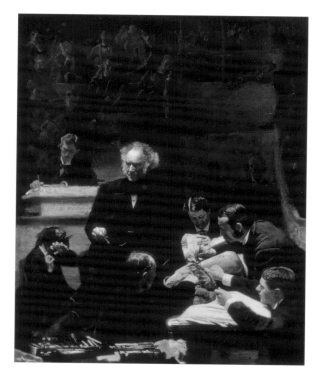

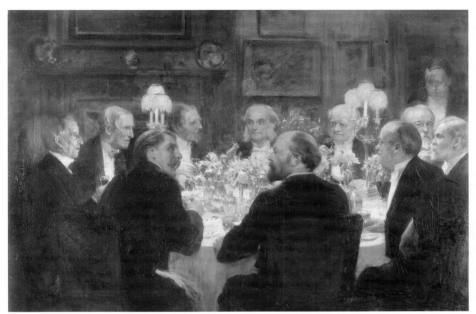

Plate 7   Solomon Joseph Solomon, *Octave for Mr Ernest Hart at Sir Henry Thompson's House*, *c*.1897, oil on canvas, 71.5 × 103.5 cm. This group portrait celebrates the work of Ernest Hart (1835–98), a medical man and editor of the *British Medical Journal*, 1867–9 and 1870–98. The *BMJ* was one of the leading medical journals of the day, and Hart's editorials on medical practice and politics helped to inform opinion within the profession. His high standing is reflected by the status and reputation of the other diners, who include Thomas Lauder Brunton (1844–1916), a pioneer in the treatment of heart disease, Thomas Spencer Wells (1818–97), a surgeon best known for his success in performing ovariotomies, and Victor Horsley (1857–1916), who researched into brain function. Wellcome Library, London

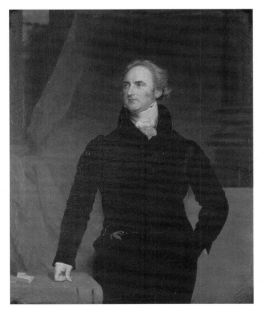

Plate 8   *Sir Astley Paston Cooper*, painting after Sir Thomas Lawrence, *c*.1830, oil on canvas, 76.5 × 63.5 cm. Astley Cooper was the most distinguished surgeon of his day. Estimates of his income vary from £15,000 to £20,000 – fabulous sums for the early nineteenth century. This painting emphasizes Cooper's high social standing and his education: his hand rests on a table with paper and an inkwell and there are classical columns (a reference to classical learning) in the background. Cooper carried enormous influence in medical circles and many of his pupils and relatives held important posts. Wellcome Library, London

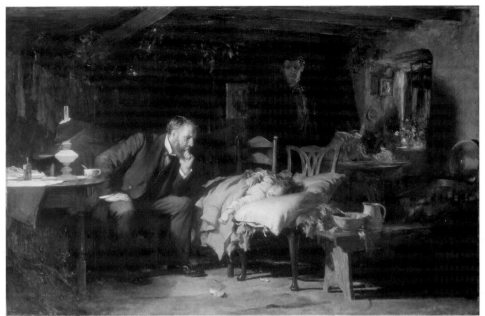

Plate 9   Luke Fildes, *The Doctor*, 1891, oil on canvas. This painting is not actually a portrait of a doctor at the bedside, but was constructed in the studio using a 'set' and artist's models. In it, a respectably dressed doctor anxiously scrutinizes the face of a sick child in a poor fisherman's cottage. In reality, such a poor fisherman would not have been able to afford the fees charged by such a doctor. The painting therefore exemplifies the public service ethos of the professional man, which medical practitioners sought to claim in the late nineteenth century. © Tate, London 2003

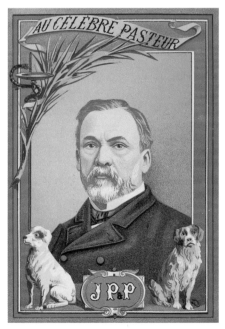

Plate 10   *Louis Pasteur*, *c.*1890, chromolithograph. This cheap print, which was produced in large numbers, shows the degree of fame enjoyed by Louis Pasteur as the result of his research into micro-organisms and his vaccines against rabies. By 1890, Pasteur had become a national hero, and the Pasteur Institute was funded largely through donations from the public. Here, as in a religious image, Pasteur is presented with symbols of his work – a palm (associated with victory), a snake and a bowl (symbols of hygiene) and two dogs (associated with Pasteur's work on rabies). Wellcome Library, London

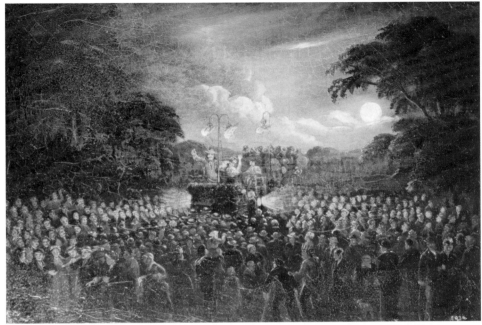

Plate 11 *Sequah on Clapham Common*, by an English painter, *c.*1890, oil on canvas, 30.3 × 40.6 cm. This painting is a reminder that irregular, as well as regular, medical practitioners gained prestige and power through their claims to possess specialist knowledge. 'Sequah' was a quack, who sold 'native Indian remedies' as part of a travelling show. This painting shows a scene that had changed little since the sixteenth century – the strangely dressed quack on a stage, aided by assistants, holding the attention of a large audience. It is a testament to a strong tradition in the methods of selling patent remedies, and to the popularity of such remedies in late Victorian England. Wellcome Library, London

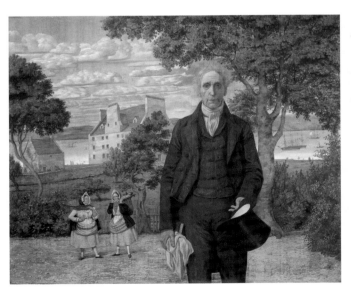

Plate 12 Richard Dadd, *Portrait of Alexander Morison*, 1852, oil on canvas, 51.1 × 61.3 cm. Richard Dadd murdered his father, was deemed criminally insane, and was committed to Bethlem Hospital and later to Broadmoor Asylum. While incarcerated, he pursued his career as a painter, and remains famous for his fairy paintings. This painting of Alexander Morison, who treated Dadd, is a rare portrait of a doctor painted by an asylum patient. Dadd takes Morison out of his social and medical context, placing him in an imaginary landscape, and thus robs the doctor of power and status. Morison becomes a tired, gentle man, whose sympathetic though rather haunted gaze meets the viewer's eye. Scottish National Portrait Gallery

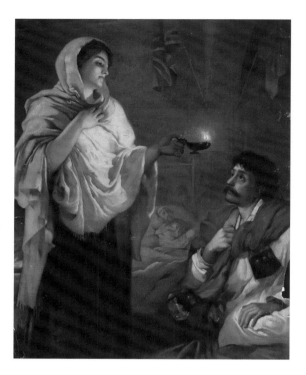

Plate 13 *Florence Nightingale with her Lamp, c.*1856, chromolithograph. This popular print – made at the time of the Crimean War – shows the heroic status accorded to Florence Nightingale in Britain as 'The Lady with the Lamp'. Here, Nightingale acquires social and political power by giving her caring skills in a patriotic cause, helping the sick and wounded British soldiers in the Crimean War. The image carries many religious overtones. The figure with the lamp (who bears little resemblance to Nightingale) is in a similar pose to that of the Madonna in a religious painting, offering succour to the patient sitting at her feet. Wellcome Library, London

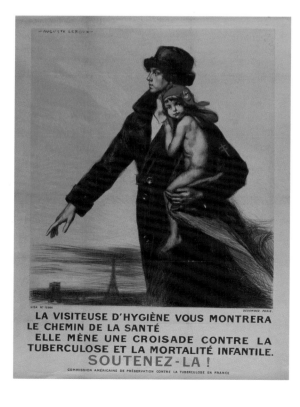

LA VISITEUSE D'HYGIÈNE VOUS MONTRERA
LE CHEMIN DE LA SANTÉ
ELLE MÈNE UNE CROISADE CONTRE LA
TUBERCULOSE ET LA MORTALITÉ INFANTILE.
SOUTENEZ-LA !
COMMISSION AMÉRICAINE DE PRÉSERVATION CONTRE LA TUBERCULOSE EN FRANCE

Plate 14   In the early twentieth century, governments across Europe launched a wide range of initiatives to guarantee the future wealth and strength of the country by improving the health of children. In this poster, which reads: 'The health visitor will show you the way to health. She leads a crusade against tuberculosis and infant mortality. Follow her!', the female health visitor is portrayed as the instrument by which these political and patriotic goals are achieved. The figure gestures forwards, suggesting progress. In her arms she holds a healthy child, who wears a red liberty cap, a symbol of France. Wellcome Library, London

reduction was the consequence of better nutrition, which helped individuals to fight off infection. Thus, an improved standard of living was the most significant factor in the decline of mortality in the late nineteenth century (MacKeown, 1976).

MacKeown's argument has in turn been challenged by Simon Szreter, a historical demographer. Szreter argued that the decline in tuberculosis deaths was not sustained throughout the late nineteenth century, and deaths from other airborne respiratory infections actually increased (as you saw in Table 7.5). He claimed that much of the overall saving of lives *was* due to a decline in water- and food-borne infections, and this decline coincided with a period of massive sanitary reform. To prove his point, Szreter analysed the huge sums lent by the British central government for sanitary improvements. Between 1858 and 1870, the government lent £11 million to local authorities, and between 1871 and 1894 it lent a further £84 million, a pattern which follows the observed overall reduction in deaths (Szreter, 1988).

Anne Hardy reached similar conclusions by looking at the issue from another angle – exploring the mortality from specific diseases rather than overall death rates. Her findings broadly agreed with Szreter: that local government action contributed to a decline in mortality. However, Hardy showed that such interventions included not only sanitary reform, but also immunization, slum clearance and education, which produced a decline in smallpox and tuberculosis as well as typhus. However, she reminded us that, even in 1900, public health measures could do little to prevent childhood diseases such as scarlet fever, measles and whooping cough (Hardy, 1993).

7.6   Conclusion

Clearly, nineteenth-century public health reform made a huge impact on the lives of Europeans. While actions against epidemics greatly reduced the numbers of deaths from diseases such as cholera and smallpox, sanitary reform not only saved lives but greatly improved the living conditions of urban dwellers. While public health reform was a massive achievement, we should not be too triumphalist: improvements were delivered unevenly across the population, and the poorer classes in greatest need of help were often the last to receive it. While governments tackled diseases that affected the adult population, children's diseases continued unchecked.

The history of public health is complex. It is tempting to think, as the early historians did, of public health as medicine on the grand scale, with national or international initiatives. But research carried out since the 1980s has shown that to understand public health we need to study the detail of reform. The views of doctors differed on the causation of different diseases, and these different views helped to shape national policy. (Although the role of practitioners in shaping sanitary reform is an area which requires further research.) National governments drew up legislation and set out programmes of action which were only partly dictated by medical ideas – they were also shaped by geography, economics, history and ideology. The local authorities who were responsible for implementing these agendas also had to respond to a further set of local contingencies –

financial, social, legal and environmental. The ultimate success of public health was not the result of big ideas, but of a myriad of local changes.

References

Ackerknecht, E.H. (1948) 'Anticontagionism from 1821 to 1867', *Bulletin of the History of Medicine*, vol.22, pp.562–93.

Ackermann, E. (1983) 'Medical care in the countryside near Paris, 1800–1914', *Annals of the New York Academy of Sciences*, vol.412, pp.1–18.

Baldwin, P. (1999) *Contagion and the State in Europe, 1830–1930*, Cambridge: Cambridge University Press.

Carroll, P.E. (2002) 'Medical police and the history of public health', *Medical History*, vol.46, pp.461–94.

Coleman, W. (1982) *Death is a Social Disease: Public Health and Political Economy in Early Industrial France*, Madison: University of Wisconsin Press.

Durey, M. (1979) *The Return of the Plague: British Society and the Cholera, 1831–32*, Dublin: Gill & Macmillan.

Evans, R. (1987) *Death in Hamburg: Society and Politics in the Cholera Years, 1830–1910*, Oxford: Clarendon Press.

Eyler, J.M. (1979) *Victorian Social Medicine: The Ideas and Methods of William Farr*, London: Johns Hopkins University Press.

Finer, S.E. (1952) *The Life and Times of Sir Edwin Chadwick*, London: Methuen.

Frieden, N. (1977) 'The Russian cholera epidemic, 1892–93 and medical professionalisation', *Journal of Social History*, vol.10, pp.538–59.

Gairdner, W.T. [1862] (2001) *Public Health in Relation to Air and Water*, facsimile reprint in K. White (ed.) *Early Sociology of Health and Illness*, vol.5, London: Routledge.

Hamlin, C. (1988) 'Muddling in Bumbledom: on the enormity of large sanitary improvements in four British towns, 1855–1885', *Victorian Studies*, vol.32, pp.55–83.

Hamlin, C. (1992) 'Predisposing causes and public health in early nineteenth-century medical thought', *Social History of Medicine*, vol.5, pp.43–70.

Hardy, A. (1993) *The Epidemic Streets: Infectious Disease and the Rise of Preventative Medicine, 1856–1906*, Oxford: Clarendon Press.

Kearns, G. (1988) 'Private property and public health reform in England, 1830–70', *Social Science and Medicine*, vol.26, pp.187–99.

La Berge, A.F. (1992) *Mission and Method: The Early Nineteenth-Century French Public Health Movement*, Cambridge: Cambridge University Press.

MacDonagh, O. (1977) *Early Victorian Government, 1830–1870*, London: Weidenfeld & Nicolson.

MacKeown, T. (1976) *The Modern Rise of Population*, London: Edwin Arnold.

Mort, F. (1987) *Dangerous Sexualities: Medico-Politics in England since 1830*, London: Routledge.

Porter, D. (ed.) (1994) *The History of Public Health and the Modern State*, Amsterdam: Rodopi.

Porter, D. (1999) *Health, Civilisation and the State: A History of Public Health from Ancient to Modern Times*, London: Routledge.

Registrar-General's Office (1857) '18th annual report', *Parliamentary Papers*, session II, vol.22.

Registrar-General's Office (1884–5) '45th annual report, supplement', *Parliamentary Papers*, vol.17.

Registrar-General's Office (1895) '55th annual report, supplement', *Parliamentary Papers*, vol.23.

Registrar-General's Office (1905) '65th annual report, supplement', *Parliamentary Papers*, vol.18.

Riley, J.C. (1987) *The Eighteenth-Century Campaign to Avoid Disease*, New York: St Martin's Press.

Rosen, G. (1974) *From Medical Police to Social Medicine: Essays on the History of Health Care*, New York: Science History Publications.

Sigsworth, M. and Worboys, M. (1994) 'The public's view of public health in mid-Victorian Britain', *Urban History*, vol.21, pp.237–50.

Smith, F.B. (1979) *The People's Health, 1830–1910*, London: Weidenfeld & Nicolson.

Szreter, S. (1988) 'The importance of social intervention in Britain's mortality decline *c*.1850–1914: a reinterpretation of the role of public health', *Social History of Medicine*, vol.1, pp.1–37.

Tomes, N. (1998) *The Gospel of Germs: Men, Women, and the Microbe in American Life*, London: Harvard University Press.

Wohl, A. (1983) *Endangered Lives: Public Health in Victorian Britain*, London: J.M. Dent.

Worboys, M. (2000) *Spreading Germs: Disease Theories and Medical Practice in Britain, 1865–1900*, Cambridge: Cambridge University Press.

Source Book readings

E.H. Ackerknecht, *A Short History of Medicine,* Baltimore: Johns Hopkins University Press, 1969, pp.210–17 (Reading 7.1).

'Report of Mr Gilbert' in E. Chadwick, *Report on the Sanitary Condition of the Labouring Population*, ed. by M.W. Flinn, Edinburgh: Edinburgh University Press, 1965, pp.80–1 (Reading 7.2i).

H. Mayhew, 'A visit to the cholera districts of Bermondsey', *Morning Chronicle*, 24 September 1849, p.4, reprinted in K. Flint (ed.) *The Victorian Novelist: Social Problems and Social Change*, London: Croom Helm, 1987, pp.165–8 (Reading 7.2ii).

C. Dickens, *Bleak House*, Boston: Houghton Mifflin, 1956, pp.167–8, 475 (Reading 7.2iii).

Editorial, *The Times*, 1 December 1865, p.6, col.d (Reading 7.2iv).

C. Hamlin, 'Edwin Chadwick, "mutton medicine" and the fever question', *Bulletin of the History of Medicine*, 1996, vol.70, pp.235–60 (Reading 7.3).

G. Kearns, 'Cholera, nuisances and environmental management in Islington, 1830–55' in W.F. Bynum and R. Porter (eds) *Living and Dying in London*, London: Wellcome Institute for the History of Medicine, 1991, pp.118–23 (Reading 7.4).

A.S. Wohl, *Endangered Lives: Public Health in Victorian Britain*, London: J.M. Dent, 1983, pp.105–7 (Reading 7.5).

Something Homely: A Fireside Chat, London: Jarrold, ?1872, pp.11–12 (Reading 7.6).

8

Colonial and Imperial Medicine

Michael Worboys

Objectives

By the end of this chapter you should be able to:

- describe the ways in which European medicine was transferred and adapted to different colonial settings;

- describe the disease control strategies developed by European colonial powers;

- understand the place of western medicine and its practitioners in the interaction between Europeans and the indigenous populations of colonial territories;

- assess the claim that medicine was a 'tool of empire';

- describe some of the views on race expressed in medical writings.

8.1   Introduction

Until quite recently, most historians saw the transfer of western medicine into colonial settings as one of the beneficial consequences of imperialism. The 'light' of progressive, improving medical science was brought by individual doctors, state services and missionary activity to 'dark' peoples on the 'dark' continents. The central notion of 'the spread of European medicine' to colonial territories led historians to adopt a simple centre–periphery model of this relationship, with a one-way flow of personnel, ideas and practices from Europe to colonial territories.

The new social history of colonial and imperial medicine is based on quite different assumptions. The impact of European medicine on the health of colonial peoples is now seen as not simply a 'good thing'. Historians today argue that while European-trained doctors in the colonies may have been more technically effective than indigenous practitioners, for the most part medicine was deployed to serve imperial policies. Many of these policies did not improve the health of colonial peoples, but directly and indirectly led to higher levels of disease. A key idea is that European medicine was a tool of empire used to support imperial expansion and rule, not least by the development of special bodies of knowledge and practice, principally tropical medicine and hygiene. Not all historians agree on the timing and extent of this deployment. Some emphasize that colonial medical policies were initially **enclavist**, prioritizing the health of European troops, traders and administrators. Others argue that medicine diffused towards subordinate peoples as a colonizing force, practically, in the control of epidemics, and ideologically, as a symbol of western cultural superiority. Also, while these 'tools' were designed by the 'colonizers', they were taken up by the 'colonized', often with unintended consequences.

Historians continue to use centre and periphery models in understanding the spread of western medicine, but they no longer understand it as a simple one-way flow. Rather, historians have demonstrated two-way flows of ideas and people – from the colonial periphery to the European centre.They have recognized, also, that centres and peripheries change over time and can be reversed, and they have shown how colonial institutions that were peripheries to European centres, were themselves centres within a colony or region. For example, the global network of Pasteur Institutes, set up in the wake of the development of anti-rabies vaccine in the 1880s, was intended to distribute the vaccines and other products of the Paris-based Pasteurian research programme. However, in time, the work of Pasteur Institutes in the colonies, for example, on the plague in the Far East, outshone that being carried out in Paris (Pelis, 1997). The Saigon Pasteur Institute, seen as peripheral to Paris, became the central research and service laboratory in French Indo-China and in the whole of south-east Asia.

In this chapter, I introduce the history of colonial medicine in a range of different types of colonies: 'settler' colonies, such as Australia and New Zealand, 'orientalist' colonies in India and 'executive' colonies in Africa. This division is very schematic (many colonies, including South Africa, do not fit readily into a single category), but it is a useful device for capturing the character of different spheres of empire. By comparing medical practice in these different types of colonies, I show how medicine was shaped not just by climate and indigenous disease patterns, but also by politics, culture and administration. (See Figure 8.1 for a map that shows the main European colonies.)

8.2   Medicine in settler colonies

Settler colonies, such as Australia, Canada and New Zealand, are characterized by large settlements of Europeans in areas where the indigenous population was small, or became small as a result of European settlement. Similarities in geography, climate and the disease environment allowed settlers to aim at the recreation of European society and culture overseas. European-style institutions were founded and were expected to remain subordinate to established centres in Europe. European practices were maintained in these institutions, but there was some adaptation to local circumstances. In some colonies, for example, distances within the colony and between the colony and Europe presented problems in the provision of medical services.

In these settler colonies, the main aim for medicine was to recreate European medical institutions, following the precedent of North America. For much of the nineteenth century, the tacit policy of the profession and of local governments was to emulate metropolitan institutions and practices, though the time lags involved often meant that settlers created the medicine of the Britain they left behind many years ago rather than that current in the metropolis. The medical profession was predominantly educated in Britain. Between 1850 and 1901, in the state of

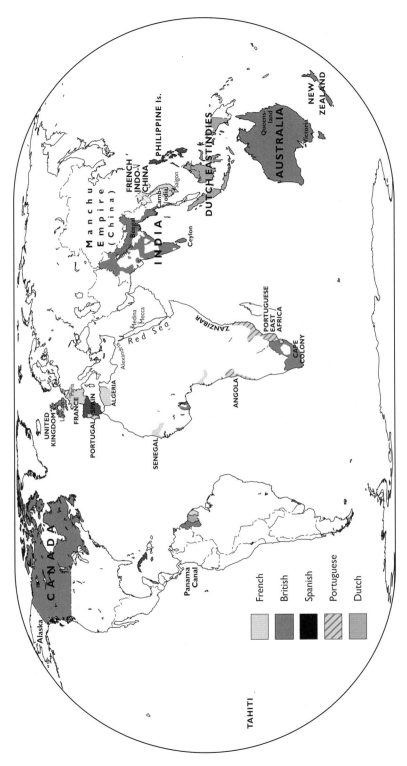

Figure 8.1 Main European possessions, 1878.

Victoria, Australia, 48.5 per cent of doctors held degrees from Scottish universities, 7 per cent from Irish and 5 per cent from English institutions. The remaining 39.5 per cent qualified in Melbourne, Victoria, although the number of colonially trained doctors increased greatly towards the end of the century. Professionally, the subordinate status of doctors working in the colonies was exemplified in the fact that national medical associations remained branches of the British Medical Association. Even in the early twentieth century, by which time both Australia and Canada had developed an impressive range of professional, clinical and public health services, doctors seeking advanced training and research opportunities went abroad to Britain or the United States. Adaptation to local circumstances can also be demonstrated. In Australia, for example, few voluntary hospitals were established because the aristocratic and middle-class groups that supported them in Britain were absent or relatively small in the colony.

As a result of their education, social connections and prestige, many doctors played a leading role in the political and social development of the new settler colonies. In South Africa, where the aim was to establish a settler colony, Sir Leander Starr Jameson (1853–1917), a graduate of London's University College Medical School, moved from being 'The Doctor' in the Kimberley goldfields to the trusted lieutenant of Cecil Rhodes. And in December 1895, he was leader of the ill-fated Jameson Raid that soured relations between Dutch settlers and the British. In New Zealand, Frederick Truby King (1858–1938), an early paediatrician, became involved in social reform initiatives that focused on maternal and child welfare and aimed to counter physical degeneration among 'the white race'. (Such schemes were used in Europe to promote the health of different nations. You will read about these in Chapter 9.)

As well as providing medical services, doctors played a leading role in changing ideas about the indigenous populations of settler colonies. In the mid-nineteenth century, they helped to elaborate on the new ideas of race, ideas which in turn were used to legitimize colonial policies. Until this time, the dominant assumption in scientific and medical circles was that human form and function, like that of other animals and plants, had been made to suit geography and climate. Enlightenment thinkers assumed that human nature was the same all over the globe: human diversity was the product of acclimatization and adaptation to different surroundings. This phenomenon could be observed in individual adaptations, such as darkening of the skin of Europeans in tropical climes, or collectively in the **seasoning** of immigrant communities in North America, where they gradually became able to withstand attacks of what were seen as indigenous diseases. However, after 1850 a new conception of 'race' emerged, in which greater stress was placed on innate or biological differences, the limits of human adaptation, the dominance of nature over nurture and an evolutionary hierarchy of human types. As a consequence, doctors became increasingly pessimistic about the possibility of European settlement of certain hostile areas in settler colonies. For example, Queensland in Australia and parts of southern Africa were recast as distinctly tropical and unsuitable for settlement.

While the notion of a switch in ideas of race around the 1840s and 1850s is useful, not just for settler colonies but for other spheres of empire, ideas of racial

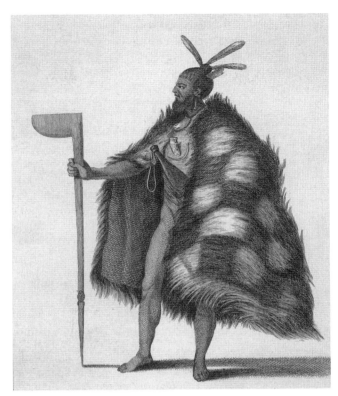

Figure 8.2   A typical image of the Maori as a Noble Savage, *c.*1723. This picture was drawn by Sydney Parkinson, who travelled on James Cook's *Endeavour* as artist to the voyage's naturalist, Joseph Banks. Parkinson drew all the different parts of nature – animal (including humans), vegetable and mineral. © Historical Picture Archive/Corbis

difference were complex. In a study of medical writings on the Maori people of New Zealand and of policies that were made concerning them, Malcolm Nicolson has identified four different views: the Noble Savage (Figure 8.2), the Romantic Savage, the Amalgamating Savage and the Dying Savage (Nicolson, 1988). Common to each view is the notion of the inherent biological and cultural inferiority of the Maoris and their culture, judged against the yardstick of Europeans and their civilization. The Maori as Noble Savage was an echo of the philosopher Jean-Jacques Rousseau's idea that people were happy and peaceful before the advent of civilization, when they were corrupted by society, and it remained current in the early nineteenth century. This optimistic view stressed that the health and physical vigour of the Maori people, along with their moral and religious sensibilities, were such that they would gain little if anything from European culture and medicine. The notion of the Romantic Savage, which Nicolson identifies as emerging in the 1830s, has certain similarities with the Noble Savage, but its advocates made more of Maori closeness to nature and their physical adaptation to the local environment. And, while they were seen as pagans who would benefit from civilizing forces, at least they had the potential to benefit from such influences, especially Christian missionary teaching and charity. The view of the Amalgamating Savage was a product of the 1840s, with Maoris constituted as people who could be incorporated into settler culture and institutions, and who would benefit from changed habits and beliefs. In fact, they would not be improved as such, but would over several generations be absorbed into the superior white race, although some of their characteristics might occasionally re-emerge many generations later. The idea of the Dying Savage entered medical discourse after the 1850s, when Maoris were portrayed not only as inferior and physically weak, but also as essentially unimprovable and likely to suffer through contact with superior white civilization. This notion was later given a Darwinian twist, when Maoris were seen as likely losers in the struggle for existence and were thought to be facing inevitable extinction. This view became dominant in the last quarter of the nineteenth century, exemplified in Dr William Buller's statement in 1884 that: 'The aboriginal race must in time give place to a more highly organized one. This seems to be one of the inscrutable laws of Nature' (quoted in Nicolson, 1988, p.91).

Exercise

Read the five quotations below and decide which view of the Maori is represented by each. Remember, there are four views – Noble Savage, Romantic Savage, Amalgamating Savage and Dying Savage – therefore one view is illustrated twice.

1   'As the Anglo Saxon settlers in New Zealand must soon outnumber the aborigines, the features of the Maori race will disappear from amongst the half-caste, although traces of their blood will occasionally be seen in families after many generations' (quoted in Nicolson, 1988, p.82).

2   'The natives of New Zealand ... are of a very superior order, both in point of personal appearance and intellectual endowment ... The men are ... well proportioned and exhibit evident marks of great strength' (quoted in Nicolson, 1988, p.68).

3   'Beyond thinning the forest of its stately inhabitants and propagating amongst natives a filthy and terrible disease, commerce ... left the country unimproved by her visitations and its aboriginal tenantry, not a little injured' (quoted in Nicolson, 1988, p.74).

4   '[Before venereal diseases were introduced Maoris were] a race of people hitherto enjoying a constitution of body remarkably sound and healthy. In a few generations, in all probability, how great will be the change – children of diseased parents ... will grow up a puny race; and in many instances both miserable and disgusting; in no respect resembling the hardy inhabitants of the island' (quoted in Nicolson, 1988, p.70).

5   'If, by the intrusion of vigorous races of Europe, smiling farms and busy markets are to take the place of the rough clearing and hut of the savage, and the millions of a populous country, with arts and letters, the matured policy, and the ennobling impulses are to replace the few thousands of the scattered tribes now

living in an apparently aimless and unprogressive state, even the most sensitive of philanthropists may learn to look with resignation, if not complacency on ... a people which, in the past had accomplished so imperfectly every object of Man's being' (quoted in Nicolson, 1988, pp.86–7).

Discussion

1   This illustrates the notion of the Amalgamating Savage. It is taken from A.S. Thomson's *The Story of New Zealand: Past and Present, Savage and Civilised* (1859). The author points to the beneficial effects of racial mixing, though it was, of course, the amalgamation of two races at different levels of evolution, as when he states that 'Caucasian blood [that] already flows in the veins of two thousand of the native population ... [was producing] another and a better class' (quoted in Nicolson, 1988, p.82).

2   This quotation from J. Savage's *Some Account of New Zealand* (1807) clearly exemplifies the idea of the Noble Savage.

3   This quotation is from a travelogue by W.B. Marshall entitled *A Personal Narrative of Two Visits to New Zealand in Her Majesty's Ship 'Alligator'* (1836). It illustrates the idea of the Romantic Savage as an admirable race damaged by contact with western civilization and its diseases.

4   Here is another illustration of the Romantic Savage. Missionaries, who worried about the damaging effects on Maoris of contact with military and secular forces, often suggested that Christianity was a superior pacifying force, not least when it was associated with Christian morality of sexual and other relations. (Note that this quotation is also taken from Savage's *Some Account of New Zealand*. The fact that two different views are expressed by Savage in this one text, proves that authors can be inconsistent and demonstrates the need for careful, critical reading.)

5   This quotation was taken from an article by W.T.L. Travers that was published in 1869 in a medical journal, *Transactions of the New Zealand Institute*. It shows the Dying Savage disappearing as the result of natural Darwinian laws, hence there was no need to mourn the loss.

Nicolson relates these different views of the Maori to the professional and political interests of the doctors that articulated them, for example, whether they were private practitioners or worked in public health, and to the presumed social role of the hospital. While the Maori were perceived to be Romantic Savages then the hospital provided not only care, but a means by which missionaries might convert them to the Christian faith. Once the Maori were thought of as Amalgamating Savages then the hospital was seen as a vehicle to educate them in western ways and behaviours while they were treated alongside European patients. When the Maori was thought of as a dying race, then hospital care served no purpose, and many of the facilities set up to treat Maori people fell into disrepair.

8.3   India: epidemics, orientalism and hegemony

In an orientalist colony, a small European army and administration was sent to govern developed cultures, such as those in India, Vietnam (Indo-China), North Africa and the Middle East. The transfer of western medicine to these colonies was more selective and adaptive than it was in the settler colonies, partly as a result of the more variable and often hostile disease environments. Medical services directly supported imperial economic and political institutions. In such orientalist colonies, European-trained doctors, often military men, worked in difficult climatic and cultural conditions to promote the health of Europeans and to control the epidemics that threatened trade and social order. Medicine also helped to legitimize the 'civilizing mission', an increasing part of which became the training of local people in western medicine and the censuring of indigenous religious and medical systems.

Until the end of the nineteenth century, most British doctors in India were military officers. Their priorities were first to maintain the health of British troops, then to look after the well-being of Indian soldiers and finally, when the need arose, to help control epidemics within the wider population. In the cities and larger towns some **Indian Medical Service** (IMS) doctors engaged in private and hospital practice, but such opportunities were limited because of the small numbers of Europeans present. The 1840s saw an apparent oversupply of doctors in Britain, which led some practitioners to seek work overseas. The IMS could afford to be selective and the educational standard of its doctors was equal to or better than the European norm. By the second half of the nineteenth century, local medical colleges and schools were producing growing numbers of Indian doctors trained in western medicine. These doctors were of two types. The medical colleges produced graduates whose qualifications were, in theory at least, equivalent to those who qualified in Britain. These colleges became local or regional training centres and were associated with large hospitals. The medical schools produced practitioners of lower rank, known as 'sub-assistant surgeons'. Their training was less advanced and was designed for those practising among the Indian people, especially in rural areas. The increasing demand among Indians for western medicine, and indeed for the elite to have their sons qualify as its practitioners, was seen at the time as recognition of its superiority over indigenous healing practices. However, such superiority had not always been assumed.

Exercise

Study these verses from a poem written in 1813. What do they indicate about British attitudes to Indian lifestyles?

> Observe the Hindoo, whose untutor'd mind,
> All false seductive luxury declines;
> To Nature's wants his wishes are confined,
> While Health her empire o'er his frame maintains.

His modes of life, by ancient sages plann'd
To suit the temper of his burning skies,
He, who the climate's rage would long withstand,
Will wisely imitate, nor e'er despise!

(quoted in Harrison, 1998, p.86)

Discussion

Indians are assumed to lack education, yet they avoid a decadent, unhealthy lifestyle and follow nature's dictates – the best route to good health. What is being suggested here is something akin to Nicolson's notion of the Romantic Savage – the 'untutor'd mind' had very simple, natural needs and a balance of body and soul. The poem goes on to show respect for Indian religious thought, with the notion that a guide to nature's ways had been set out in ancient wisdom, particularly ways of avoiding the effects of climate. Finally, the poet suggests that British colonists should copy Indian ways and that they should not look down on them.

The humoral system is described in the section on bedside medicine and the new ideas that followed in Chapter 1.

Before 1850, many British doctors felt they had much to learn from the medical systems of India and an exchange of ideas was common. European and Indian medicine shared a similar humoral model of the body: in both systems disease was linked to 'imbalances' within the body and body and soul were inextricably linked. Contemporaries observed that neither system enjoyed decisively superior therapeutic results. Western doctors assumed that many diseases were associated directly with places or were affected by local circumstances, thus, indigenous practitioners would have greater knowledge of local diseases and their ecologies. Many British doctors in India advised people to follow Indian diets, dress and lifestyles. Western doctors also believed that God's providence had provided natural remedies for most afflictions and that these would also be local.

The gulf that appeared between European and Indian medicine during the second quarter of the century was part of a wider shift in attitudes towards indigenous cultures and people. This saw, for example, the establishment of English as the official language of government and education in India, and the emergence of modern racial categories. As the racial superiority of Europeans and of their civilization was increasingly defined in terms of technology, industrialization was seen to have put Britain and then other western countries at a higher level of civilization (Adas, 1989). The rise of 'hospital medicine', with the eclipse of the humoral model and the development of ideas of disease as a process localized within certain organs or tissues, meant that European and Indian medicines were based on completely different understandings of the body. At the same time, the drive for improved professional status among rank-and-file practitioners led to attacks on the competence, effectiveness and ethical standards of every other type of medical practice in Britain (as you have read in Chapter 5). A similar process went on in India, with western practitioners attacking irregular and unorthodox Indian healers.

Medicine as a tool of empire

Many historians have seen medicine in India as shaped by its function as a tool of empire, used by states to support imperial expansion. Just as establishing a hospital in a town in northern England or demolishing slum housing in Paris (described in Chapter 7) served not only to improve health but also to control social unrest, medicine served the interests of colonial rulers by protecting the health of their armies and administrators. In India, throughout the nineteenth century, the overwhelming preponderance of doctors was engaged in looking after army personnel. Military doctors were employed to combat the high disease and death rates among European troops, who suffered mainly from malaria and dysentery. These were tackled using the sanitary reform practices described in Chapter 7, rather than through clinical practice, which markedly reduced the mortality rate over the century, though **morbidity rates** (levels of disease and illness) remained high. The success of sanitary reform was made possible by the post-1850 pattern of settlement. The British in India became more enclavist, they lived in camps or cantonments where they benefited from improved water supplies, safe sewerage systems and reduced contact with indigenous communities. They also received better advice on individual precautions, for example, taking quinine to prevent malaria.

Medicine also served as a tool of empire when applied to indigenous populations. European doctors in India assisted municipal and state authorities in combating the many epidemics. This not only helped to protect the lives of British and Indian soldiers, but also helped to safeguard internal and external trade and maintain social and political order. In the early nineteenth century, just as in Europe, the **East India Company** (the commercial company which effectively ruled India) attempted to control smallpox with a vaccination programme for all children. However, the scheme met with difficulties. There were problems in the transfer of the technology, especially in maintaining a viable vaccine in the heat of an Indian summer. Also, many Indian people objected to having their infants vaccinated with fluid taken from pustules of a previously vaccinated child, if that child was of a lower **caste**. Another problem arose as a result of different understandings of the vaccination procedure. British officials assumed, wrongly in many instances, that Hindus would not object to a vaccine originally derived from the cow, the sacred animal of their religion. It was thought that they would see vaccination as an improvement on the indigenous practice of variolation or inoculation (deliberately infecting a child with a mild strain of smallpox). However, Indians did not experience variolation or vaccination as purely medical procedures, but rather associated them with religious ritual and appeasing Sitala – the goddess of smallpox. Thus, what to European medical eyes was a choice between medical techniques was to Indians something invested with cultural, religious and political meanings.

After the **Indian Mutiny** of 1857, when the governance of India shifted from the East India Company to the British crown, a period known as the Raj, there followed more attempts to extend public health measures to the Indian population, partly in an effort to prevent further civil unrest (Figure 8.3). Sanitary commissioners were appointed to the main regions, but day-to-day responsibility rested with local authorities, whose officials struggled against permissive legislation, low revenues and the absence of funds for large capital schemes, such as sewerage. You may have realized that there are many parallels between Indian sanitary reform described here and sanitary reform in Europe, described in the previous chapter. In both cases, local officials struggled to implement practices; the wealthiest classes and western communities were the first to benefit, while the poorest people and indigenous peoples were subjected to sanitary practices regardless of whether they approved of them.

While historians agree that medicine did serve as a tool of empire, they differ in their interpretations of the functions it served. Some Indian historians have argued that European medicine remained essentially enclavist – primarily serving colonial armies and administrators – and that Indians did not benefit from the spread of medical expertise. Others, such as David Arnold (1993), have argued that European medicine was spread to the Indian population, albeit unevenly, and became a significant colonizing force. Arnold argues further that medicine and preventive programmes had a second function. As well as directly tackling disease, they helped to secure the consent of Indians to British rule by symbolizing the humanitarian intent of the government in bringing advanced science and technology to the sub-continent.

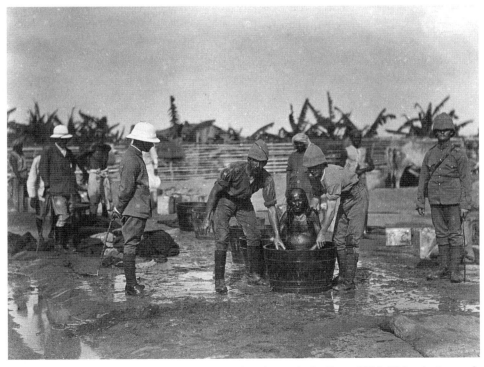

Figure 8.3 Disinfection of patients with the plague in India, c.1896. This photograph portrays passive Indian people receiving the 'benefits' of modern sanitation. From the perspective of the Indian community, of course, many of these measures were coercive, intrusive and may have been contrary to what they thought were the best ways to combat the disease. Wellcome Library, London

A useful test of these interpretations is the policy of the government of India in the control of cholera. As you read in Chapter 7, from the 1830s, this high-profile disease spread around the world causing high mortality and public panic. Governments were prompted to develop short- and long-term programmes of sanitary reform to deal with the epidemics. Long-running debates on whether the disease was contagious and on how to halt the epidemics highlighted the key policy issue of whether to institute quarantines and other medical police measures. There was general agreement that all of the epidemics spread out from the Bengal and Ganges river basin, the home of Asiatic cholera. And, from the 1860s, governments in the Middle East and the Mediterranean imposed quarantines on ships from India when epidemics threatened. These measures were opposed by the government of India because of their effect on trade and the administrative and political difficulties they created. The government's experts remained anticontagionist, being wedded to the idea that cholera was a disease of specific localities, and that it was airborne and could arise spontaneously. When quarantines were imposed on Indian shipping in the Red Sea, pilgrimages to Mecca and Medina were affected, leading religious leaders to blame the British for the delays, restrictions and higher costs. Despite international pressures and the interruption of trade, the government of India did little to tackle the problem of cholera directly. The effects of the epidemics were sporadic and relatively short-lived, so rather than plan nation-wide improvements, blame was cast on the 'filthy habits' of the Indian people and any measures against the disease were left to the poorly funded local sanitary authorities.

Historians have explained this lack of action in a number of ways: enclavism, and hence indifference to the suffering of Indians; medical uncertainties, leading to policy paralysis; financial and legislative constraints on sanitary authorities; the complex internal and external geography of the epidemics; and fear of the political consequences of intervening in the social and cultural practices of the Indian people. All of these factors were significant, and the latest research suggests that the balance of factors varied between epidemics, across time and in different localities. At certain times and places, especially if imperial interests were not threatened, the policies of the Raj were enclavist, but at other times and places, especially if trade or the social order was at risk, then intervention could be swift, as with quarantines in the case of the plague.

While Arnold supports the contention that medical and public health services in India were tools of empire, he questions the extent to which medical and public health measures were necessarily coercive in the ways they were deployed. Instead, he suggests that to a large extent western medicine spread by consent and was adapted and assimilated into Indian society and culture, especially by Indian elites.

Exercise

Read 'Health, race and nation' (Source Book 2, Reading 8.1). In what ways does Arnold show the ambivalence of Indian elites to western medicine with regard to race and nationalism?

Arnold presents an array of examples – from cases where Indians appear wholeheartedly to adopt the views of western practitioners, to instances where Indians reject western medicine on political rather than medical grounds. He points out that it was common in British discussions of the sub-continent to portray India as a country of many races and to place these on a hierarchy. In many respects this reinforced the caste-based ideas of human difference already current in India. Thus, in the twentieth century, Hindu critics of child marriage drew on the notion of degeneration that was current in western medical discourses on a range of disease problems, which itself drew on ideas from Darwinism and eugenics. The racial decay of Indians was firmly blamed on the changes and dislocation wrought by British rule, with many Indians imagining a 'golden age' of health and prosperity before colonization. The key to an Indian revival was not simply to throw off the yoke of British rule, but for Indians to regenerate their culture in a new way that reflected their spiritual values over the materialism of the west. Thus, while the sanitary technologies of Europeans might produce water that was clean and **pathogen**-free by scientific criteria, Indians should aim to produce healthy, pure water. Mostly, this involved the selective adoption and adaptation of western science and medicine, though in the case of Mahatma Gandhi there was outright rejection. Nonetheless, Arnold suggests that the vehemence of Gandhi's attack on western medicine is perhaps revealing of the influence and power that doctors were achieving among Indians. Arnold's work is underpinned by the notion of 'hegemony', which emphasizes the ways in which power was exercised through cultural agencies that win the assent of the ruled by defining what is and what is not possible and by establishing dominant values.

8.4   Africa: tropical medicine and executive power

A third type of administration was evident after 1880 in the newly annexed colonies of Africa and the older colonies in the West and East Indies (Figure 8.4). In these mostly tropical colonies, a relatively small European military and political administration had executive power over often sparsely populated regions, with cultures that varied from those termed 'primitive' to those that were highly developed. European medicine had only a meagre presence in tropical areas before the twentieth century. The few doctors present were attached to the military, served in ports and large towns or practised as missionary doctors. The dearth of doctors reflected the very small number of Europeans.

Disease presented a major problem for imperial powers. The dominant image of Africa in the nineteenth century was that of the 'white man's grave', a view that many commentators see as continuous with the modern notion of Africa as the 'sick' continent (Prins, 1989). The reported mortalities among those involved in slave and commodity trading were very high, for Africans especially but also for Europeans. There were high rates of death and invalidism among the European military, administrative and commercial personnel resulting from so-called 'tropical' diseases. For example, between 1830 and 1840, six successive governors

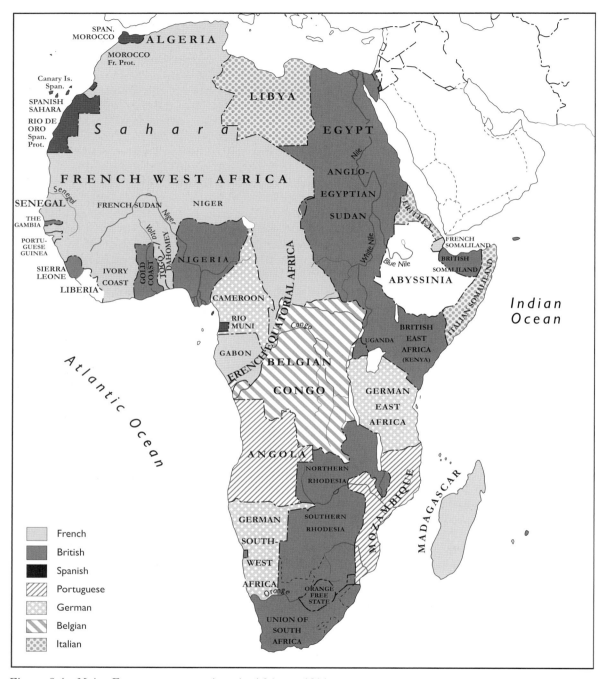

Figure 8.4   Major European possessions in Africa, *c*.1914

of the Dutch settlement of Christianborg (near Accra in modern Ghana) died, a key factor in the decision of the Dutch government to sell their possessions in West Africa to the British. The British expeditions to find the course and source of the Niger, that ran from 1832 to 1854, were described by contemporaries as 'little short of murder'. However, it would be wrong to extrapolate the experience of the west coast to the whole continent; the north and south had established European settlements and the east had a mixed record. Also, many explorers expected there to be healthy regions within the continent where European settlement would be possible. Indeed, the earliest travels of David Livingstone (1813–73) aimed to find areas free of dangerous fevers where new missionary stations might be established. Such hopes reflected the wider ambivalence of European culture towards the tropics, where along with the fear of death and darkness and the threat of the unknown went the excitement of discovery and possibilities of great wealth from abundant plants and untapped mineral sources (Curtin, 1964, pp.58–87; Stepan, 2001, pp.11–30). This ambivalence was nowhere better seen than in West Africa, where the notion of the 'white man's grave' coexisted with that of the wealth of the Gold Coast and Ivory Coast.

For much of the nineteenth century, the health problems that Europeans faced in Africa were not seen to be wholly unique to tropical latitudes – after all, the health of Europeans living on equatorial Pacific Ocean islands was good. The problem in large parts of Africa was seen to be a combination of climate, topography, vegetation, fauna and flora, and human ecology. New ideas of race implied that European bodies were unfit for African conditions. While early settlers in North America, South America, Australasia and elsewhere in Africa had experienced high rates of death and disease, these eventually fell as migrants became seasoned to their new environment. In equatorial Africa, after 1850, many doctors and experienced travellers argued that the limits of acclimatization had been reached, partly because environmental conditions were so extreme and partly because their accepted ideas of race seemed to set biological limits on the mutability of European bodies. Underlying such views was an assumption, undoubtedly false, that the indigenous population enjoyed rude good health because of their inherited and acquired racial features (such as dark skins and particular statures), which fitted them for African conditions.

Philip Curtin has recently revised the pessimistic view of the health of Europeans in tropical Africa in the nineteenth century. His research uses the concept of relocation costs: the difference between soldiers' death rates in Europe compared with those in tropical stations. His conclusion is that soldiers posted overseas actually gained more from the 'mortality revolution' of the nineteenth century than soldiers posted in Europe. The improvement was only a relative one, however, as by the end of the century, troops were still more likely to die of disease if they were posted abroad. But, their chances of survival were much better than those of soldiers in the early part of the century. And there was an exception to the rule among French troops in Tahiti. They had a higher life expectancy than soldiers at home, because food and hygiene was better on the South Pacific island than it was in France. Curtin attributes the reduction in relocation costs to changes in medico-sanitary ideas and practices. In 1964, he wrote that the mortality decline was a result of 'tropical medicine and the triumph of empiricism', with two main periods of innovation and improvement. The first was an empirically driven phase from the middle decades of the nineteenth century, based on the application of sanitary principles, such as the compilation of vital statistics on the health of particular stations, better advice on behaviour during seasoning, the adoption of the lessons of medical topography, especially the building of settlements on high ground and the seasonal use of hill stations, and the adoption of quinine prophylaxis for malaria (Figure 8.5). Many of these policies were imported directly from European public health schemes, but others were developed locally. The second phase came towards the end of the century and centred on campaigns against mosquitoes and on segregation in towns, both measures that were developed in the light of new findings on the causes of tropical fevers (Curtin, 1964, pp.343–62; Curtin, 1989, pp.40–61, 104–29).

The emergence of tropical medicine

The claim that tropical diseases represented a distinct area of medical practice was first made in 1897 by Patrick Manson (1844–1922), then a physician at the Seaman's Hospital, Greenwich and medical adviser to the Colonial Office (Haynes, 2000). Manson had emerged as Britain's leading expert in this area of medicine, from his experiences and research in China and Hong Kong in the 1870s and 1880s, and from his work as a consultant in London in the 1890s. His wish that specialist training in tropical medicine be institutionalized was granted in 1898. Rather than tropical medicine becoming a regular specialty with lecturers in every medical

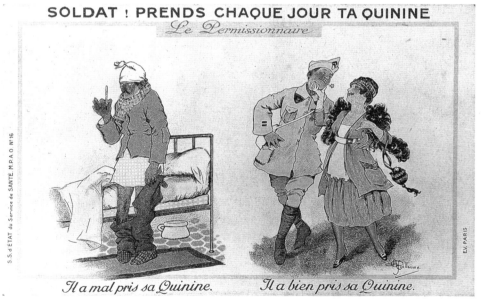

Figure 8.5   This poster, by Albert Guillaume, *c*.1900, was aimed at the French soldier on leave ('le permissionnaire'). It reads: 'Soldier! Take your quinine every day', and contrasts the pain of not taking quinine regularly with the benefits of doing so. These posters were widely disseminated, as the army had trouble getting soldiers to stick to a regular quinine regime. Wellcome Library, London

school, two dedicated institutions were founded – the London School of Tropical Medicine and the Liverpool School of Tropical Medicine. Manson was appointed head of the London school (Figure 8.6).

The crucial research which set the agenda for the new specialty was undertaken by Ronald Ross, who spent many years in India. His work culminated in 1897, when he was able to demonstrate that malaria was caused by a **protozoan** parasite and spread by mosquitoes. (The mosquito was the vector, transmitting the disease-causing parasite.) This parasite–vector mechanism, first discovered in malaria, became the model for researchers. It was discovered in many other important tropical diseases, for example, sleeping sickness (caused by the parasite trypanosoma and transmitted by tsetse-flies), yellow fever (caused by a virus and transmitted by mosquitoes), **leishmaniasis** (caused by protozoa and transmitted by sandflies) and **bilharzia** (caused by parasitic flukes and transmitted by water snails). The investigations also spawned new biological specialties – parasitology (the study of parasites, which range from single-cell organisms to tapeworms) and helminthology (the study of worms). It also transformed entomology (the study of insects) from an amateur pastime to a subject of systematic scientific investigation. The spectre of parasite-carrying insects did much to popularize the germ theory of disease and to suggest that the best way to control communicable diseases was to destroy disease agents or their carriers.

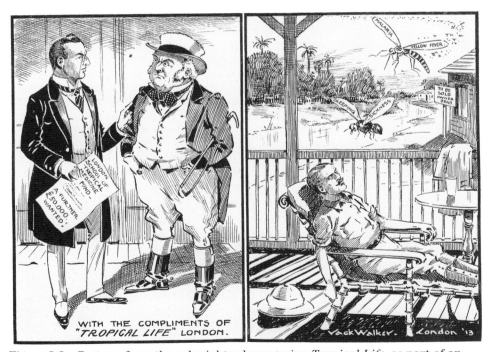

Figure 8.6   Cartoon from the colonial trade magazine *Tropical Life*, as part of an appeal for funds for the London School of Tropical Medicine, 1913. The drawing highlights how insects, and especially the mosquito, loomed large in the public and scientific perception of tropical medicine. By permission of the British Library, shelfmark: (P)CA711-E (2)

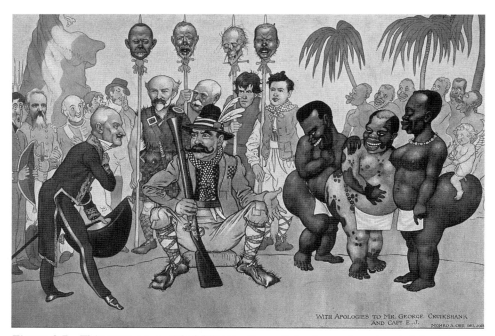

Figure 8.7   This cartoon, entitled *Mission Parasitologique*, almost certainly dates from the International Congress of Tropical Medicine in 1913. The two main figures are Professor Louis Blanchard (left), a leading French expert on tropical medicine and parasitology, and Louis Sambon, an Italian scientist, portrayed as a Neapolitan bandit, who had worked with Patrick Manson on the confirmation of the mosquito–malaria hypothesis. The racism and sexism that was characteristic of tropical medicine at this time is evident in Sambon's presentation to Blanchard of three Hottentot women. Blanchard was researching the anatomical features of different ethnic groups, hence one woman has an unusual pattern of skin pigmentation and another has large (steatopygous) buttocks. The four 'hunters' in the centre and the impaled heads they carry represent leading British figures. The hunters are, from left, James Cantlie, Patrick Manson and two unknown men. The impaled heads are, from left, Rickard Christophers, an unknown man, possibly Sir William Macgregor, Robert Leiper and Ronald Ross (Bruce-Chwatt, 1979, pp.353–5). Wellcome Library, London

Imperial ambitions and rivalries among European nations ensured that these discoveries attracted international political and scientific attention. This was the time of the 'scramble for Africa', as European governments sought to establish new territories. The tropics were seen as a source of knowledge, and there was an international competition to make new discoveries (Figure 8.7). The understanding of transmission mechanisms opened up three possible means of controlling the spread of disease: to kill the parasite; to kill the vector; or to break the cycle of transmission by separating the human host and insect vector. Many of the parasites producing tropical diseases were found to be vulnerable to chemotherapy, and a variety of quinine- and arsenic-based products were used in prevention and therapy. Research into chemicals to control tropical diseases was an important foundation for the work that produced antibiotics in Europe in the 1930s and 1940s. This is an example of how research can shift back and forth between centre and periphery. Colonial medical agencies tended to either attack disease vectors or attempt to break the chain of disease transmission, strategies which often overlapped. The measures taken ranged from individual protection, such as avoiding contact with flies by wearing protective clothing and sleeping under insect nets, to a complete change of lifestyle. After 1900, for example, many Europeans lived in settlements, segregated from the indigenous population who were assumed to be reservoirs of infection. Attempts to control disease were also made through total ecological management schemes that required the relocation of populations or the reshaping of local environments. The direct assault on vectors with pesticides had only limited success before 1939, because the chemicals and methods of delivery used were inefficient. The only viable vector-oriented approach, which also promised a once-and-for-all solution, was 'species sanitation' – that is, to deny particular insect vectors their required habitats for breeding and feeding by changing the landscape (through deforestation, for example), the land use (perhaps with the installation of drainage) or by otherwise altering the local ecology of towns. This approach had its most spectacular success in the 1900s during the construction of the Panama Canal, when General William Gorgas (1854–1920) used his military authority to introduce engineering, sanitary and ecological methods to control both yellow fever and malaria.

Tropical medicine as a tool of empire

From the start, research into tropical diseases had been presented as a potentially valuable tool of empire. Manson set out the agenda for the London School of Tropical Medicine thus:

> The school strikes, and strikes effectively, at the root of the principal difficulty of most colonies – disease. It will cheapen government and make it more efficient. It will encourage and cheapen commercial enterprise. It will conciliate and foster the native.
>
> (Manson-Bahr and Alcock, 1927, p.217)

Alfred Jones, a shipping magnate who raised the funds to found the Liverpool School of Tropical Medicine, stated that 'the money spent in our School is an investment, and we expect dividends from it' (quoted in Lyons, 1992, p.70). The hope was that investment in the latest laboratory-based medicine would provide new approaches to prevention and treatment, which, being focused on disease-agents and individual sufferers, would offer quick fixes to diseases such as malaria, that had previously seemed extraordinarily complex.

According to some historians, the characteristics that tropical medicine developed in the 1900s endured until decolonization and beyond. John Farley has termed the specialty 'imperial tropical medicine' and defines its main features as 'definition, imposition and non-involvement'. Farley argues that 'the medical problems of the tropical world and solutions to them were defined and imposed by practitioners of western-style medicine without involving the indigenous populations in these decisions and with little reference to the culture and social milieu in which they practised' (Farley, 1991, pp.4, 293). Farley makes the following trenchant observations about tropical medicine at the turn of the twentieth century:

> [T]ropical medicine was an important part of empire building and empire maintenance. As stated consistently at the time, the basic goal of tropical medicine was to render the tropical world fit for white habitation and white investment. Its practitioners were members of colonial services, armies of occupation, and mining and fruit companies. What, if anything, should be done about the health of the native inhabitants was determined by the policies of these Western agencies without reference to the needs of the indigenous communities. Not surprisingly their health needs became a priority only when their diseases were felt to threaten the health or profits of the white man, or when imperial policies demanded that the health needs of the populations be addressed. The imperial nature of tropical medicine was most cogently displayed during the imposition of desired solutions ... All experts were Western and Westernised ... [Vector] killing was viewed as the most satisfactory method precisely because it could be done without upsetting the political and social status quo and without the participation of the indigenous populations.
>
> (Farley, 1991, p.296)

We can test Farley's ideas through a case study of responses to sleeping sickness in east and central Africa in the early 1900s. In some respects this is an unusual case, because sleeping sickness was a major disease problem among the indigenous population of Africa. The effort devoted to this condition therefore seems to challenge any simple notion of medicine as a tool for western interests only.

The epidemic was first recognized in Uganda in 1901, and was thought at the time to be linked to the increased movement of the indigenous population that was the result of pacification, migration and the growth of trade following the establishment of colonial rule. By 1902, the situation had become serious enough for the local administration to call for assistance from Britain. The outbreak was seized upon by the supporters and personnel of tropical medicine as an opportunity to show what the new specialty could do. And the Malaria Committee of the Royal Society despatched a research commission. Although sleeping sickness was a recognized condition, little was known about its nature and cause, and it had not been previously reported in epidemic form. The task of the British commission was to investigate the pathology and aetiology of the disease – it being assumed that a preventive or curative strategy would necessarily follow. The initial judgement of British experts was that the disease was contagious and they recommended the isolation of sufferers. However, a second commission under David Bruce (1855–1931), another leading tropical disease expert, undertook investigations which found that the disease was caused by a trypanosome parasite, spread by a tsetse-fly vector. The initial presumption was that the fly acted as a mechanical carrier and that transmission was through its bite. It followed that, like malaria, sleeping sickness was not ordinarily contagious and that it could be controlled by killing tsetse-flies and preventing contact between human and fly.

In 1903, officials reported that the epidemic had spread to the Belgian Congo, and, with the recent Ugandan experience an unwelcome portent, the authorities in Brussels gave the matter prompt attention. They sought advice from the Liverpool School of Tropical Medicine and were initially advised to isolate sufferers. In an attempt to find out more, the school mounted an expedition to the Congo that ran from September 1903 to February 1905. The expedition carried out research on the cause of the disease, and prepared a sanitary report and an epidemiological survey. The latter turned out to be of great significance: it showed that the Congo could be divided into areas in which sleeping sickness was endemic or epidemic or absent. They recommended that attempts be made first to contain sleeping sickness within epidemic and endemic areas by restricting migration and trade, and then to eliminate it in these areas by the isolation of sufferers and carriers.

Exercise

Read 'La lutte: the campaign against sleeping sickness' (Source Book 2, Reading 8.2). Does this account fit with Farley's typology of definition, imposition and non-involvement?

Discussion

There can be little doubt that Maryinez Lyons describes examples of definition and imposition. The construction of the epidemic was congruent with civil and military perceptions of the colony as either areas to be governed or defended. This reflected two key features of Belgian colonialism at this time: one, that policy-making was centralized in Brussels; and two, that policy was implemented through a local administration dominated by the army. While military metaphors were common in all discussions of disease and its control around the turn of the century, it is not without significance that the Belgian campaign against sleeping sickness was known as 'la lutte' – the fight. Lyons observes that after 1903–4, when the cause of the disease was understood, trypanosomes and tsetse-flies could be targeted for attack. However, she goes on to show that trypanosomes were not 'engaged' directly in any major way, even though chemotherapy with atoxyl was available. Instead, what characterized the Belgian approach were the attempts to break contact between human and fly. The control of transmission was to be achieved first and foremost through the human factor, by isolation and incarceration of sufferers, and by the use of medical passports to monitor and control population movements.

Belgian colonial officials were concerned about their own vulnerability to an unknown disease, and its threat to the social order and the economic exploitation of the colony. The solutions adopted were imposed by military methods. This in turn created new threats to the social order because of resistance by the indigenous population to incarceration in **lazarets** and controls on their movement. However, the Belgian policy cannot really be seen to show non-involvement – control measures focused not only on parasites and vectors but also on human sufferers and potential carriers. Although this was an extreme case, it may point to a contradiction in Farley's triad. Can there have been imposition alongside non-involvement with the indigenous population? Perhaps the Congolese suffered the pains of imposition as they had no choice in becoming residents in a medical police state, and most imposed solutions required passive involvement, if not the experience of exclusion.

Missionary medicine

The development of imperial tropical medicine occurred at the same time as a general reform of medical services in the colonies. In the British colonial empire, all medical departments changed from military to civil control between 1880 and 1910. There were also reforms in conditions of service, salaries and facilities, all of which aimed to make it easier to recruit and retain colonial medical officers. For example, in 1902, the four British African territories of the Gambia, Gold Coast, Nigeria and Sierra Leone formed the West African Medical Service. This agency was a point of contact and exchange for local doctors who were dispersed over thousands of square kilometres, providing them with a common identity and a journal. Several hundred doctors were employed by the service, which increased the opportunities for job mobility and specialization. However, the work of the reformed colonial medical service continued to concentrate on supporting the health of British expatriates and on surveillance for epidemics. The number of medical personnel remained very small. In Kenya, a colony with a relatively large British settler presence, the medical department in 1910 consisted of one principal officer, three senior officers, fifteen district officers, one bacteriologist, four assistant surgeons, eighteen sub-assistant surgeons, twenty-two dispensers, one matron and six nursing sisters (a grand total of seventy-one people). Such departments showed racial hierarchies, with Britons occupying the senior medical and nursing positions, while sub-assistant surgeons were often from India and the lowest ranks were staffed by Africans. Hospitals and dispensaries were established in the main towns, and attempts were made to safeguard the health of Britons by a mixture of urban improvements and residential segregation (Curtin, 1985).

In writing the history of imperial tropical medicine, historians have tended to concentrate on public health, disease control measures and the activities of the state and its medical agents. The development of clinical medicine, which was mainly diffused by medical missions, has largely been ignored. During the nineteenth and early twentieth centuries, the ever-growing number of urban Africans had some access to government hospitals and many more would have encountered medical inspections and services as employees – for example, as house-servants, miners, plantation workers, soldiers or in other state employment. But, before 1920, the main form of western medical care that Africans would have encountered directly was missionary medicine. And this was despite there being relatively few missions in Africa in comparison with other parts of the world. Between 1838 and 1914, the London Missionary Society sent 987 missionaries abroad. A mere eighty-two of these were doctors, of whom forty-eight went to China, twenty to India, six to Madagascar and eight to central Africa.

The most well-known medical practitioner to visit Africa in the nineteenth century was, of course, David Livingstone. He had been inspired to train as a doctor by Karl Gutzlaff (1803–51) of the Netherlands Missionary Society, who suggested that medicine might help secure conversions by demonstrating the Christian tradition of healing and caring. In the event, Livingstone never practised as a medical missionary, because after his first expedition (1841–52) he became a full-time explorer. This was unsurprising because Africa was not regarded as favourable terrain for missionary activity at all, let alone for medical missionaries.

In certain ways, missionary medicine was the opposite of tropical medicine: clinical rather than laboratory-based, patient-centred rather than disease-centred and local rather than imperial. The services provided by missionaries complemented state medical provision. In many colonies, missionaries developed curative clinical services working with individuals, while governments concentrated on preventive public health measures. Whereas medical missionaries had to gain the support of indigenous peoples, colonial states could use coercive powers. Where state medical services used male practitioners (often attached to the military), medical missions were commonly seen as women's work, especially as men found it very difficult to win the trust of female patients or to gain a foothold in midwifery. While most missions aspired to have a hospital with inpatients, typical missionary practice was through dispensaries. Here, female nurses played a key role in delivering routine treatments and care, with many of the women being converted **indigenes** (Figure 8.8).

Medical missionary work had many functions, but four main aims developed in the nineteenth century:

- to continue the work of Christ the healer;

- to protect the health of missionaries themselves;

- to provide an opening into alien cultures and facilitate conversions; and

- to represent the superiority of western civilization, which was presented as wholly Christian.

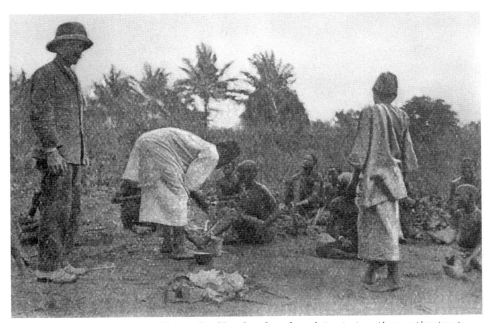

Figure 8.8   Missionary medicine: Dr Shepherd and assistants treating patients at Muhaka, Digo Country. Wellcome Library, London

The first British organization exclusively to promote medical missionary work was formed in Edinburgh in 1841. Protestant missions embraced medicine before Catholic missions, and more wholeheartedly, reflecting their less fundamentalist stance on conversions. Medical missionaries were used more frequently in societies with developed indigenous cultures. According to Andrew Walls, they were the 'heavy artillery' of missionary work, mobilized in societies where conversions were more difficult because of existing organized religions, and where the church sought to utilize the technical superiority of western culture to bolster evangelism, hence their concentration in China and India (Walls, 1982). From 1893, medical courses were taught at the Livingstone Medical College in London by the Church Missionary Society. The courses provided basic medical training for new lay missionaries and for old hands at home on leave. The three-term course taught self-preservation, first aid and nursing skills. Factors of supply were also at work in the development of medical missions. Women medical graduates found it hard to gain hospital or practice appointments in Britain, so overseas service was a more accessible career. How effective medicine was as a weapon of conversion has been questioned by historians, because for much of the nineteenth century, and especially in foreign parts, western medicine may not have been obviously more effective than indigenous systems. Livingstone, along with many other travellers, often preferred local healers and their remedies. There was much debate about the possible conflict between saving bodies and saving souls, and it was generally incumbent on medical missionaries to build a chapel before a hospital (Williams, 1982).

The opening that modern medicine promised to provide into African cultures was paradoxical. The ideal was for Africans to try western medicine, to be impressed by its curative powers and superiority over indigenous healing systems and then to try the religion that had brought them their cure. The feature of western medicine that most impressed Africans was surgery, especially the removal of tumours and cataracts. The way in which the latter operation enabled the blind to see was often portrayed literally as miraculous. Africans were also quite willing to try western drugs, many of which were plant- and mineral-based in the same vein as indigenous African remedies. In some ways, therefore, western medicine did not appear that strange: 'Mission medicine demanded belief in both the scientific and the supernatural' (Vaughan, 1991, p.60). In terms of religion, missionaries were inviting Africans to convert from a primitive belief about the supernatural to the advanced Christian form. Yet, the mixing of healing and religion was one of the features of African 'primitive' cultures that was most criticized. The combination was symbolized, even demonized, in the figure of the 'witch doctor'. In Europe, medicine often seemed to be at the forefront of secularization, as its assumptions became more materialist and many doctors were regarded as atheistic. Given all these contradictions, it is unsurprising that Africans might have seen medical missionaries, not as apostles of rationality with a different type of healing, but as 'European witch doctors'.

Colonial medicine, western diseases

Doctors across all European empires knew that the colonizers and colonized suffered from illnesses other than the classical tropical diseases of malaria, yellow fever, bilharzia, leishmaniasis, cholera, plague and leprosy. The influenza pandemic of 1918–19 affected tropical and non-tropical regions alike, as had cholera in the nineteenth century. Colonial medical reports showed that respiratory infections, childhood infections and degenerative diseases were common across all peoples. Clinicians did, however, routinely report variations in the forms and intensity of these conditions in different environments and also different susceptibilities across racial groups. Significantly, the fact that cholera, plague and leprosy were by the 1930s regarded as tropical diseases led some practitioners to reflect that these once globally prevalent conditions were now confined to these latitudes, not because of their tropical climate, but because of their economic and sanitary backwardness (Hamilton Fairley, 1936, pp.985–1114).

From the 1920s, there was growing evidence across European empires that the health of the indigenous population of many formal and informal colonies was poor. There was also a conviction, among both imperialists and their critics, that the situation was deteriorating and many critics were arguing that the main reason was colonialism itself. They declared that European penetration had disrupted established communities and social networks; it had created burgeoning, unplanned towns; it had led agricultural production to be switched from food to export crops; it was associated with new forms of labour in mines, processing plants and plantations; and, paradoxically, the importation of western clinical medicine and hygiene had made matters worse by saving lives and increasing the native populations. Growing social unrest and calls for political independence ensured that health became linked with welfare in what became a major crisis of colonialism (Hetherington, 1978). Surveys showed that indigenes did not even enjoy racial or adaptive immunities to tropical diseases. There was also evidence that their nutritional status was poor and that this was compromising their health (Worboys, 1988). Some doctors began to ask about the value of medical and disease prevention programmes in malnourished communities and, in debates that mirrored those in Europe, the extent to which malnutrition was the result of ignorance or material poverty. The discussion of these issues was cast in the context of the dual mandate which most colonial powers felt they had now to pursue – namely, policies that offered both protection and development. The contradictions of a policy which aimed at the same time to protect (preserve) and develop (change) were evident in almost every sphere of colonial policy between the wars.

The rising incidence of mental illness in Africa exemplified anxieties about the health of colonial peoples and the mixed impact of colonial rule. As Megan Vaughan has set out, the main explanation of the problem was the impact of civilization on 'tribal' culture and the extent to which the primitive 'African mind' could adapt to new social relations and ideas. A key issue was to what extent was the 'African mind' a product of culture or inheritance? Practically, this issue influenced decisions on whether or not to build asylums, and how to treat Africans suffering from mental illness. Interestingly, colonial psychiatry was quick to adopt Freudian ideas and assumed that most mental illness was produced by socialization and culture, and could be 'cured' with appropriate therapy and changes in social relations. However, the debates about the causes of mental illness among Africans were complicated because psychiatrists no longer worked with an undifferentiated notion of madness. Instead, they distinguished many forms of mental illness and were interested in comparative studies between Europeans and Africans, and of Africans in different conditions (for example, African Americans compared with urban and tribal Africans).

Read 'The madman and the medicine men' (Source Book 2, Reading 8.3). Why did the theories of the 'African mind' developed by British doctors stress culture (that is, social environment) rather than inherited racial features as the cause of the rise in madness in colonial Africa?

Perhaps the most important reason for the emphasis on culture was that this was the dominant approach in British psychiatry, showing that centre and periphery were engaged in a single discourse. The influence of Freudian ideas was one of many factors pointing to the importance of individual biography and socialization in the incidence of depressive and psychotic conditions. A second factor was the wider situation in colonial medicine, where doctors were finding as many similarities as there were differences between health and disease in different groups and in different societies across the world. Also, in the 1930s, biologists began to question the very validity of the biological concept of race. The clinical experience of colonial doctors was, of course, that rates of insanity were highest among those indigenes who had most contact with Europeans. Though, it is surprising that this was immediately seen in terms of 'detribalization' or cultural change, and not explained simply as a result of colonial medicine revealing a previously submerged problem. As Vaughan argues, one factor that seemed to point to the influence of culture was the content of delusions, and the distinction that psychiatrists made between western and non-western delusions. Though here, the distinction between delusions and spiritual possession proved difficult terrain for colonial psychiatrists.

8.5   Conclusion

This chapter has provided a glimpse of the extraordinarily varied character of colonial medicine. The agenda of colonial medicine has changed over time. European doctors used all the means at their disposal to combat disease, which in the early nineteenth century included indigenous medical practices. Later in the nineteenth century, they turned to the theories and products of laboratory medicine, though preventive measures through sanitary reform remained important, especially in India. The disease control strategies developed by European medical officers tended to follow vertical approaches – that is, measures adopted to target a single disease at a time – rather than setting up horizontal services that aimed to promote health more generally. The latter approach began to take precedence after 1920, when colonial state medical services turned their attention to the health of indigenous people. This was in part due to the recognition that their health was poor and perhaps deteriorating, which fed into wider unease about colonial policies.

The transfer of European medicine into colonial settings was equally complex. It was not a 'one size fits all' policy – spreading enlightened medicine to dark continents. Medical institutions and practices reflected the medical problems encountered in particular geographic areas. They also reflected the social and political context of each colony. While centre–periphery models of medical relations are useful when studying colonial medicine, they need to be considered in a framework of wider power relations between centre and periphery. Similarly, while it is easy to see that western medicine was used as a tool of empire, it is important to think about how medicine functioned within particular contexts, and to explore how different people resisted or accommodated colonial power – rather than simply accepting its direct imposition.

A further complicating factor was the attitudes of native people to European medicine. These attitudes were determined by many influences, not least the medical missionaries who were the main agency for the spread of clinical services. While there were some overt conflicts between European and indigenous medical practitioners, the users of medical services, both colonists and indigenes, tended to pick and mix their therapies – using different practitioners to treat different conditions at different times.

References

Adas, M. (1989) *Machines as the Measure of Men: Science, Technology and Ideologies of Western Dominance*, Ithaca: Cornell University Press.

Arnold, D. (1993) *Colonizing the Body: State Medicine and Epidemic Disease in Nineteenth-Century India*, Berkeley: University of California Press.

Bruce-Chwatt, B.L. (1979) 'Tropical medicine: historical cartoon', *Transactions of the Royal Society of Tropical Hygiene and Medicine*, vol.73, pp.353–5.

Curtin, P.D. (1964) *The Image of Africa: British Ideas and Action, 1780–1850*, Madison: University of Wisconsin Press.

Curtin, P.D. (1985) 'Medical knowledge and urban planning in tropical Africa', *American Historical Review*, vol.90, pp.594–613.

Curtin, P.D. (1989) *Death By Migration: Europe's Encounter with the Tropical World in the Nineteenth Century*, Cambridge: Cambridge University Press.

Farley, J. (1991) *Bilharzia: A History of Imperial Tropical Medicine*, Cambridge: Cambridge University Press.

Hamilton Fairley, N. (1936) 'Diseases of the tropics' in E.P. Poulton, *Taylor's Practice of Medicine*, 18th edn, London: J. & A. Churchill.

Harrison, M. (1998) *Climates and Constitutions: Health, Race, Environment and British Imperialism in India*, New Delhi: Oxford University Press.

Haynes, D.M. (2000) *Imperial Medicine: Patrick Manson and the Conquest of Tropical Disease*, Philadelphia: University of Pennsylvania Press.

Hetherington, P. (1978) *British Paternalism and Africa, 1920–1940*, London: Cass.

Lyons, M. (1992) *The Colonial Disease: A Social History of Sleeping Sickness in Northern Zaire, 1900–1940*, Cambridge: Cambridge University Press.

Manson-Bahr, P.H. and Alcock, A. (1927) *Sir Patrick Manson*, London: Cassell.

Nicolson, M. (1988) 'Medicine and racial politics: changing images of the New Zealand Maori in the 19th century' in D. Arnold (ed.) *Imperial Medicine and Indigenous Societies: Disease, Medicine and Empire in the Nineteenth and Twentieth Centuries*, Manchester: Manchester University Press, pp.66–104.

Pelis, K. (1997) 'Prophet for profit in French North Africa: Charles Nicolle and the Pasteur Institute of Tunis, 1903–1936', *Bulletin of the History of Medicine*, vol.71, pp.583–622.

Prins, G. (1989) 'But what was the disease? The present state of health and healing in African studies', *Past and Present*, vol.124, pp.159–79.

Stepan, N.L. (2001) *Picturing Tropical Nature*, Oxford: Reaktion Books.

Vaughan, M. (1991) *Curing their Ills: Colonial Power and African Illness*, Oxford: Polity Press.

Walls, A.F. (1982) 'The heavy artillery of the missionary army: the domestic importance of the nineteenth-century medical missionary' in W.J. Sheils (ed.) *The Church and Healing*, London: Basil Blackwell, pp.287–98.

Williams, C.P. (1982) 'Healing and evangelism: the place of medicine in later Victorian Protestant missionary thinking' in W.J. Sheils (ed.) *The Church and Healing*, London: Basil Blackwell, pp.271–87.

Worboys, M. (1988) 'The discovery of colonial malnutrition' in D. Arnold (ed.) *Imperial Medicine and Indigenous Societies: Disease, Medicine and Empire in the Nineteenth and Twentieth Centuries*, Manchester: Manchester University Press, pp.206–25.

Source Book readings

D. Arnold, *Colonizing the Body: State Medicine and Epidemic Disease in Nineteenth-Century India*, Berkeley: University of California Press, 1993, pp.280–8 (Reading 8.1).

M. Lyons, 'Sleeping sickness epidemics and public health in the Belgian Congo' in D. Arnold (ed.) *Imperial Medicine and Indigenous Societies: Disease, Medicine and Empire in the Nineteenth and Twentieth Centuries*, Manchester: Manchester University Press, 1988, pp.105–23 (Reading 8.2).

M. Vaughan, *Curing their Ills: Colonial Power and African Illness*, Oxford: Polity Press, 1991, pp.100–23 (Reading 8.3).

9

From Germ Theory to Social Medicine
Public Health, 1880–1930

---------------------- *Paul Weindling* ----------------------

Objectives

When you have completed this chapter you should be able to:

- describe the shift in public health policy from strategies based on the germ theory to social medicine;

- explain the multiplicity of factors that shaped health outcomes in a period of rapid social transformation, industrialization and changing family structure;

- understand the complexities involved in an assessment of the impact of both bacteriology and social medicine on levels of disease.

9.1   Introduction

The period 1880–1930 was one of immense social upheaval. It saw continued rapid urbanization and industrial expansion, the catastrophe of the First World War with its aftermath of famine and political convulsions and the devastating international financial crash of 1929. These events took their toll on the health of European populations, but, nonetheless, this period is generally seen as one marked by improved standards of health. Europe began to experience the 'epidemiological transition', when deaths from infectious diseases declined (discussed in Chapter 7). This was partly offset by a rise in degenerative conditions – such as cancer and heart disease – but, overall, life expectancy rose.

In the past, historians have ascribed this improvement to the application of scientific medicine, especially bacteriology. They assumed that the development of the germ theory allowed disease increasingly to be brought under control. This was achieved by the application of knowledge that was devised in the laboratory and delivered through clinics and by health professionals. More recently, however, historians of medicine have questioned whether scientific medicine really led to better health. Instead, they suggest, it may have resulted from health programmes aimed at social factors, such as housing, hygiene and diet. They have shown that between 1880 and 1930, the role of the state in health care was greatly expanded. Until this time, the main concern of states had been to control epidemics of infectious disease. They also played a limited role in providing health care to the very poor. In this chapter, I explore the shift from public health programmes that aimed to control disease to **social medicine**, a wide range of policies that aimed to improve social conditions and provide health education and new medical services.

I also examine the impact of the First World War on the development of health policy and explore the close relationship that developed between medicine and politics after 1918.

9.2   European experiences

Before exploring these questions, we need to review the condition of Europe in the late nineteenth and early twentieth centuries. Although this chapter focuses mainly on health-care policies in Germany, France and Britain, the sphere of influence of these imperial powers reached out to eastern Europe and the Near East. We often think of Europe as a single entity with similar social conditions, and between 1880 and 1930 there were some important common factors. All areas of Europe experienced the epidemiological transition. There was a pronounced convergence in demographic patterns, with a tendency towards a nuclear family. Many governments followed a similar path towards the construction of a modern welfare state. Practitioners in different countries shared the same medical knowledge, an exchange that was aided by international meetings. The organization of medical services also was broadly similar.

You may find it helpful here to refer to Plates 1 to 3.

But, while there was a general decline in epidemics, the patterns of disease in European countries were diverse, and there were immense disparities in life expectancy and health. In terms of disease, central Europe was split between east and west. In western Europe, in regions such as the Ruhr in Germany, the population was relatively healthy, despite the strains of industrial labour. However, in eastern Germany (now the Russian exclave of Kaliningrad and parts of Lithuania and Poland), infant mortality was high and infectious disease was prevalent. Differences were clear at the regional as well as the national level. There was a sharp contrast between the improving health in industrializing Bohemia and the persistently poor health in the adjoining more easterly areas of Slovakia and Ruthenia. Pockets of infectious disease also continued to lurk on Europe's margins. Insect-borne infections such as malaria and typhus remained endemic in the Balkans, while leprosy was endemic in Norway and in the eastern Baltic. Particular events also affected the health of populations. The First World War devastated central Europe and led to outbreaks of infectious disease, while other countries, notably Scandinavia and Switzerland, were left unscathed (Vögele, 1998).

The most important factor contributing to these variations in health was socio-economic change. Europe was still in the process of industrialization, but the rate and degree of socio-economic change varied widely. For example, in the nineteenth century, France underwent a gradual process of urbanization and industrialization. Large numbers of people flocked to the cities to work in factories. Although this was initially associated with increased mortality, by the beginning of the twentieth century the disparities between urban and rural health were diminishing and health and life expectancy had improved overall. In Prussia, differentials in urban and rural mortality had evened out by the 1890s. In Russia, by contrast, there was limited industrialization. The rural population continued to be ravaged by epidemics. The majority of peasants lived in abject poverty and their health was poor. In 1885, infant mortality was more than double the rate in Russia than it was in England. In Russia, the death rate for infants under 1 year old was

301 per thousand births; in England, it stood at 141 per thousand births (Mitchell, 1985, p.139).

It is important to see Europe not in static terms of fixed borders and national units, but as an area of population flows. The period from the 1860s to the First World War was one of mass emigration – notably from east to west in Europe, from the countryside to the expanding cities and from Europe to the colonies and the Americas. In addition, there were seasonal movements of agricultural labourers, with large numbers of workers crossing from Russia to Germany. Europe was a highly mobile society, which meant that travellers on all means of transport – particularly shipping and railways – posed health risks and were subject to health controls. It was thought that emigrants crossing from eastern and southern Europe might introduce disease to major metropolitan centres such as Berlin and Hamburg. Western European states were anxious about the possible importation of epidemics of plague, cholera and typhus from the east. Particular groups were blamed for spreading disease. In the Hamburg cholera epidemic of 1892, anti-Semites assumed that Jews spread the disease, although there was no basis for this assumption.

Family size was a major factor that influenced health outcomes: in general, smaller families meant healthier children. The move away from large families brought a steady decline in infant mortality, although maternal mortality remained a serious problem. Here, again, there were sharp European disparities. In western and northern Europe, family size diminished. The birth rate plummeted in France, from more than 26 births per 1,000 population in 1876 to 22 births per 1,000 at the turn of the century. In eastern and southern Europe, while families remained larger, the birth rate also fell. In Austria-Hungary, there were more than 44 births per 1,000 population in 1876, falling to 39 births per 1,000 at the turn of the century (Dwork, 1987, p.5). Again, variation occurred at the regional as well as the national level. Westphalia in western Prussia had a relatively low child mortality in contrast to persistent high mortality on the large estates of eastern Prussia.

9.3   The impact of bacteriology

The work of Pasteur, Koch and the development of laboratories is discussed more fully in Chapter 4.

In the past, the decline of epidemic disease was usually attributed to the rise of bacteriology, the remarkable achievements of which are well known. In the late 1870s, the French chemist Louis Pasteur isolated several disease-causing 'microbes'. In July 1885, in a blaze of publicity, he announced the first successful treatment of rabies infection using a vaccine. Pasteur's rival was a German doctor, Robert Koch, who worked in a remote location in eastern Poland. Koch made advances in microscopical techniques, using new dyes and stains to observe bacteria, and he established a procedure to prove that a particular micro-organism caused a disease. Pasteur and Koch are both seen as founding figures in the field of bacteriology, but they had different strengths. Pasteur was successful in introducing new therapies, whereas Koch excelled in isolating the causal bacteria. Following Koch's breakthrough, there was a scramble for a stake in the hitherto uncharted and invisible world of bacteria and microbes. A stunning sequence of discoveries was made by Koch, his assistants, who included Friedrich Loeffler (1852–1915) and Georg Gaffky (1850–1915), and by others using his methods of cultivation and isolation of bacteria. These discoveries included the identification of the bacteria responsible for diphtheria, typhoid, tetanus and cholera.

The work of Pasteur and Koch led to the establishment of grand research institutes, which were independent of universities and were oriented to public health and hospital therapy. The Pasteur Institute, which opened in March 1886 in Paris, became an international model for such facilities. By the mid-1890s, each European metropolis could boast of a central bacteriological laboratory, where advanced research took place alongside routine testing to determine the prevalence of infections and contamination of food, water and the environment.

The foundation of such institutes was spurred on by the hope that bacteriology would provide a solution to the problem of infectious disease in the burgeoning cities of Europe. By the 1880s, extensive programmes of sanitary reform had been implemented, but there was still a demand for new and better disease control measures, especially in major metropolitan centres and industrial areas such as Berlin, Paris and Vienna. It was thought that controlling disease would not only preserve lives, but also diminish social unrest. Military and colonial services had similar hopes and saw bacteriology as a potential means of maintaining order. As you read in Chapter 8, military medical officers were trained to apply bacteriology to disease control among soldiers and native populations in the colonies. It is no coincidence that bacteriologists spoke of 'colonies' and 'cultures' of bacteria, words borrowed from colonialism that reflected the close connections between bacteriology and imperialism (Figure 9.1).

Earlier public health strategies and their effects are discussed in Chapter 7.

Bacteriology offered two quite separate means of controlling disease. First, the discovery of the identity of disease-causing pathogens gave rise to hopes that particular complaints could be prevented and treated by new vaccine therapies, similar to those used against smallpox or rabies. The disease pathogen would be cultivated, rendered less virulent and injected so as to produce immunity. Later, researchers showed that *some* diseases were the result of toxins produced by bacteria, and they developed antitoxins to cure infections. However, optimism that these techniques would prove effective against all diseases was short-lived. Even where micro-organisms were discovered, as for gonorrhoea and syphilis, a vaccine proved elusive. Hopes were further dashed when researchers wrongly claimed that diseases as varied as influenza and cancer were caused by bacteria.

The second means of disease control offered by bacteriology was the isolation of infected persons, thus ensuring that pathogenic bacteria were not transmitted to others. Quarantines and isolation had long been a crucial part of state public health policy, and were used as a way to exclude disease and control its spread. But better knowledge of the organisms responsible for a disease offered the possibility of a more targeted response. Rather than closing borders and inspecting all travellers – a huge task in a period of large-scale migration – bacteriological tests gave state authorities accurate knowledge of the identity and presence of disease and allowed them to focus their efforts on those areas and individuals that presented the greatest threat to public health. The same techniques offered a way of monitoring disease in urban settings. From the mid-1870s, there were attempts to provide early warning of Asiatic cholera with the establishment of monitoring stations in Alexandria, Egypt, and the imposition of

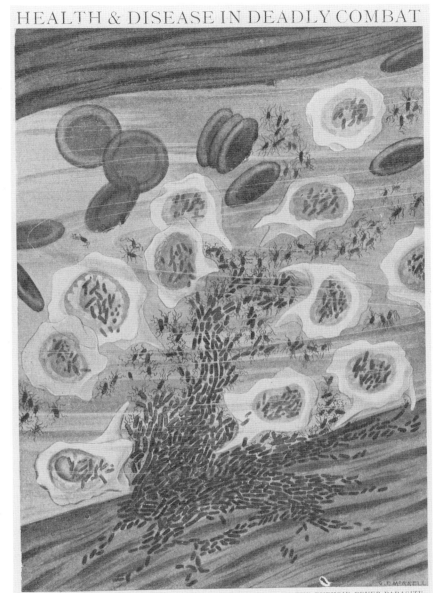

Figure 9.1 *Health and Disease in Deadly Combat*, 1912. This image appeared in a science magazine aimed at a general audience. It demonstrates how military metaphors pervade descriptions of bacteriological phenomena. Here, the white blood cells engage in 'deadly combat', 'killing' typhoid bacteria. If the white cells 'win' the battle, the patient will live. Bacteria were often described as 'foreign invaders'. The use of such military metaphors in medicine is explored in more depth in Chapter 12. Wellcome Library, London

medical controls on pilgrims to Mecca. Special sanitary facilities were developed for migrants from eastern Europe at ports and on railways. All passengers were subjected to medical inspection, and any suspected of harbouring disease were isolated, monitored and their goods were disinfected or fumigated. International agreements required fumigation of shipping to eradicate rats and other disease-carriers.

The rise of the science of bacteriology did not spell the end of infectious disease. Europe remained susceptible to epidemics, especially during periods of socio-political disruption. In Russia, famine in 1891 was followed by devastating epidemics of cholera and typhoid in 1892–3, which, in turn, were accompanied by riots and violence. And, throughout the years of the Revolution, there were epidemics of typhus. Cholera spread westwards as far as Hamburg in 1892, and influenza ravaged Europe in 1918 and 1919. Malaria remained endemic in a belt of countries in southern Europe, stretching from south-west Spain to the Black Sea. However, mortality statistics show that epidemics had become less frequent and less deadly by the end of the nineteenth century. Cholera disappeared from Europe in the twentieth century, mortality from typhoid diminished and there were fewer outbreaks of typhus.

The extent to which this decline in epidemic disease was the result of bacteriological science is very hard to assess. Bacteriological research clearly did offer breakthroughs in the control of some diseases. Pasteur's new vaccines helped to reduce the spread of infection by treating illness. A young German military doctor, Emil Behring, and a Japanese researcher, Shibasaburo Kitasato (1851–1931), developed antitoxins against diphtheria in 1890 and tetanus by 1914. Rapid diagnosis and access to diphtheria antitoxin was recognized as a way of saving children's lives, and the new treatment was distributed through children's hospitals. However, Koch's new vaccine for tuberculosis, which he called tuberculin and introduced in 1891 in a blaze of publicity, was a spectacular failure.

Bacteriological testing did provide accurate information about who was infected with particular diseases, even if they had no symptoms. But it was of limited value in controlling disease. It was impossible to collect and culture specimens from the thousands of travellers crossing Europe. Testing was used to identify sufferers from tuberculosis, but until the middle of the twentieth century, when mass X-ray screening schemes were introduced, people were tested only when they had well-developed symptoms. There was little that known sufferers could do to prevent the disease from being passed to others, although they were advised not to spit or to share cutlery. Only a minority of patients were isolated in sanatoria.

It is very difficult to assess the impact of these new germ practices because they were used alongside old sanitary reforms. Although bacteriology brought an entirely new understanding of the causes and transmission of disease, medical practitioners already had a set of ideas and practices which had been used successfully to control epidemics. Bruno Latour's work on the reception of Pasteur's ideas shows how different groups of practitioners gradually came to adopt the germ theory.

Read 'Responses to laboratory medicine' (Source Book 2, Reading 9.1).

1   How would you summarize Latour's interpretation of Pasteur's discovery of the role of micro-organisms in disease?

2   How does this fit with the more usual account of Pasteur's work as a great breakthrough in medical science?

The work of the hygienists in public health is discussed in Chapter 7.

1   Latour's account focuses on the reception of Pasteur's ideas among medical practitioners. They do not all hail the news as a great breakthrough (as many histories suggest). Rather, their reaction to the new information depends on whether they find it helpful to their own established practice. Thus, those who were interested in understanding disease in populations per se, such as the hygienists, view Pasteur's work as a breakthrough. Whereas general practitioners, used to working with individual patients rather than populations, see Pasteur's discoveries as either useless or a threat to their authority and their practice. Latour suggests that they subsequently downgrade Pasteur's achievements by emphasizing continuities with earlier practice.

2   Latour's interpretation is at odds with the older, more heroic accounts of Pasteur's work, which emphasize the novelty of his achievements and assume that his work was universally embraced by medical practitioners. He reminds us of the need to think about the context in which new ideas appear, and the importance of continuities and discontinuities with established medical practice.

As you read in Chapter 7, before 1880, sanitary reform had already resulted in a decline in deaths from infectious disease. Reform continued in the last decades of the century. By the 1890s, in rapidly growing cities such as Berlin, there were concerted attempts to remedy the worst overcrowding and to demolish slum tenements. In the Austro-Hungarian empire, governments promoted sanitary controls and introduced measures to improve the environment in the large metropolitan centres of Vienna and Budapest. Bacteriology did provide a new focus for sanitary reform: rather than simply trying to clean up dirt in the environment, the aim now was to halt the transmission of germs. So, householders switched from buying cleaning products that promised to make the home 'fresh' and 'sweet-smelling' to those that 'killed germs' and 'disinfected'. The importance of general cleanliness was thus underlined by bacteriology, and better knowledge of the role of pathogens in spreading disease was used to modify existing techniques of disease control. New strategies, or 'germ practices', were introduced to improve sanitary technologies. Water filters eliminated cholera germs. Baths and showers became more generally available in homes and public wash-houses. This helped to combat a range of infections, as did the steam laundering and ironing of clothes (Figure 9.2). New bacteria-killing disinfectants became widely used (Worboys, 2000, pp.108–48).

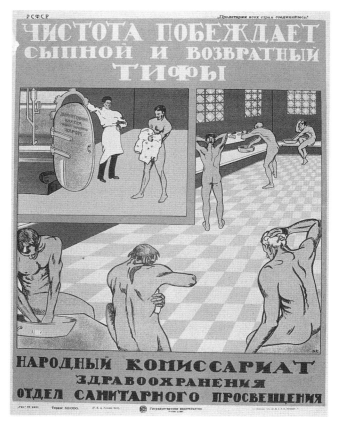

Figure 9.2   Men washing at a public facility, poster, 1921. This poster dates from the time of the Revolution, when typhus killed more than two million Russians. The caption reads: 'R.S.F.S.R. [Russian Soviet Federative Socialist Republic], workers of all lands unite, cleanliness will defeat typhus and relapsing fever, People's Commissariat for Health Care, Department of Sanitary Education.' The poster was produced in bright colours – yellow and orange – to enhance its positive message. Note the large machine used to disinfect clothing shown in the top left. Wellcome Library, London

Some contemporary commentators cast doubt on the impact being made by bacteriological knowledge, and advocated community, environmental and economically based approaches to hygiene as a more effective means of disease control. As you have read, in Bavaria, in the mid-1860s, Max von Pettenkofer correlated the incidence of disease with environmental factors such as ground-water and damp. He stressed that greater personal hygiene was a key factor in the healthiness of the English population when compared with the inhabitants of the German states (D. Porter, 1999, pp.107–9). Practitioners were divided over the relative merits of Pettenkofer's environmentalism and Koch's germ theory. In the 1890s, Pettenkofer's approach was given a boost by new theories of social hygiene in Germany that suggested it was poor socio-economic conditions that generated disease. Medical researchers established that diet and living and working conditions were significant factors in determining the response of the immune system and the metabolism to infectious disease. The medical literature swelled with debates on the mechanisms of disease transmission and immunity. Was it not better, argued socialists and radical physicians, to reduce high rates of disease through social measures, such as improved diet and living conditions for children? Moreover, all were agreed that better health education as well as exercise, to build up the body's capacity to resist disease, would prove beneficial.

By the end of the nineteenth century, there was disenchantment with the germ theory – at least in its original formulation. Bacteriology was not providing the answers that people had assumed it would. The stage was set for a conflict between the supporters of bacteriology and those who argued for social medicine, not just over the best means to combat disease, but in order to protect and enhance their authority.

Exercise

Read 'A bacteriological approach to controlling typhoid' (Source Book 2, Reading 9.2).

1   How does Mendelsohn portray the motives behind Koch's call for a campaign against typhoid?

2   How does Koch's proposed strategy differ from that of the environmentalists?

Discussion

1   Mendelsohn suggests that Koch's eagerness to launch a new campaign against typhoid had nothing to do with the prevalence of the disease, which did not present any real threat to public health. Rather, it was inspired by Koch's desire to improve his own standing at a time when other researchers were achieving breakthroughs using his techniques. He also hoped to raise the status of the whole field of bacteriology.

2   Koch's strategy against typhoid was to target individuals found to be carrying the bacteria, including people who had recently recovered as well as those suffering from the symptoms of the disease. His approach also required him to present typhoid as a problem which could not be adequately addressed by improvements to water supplies, a technique which was effective only in the long term.

9.4   The rise of social medicine

Throughout Europe, the last two decades of the nineteenth century saw fundamental innovations in public health policy. In the 1880s, the state played a very limited role in the provision of medical services. But, by the 1920s, with the decline in deaths from infectious disease, governments' priorities had shifted to improving the general health of populations. Public health experts now saw social issues as the prime determinants of health and they debated the effects of diet, unemployment, hygiene, housing and lifestyle on levels of disease. Medical authority was backed by the new science of hygiene and was used to justify policies that affected everyday life and consumption patterns. Among other things, these policies provided improved access to general practitioners, free treatment for tuberculosis and venereal disease and education about diet and hygiene. At the turn of the century, working adults were no longer the sole target group of preventive medicine. It had expanded to include mothers, infants and school-children. The health of the rural population gained attention in the late 1920s, not least because of the depressed agricultural sector. But not all groups were subjects of concern, and the health of the elderly continued to be neglected.

These services and the inequalities in their provision are considered in Chapter 13.

These new health priorities set in motion a comprehensive reform of the public provision of medicine by the state, local government and charities. Medicine became a political issue and part of a wider landscape of public policies. It also brought about a fundamental change in the relationship between the state and the people. Health was no longer the responsibility of the individual: governments had a duty to protect and promote the public's health. It should be noted, though, that it is far easier to characterize policy shifts than actual health experiences. In practice, the provision of some new services was fragmentary and reform would achieve a measure of integration only in the welfare states that came about after the First World War.

During the nineteenth century, the poor could apply for help from various sources. Some provided satisfactory treatment and relief while others did not. The Assistance Publique in Paris provided a model system of dispersed and specialized hospitals, which offered up-to-date therapies and were located so as to serve the needs of the expanding populations on the city's periphery. Berlin and surrounding municipalities also developed an impressive network of municipal hospitals, dispensaries and convalescent homes. These hospitals were no longer institutions in which to contain the indigent and infectious poor, but places where all people could receive treatment. An important turning point came in the 1890s, when the introduction of diphtheria serum therapy helped to bring the sick into these hospitals for rapid and effective treatment. Not all German hospitals were exemplary, however, and in 1896 patients boycotted the state and military hospital in Berlin, the Charité, because of its prison-like regime. In Russia, *zemstvos* (local councils) provided a community-based system of free rural medical care and health monitoring. This innovative system, supported by committed and well-trained physicians, benefited some communities, but had little effect on overall health because of the harsh conditions of life in rural areas and the lack of education and a sanitary infrastructure (Frieden, 1981). Elsewhere in Europe, state care was inadequate and often demeaning. In Britain, for example, the sick poor were cared for in Poor Law hospitals, where they lost some of their rights as citizens. Provision of public health by the state was augmented by charities and by paternalist employers like the German iron and steel manufacturer Alfred Krupp (1812–87), who promoted model housing and medical services for his workers.

One of the most important new health policies to be developed in the late nineteenth century was state health insurance. This provided working men with access to medical services. From 1883, state governments gradually began to replace direct aid to the sick poor with insurance. The first compulsory sickness insurance was introduced in Germany under Chancellor Otto von Bismarck in 1883 as part of a package of reforms that included the introduction of pensions and accident insurance. Small, regular contributions from employers and employees were paid into autonomous funds, the *Krankenkasse*, and in return workers received benefits to support them if they were unable to work and free medical treatment from a designated practitioner. Initially, insurance was compulsory only for the lowest paid categories of manual workers, but, over time, more groups were brought into the system and increasingly members of the insured worker's family were allowed to claim. Health insurance facilitated greater contact between physicians and the general population, and eventually it financed not only the treatment of individuals in hospitals, but also the building and modernizing of hospital facilities. The German model proved highly influential. Similar systems of insurance (although with varying levels and forms of benefit) were introduced in Sweden in 1891, Denmark in 1892 and Britain in 1911 (Hennock, 1987; D. Porter, 1999, pp.198–208).

The German government did not institute health insurance for medical reasons alone. There was a political motive for improving the welfare of workers. Although we tend to associate state medicine with socialism, Bismarck introduced sickness insurance as an anti-socialist measure, during a period when the German Socialist Party was banned. He recognized that investing in medical research and health care provision could provide a basis for social cohesion and would help to defuse political unrest among the working classes. Ironically, many socialist politicians were employed as sickness insurance administrators. They used their positions to provide evidence of social deprivation and to demonstrate the effects of poverty on health, which in turn led to the extension of sickness insurance to more and more workers.

The decade before the First World War saw the emergence of a new culture of hygiene and disease prevention. Various public associations complemented the efforts of the state by supporting medical advice centres and clinics, where public-spirited physicians deemed it their duty to educate the public about the hazards of disease. Health education was boosted by the International Hygiene Exhibition held in Dresden in 1911. Millions flocked to see the main exhibit, the 'visible man' – a transparent figure that revealed the body's internal organs. The organizers of the exhibition hoped that people would learn the laws of hygiene from such dramatic displays. All aspects of life became transformed by the rationalizing and reforming efforts of public health experts: diet, hygiene, exercise, work and rest. 'Air, sun and light' became the slogan of environmental approaches to preventive medicine. Even death became 'hygienized' with the introduction of cremation, which reformers supported as a means of halting groundwater pollution from overflowing cemeteries. There was a rapid take-up of cremation in Germany, where it was much favoured by secularists and free-thinkers. Even so, the police and medical authorities imposed elaborate routines to control cremation, and families were not able to freely dispose of the ashes of their relatives.

At the end of the nineteenth century, most new health policies targeted specific social groups or particular diseases. Everywhere in Europe, governments and charities attempted to reduce high levels of infant mortality (Figure 9.3). In Britain, infant mortality was relatively low by European standards. But still, in 1900, more than 150 of every 1,000 babies born died in their first year. The levels of infant and child mortality in Europe are well illustrated by the family of Adolf Hitler. Hitler was born in 1889 to a family in rural Austria, with illegitimacy and cousin marriage – both factors associated with poor health – in his parents' generation. Hitler's mother was one of only three children who survived to adulthood from a family of eleven. She had six children, of whom only two – Adolf and a younger sister – survived. Two boys and a girl died in infancy (two from diphtheria) and another boy died aged 6. The large number of deaths among young children was associated with overcrowded housing and a general lack of domestic hygiene. But poor diet was singled out as a particularly important factor.

Concern about infant welfare led to the foundation of mother and baby clinics that dispensed medical advice and dietary supplements. In northern France, an initiative launched in 1894 at a dispensary in Fécamp was the model for the

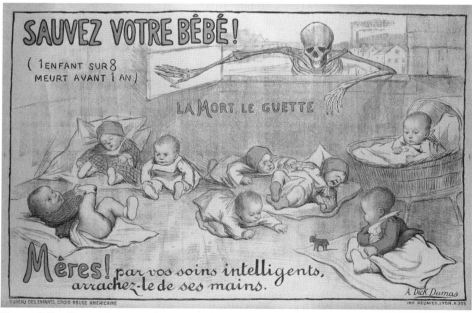

Figure 9.3   Campaign to reduce infant mortality, poster, *c.*1918. This poster was issued by the American Red Cross and shows a group of healthy babies threatened by the figure of death, who slips in unnoticed through a window. The text reads: 'Save your baby! (One in eight die before they are 1 year old.) Death is waiting his chance. Mothers! By your intelligent care you can snatch him from Death's hands.' The message is one of ever-present danger – all babies, however healthy, are under threat. Mothers who take advice from health professionals about how best to care for their infants will be able to save them. Note the industrial landscape behind the figure of Death. In this type of visual material, the city was associated with disease and the countryside with health. Wellcome Library, London

gouttes de lait (infant welfare clinics). These clinics encouraged mothers to breastfeed their babies, offered pasteurized dairy milk for those working mothers who could not breastfeed and provided regular infant health checks (Figure 9.4). Similar clinics were set up in Germany, and by 1907 there were more than a hundred *Auskunfts- und Fürsorgestellen* ('information and care clinics'). Even infant health became the subject of politics. German commentators stressed the benefits of the 'German method' of breastfeeding as combining the virtues of what was natural with what was patriotic. And they drew a contrast with the socially progressive but decadent French support for artificial feeding – although, in fact, French clinics also encouraged mothers to breastfeed whenever possible (Weindling, 1989, pp.188–209). In Britain, governments and charities were reluctant to provide free food, fearing that this would usurp the responsibility of the family breadwinner and encourage dependency. Around 1900, a few 'milk banks' were set up, offering subsidized rather than free milk and no health checks. But working mothers found the milk too expensive, and most facilities closed within a few years. Instead, charities focused their efforts on educating working-class mothers, who were seen as ignorant but eager to learn. Clinics and clubs were established where children were weighed and monitored, and women attended lectures and demonstrations on mothercraft – feeding, clothing, bathing and caring for infants (Figure 9.5). Health visitors and district nurses, funded by local authorities and charities, visited homes and dispensed advice on diet and hygiene (Dwork, 1987, pp.93–166).

Debates about the causes of such 'degeneration' and alternative means of tackling it are discussed in Chapter 10.

A small number of chronic diseases, including tuberculosis, venereal disease and alcoholism, were singled out for attention by health reformers. These diseases were thought to be undermining the fabric of society and acting as 'racial poisons' because they threatened not only the health of the present population but also that of future generations. Reformers portrayed a process of degeneration: chronic illnesses and industrial hazards would damage the innate strength of the body to

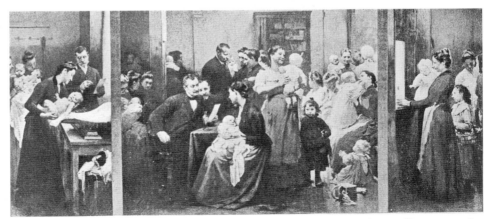

Figure 9.4   Opening of a *goutte de lait*, Paris, 1905. This image shows all aspects of the work of the *goutte de lait*: weighing babies to monitor their growth rate, consultation with a doctor and the distribution of pasteurized milk. Doctors are given pride of place, but the mothers and healthy babies who surround them emphasize the benefits of attending these centres. Wellcome Library, London

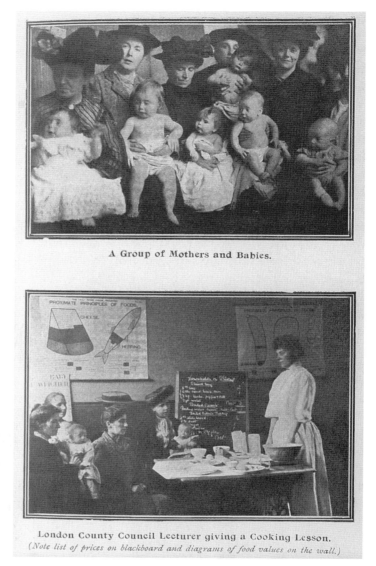

A Group of Mothers and Babies.

London County Council Lecturer giving a Cooking Lesson.
(Note list of prices on blackboard and diagrams of food values on the wall.)

Figure 9.5   Mothers and babies attending a cookery lesson, London, 1907. As in the previous image, the results of attendance at this centre are shown to be happy mothers and healthy babies. In Britain, however, this was achieved not by providing free milk and the services of doctors, but by teaching mothers how to care for their babies. Wellcome Library, London

resist infections, and would render working people unable or unfit to have healthy children. There were fears of a new generation with curved spines, flat feet, rotting teeth and obesity, and that these physical qualities would be linked to 'feeblemindedness' and insanity.

Despite the failure of Koch's tuberculin therapy, measures against tuberculosis intensified during the 1890s. An international anti-tuberculosis movement swept

Europe, and charitable societies that aimed to combat the disease were founded in France, Germany, Belgium, Italy and Britain. One strategy used against the disease was to isolate and treat infected people in special institutions. Known as sanatorium therapy, this treatment was developed in Germany in the 1860s. The exact regime varied between institutions, but all shared the same basic features. Patients were required to spend as much time as possible in the open air, in summer and in winter, even sleeping in well-ventilated rooms or on balconies (Figure 9.6). They were also given copious amounts of food, including milk, to counteract the wasting associated with the disease (Smith, 1988, pp.97–130).

Many of the sanatoria providing this fresh-air therapy were vast institutions in remote areas such as the Swiss Alps and the German Black Forest. These sanatoria were immortalized by the German writer Thomas Mann, who used them in his novel *The Magic Mountain* (1924) as a metaphor for the sickness of European society. But while Mann portrayed a private sanatorium catering to a prosperous set of patients, places were also available to less wealthy patients and were paid for by sickness insurance. Fresh-air therapy was also provided for schoolchildren

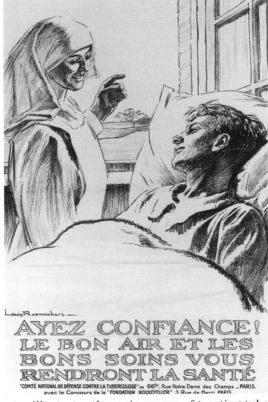

AYEZ CONFIANCE!
LE BON AIR ET LES
BONS SOINS VOUS
RENDRONT LA SANTÉ

"COMITÉ NATIONAL DE DÉFENSE CONTRE LA TUBERCULOSE"= 66ᵉ. Rue Notre Dame des Champs _PARIS.
avec le Concours de la "FONDATION ROCKEFELLER" 3 Rue de Berri PARIS

Figure 9.6 This poster illustrates the main means of treating tuberculosis – fresh air, rest and nursing care. The caption reads: 'Have faith! Good air and good care will return you to health.' Despite this positive message, such treatment was often ineffective, especially in patients with advanced cases of the disease. Courtesy of the Rockefeller Archive Centre

with chest conditions. The open-air school movement was pioneered at Charlottenburg (a municipality covering western Berlin) in 1904, and by the 1920s it had spread across Europe.

Apart from being expensive, sanatorium therapy proved ineffective, both in isolating patients (since they were usually admitted when the disease was well established) and in treating them. A far less costly strategy was to provide primary care on an outpatient basis. In Germany, France and Britain, tuberculosis dispensaries and clinics were established. These were centres for diagnosis where patients were offered advice and monitoring of their living conditions. Only minimal therapy was offered, in part so as not to deprive local doctors of lucrative patients. The advice given to patients was not to cross-infect within the family (thus plates, cutlery and beds should not be shared), to eat a healthy diet and to keep windows open. Although public health reformers agreed that damp and overcrowded housing contributed to the high incidence of tuberculosis, there was little effort to improve the housing stock. Instead, national associations, headed by royalty and the aristocracy, but dominated by the professional classes, organized home visiting and voluntary nursing. These efforts against tuberculosis illustrate two points of more general relevance to health provision. First, that mobilizing support for philanthropic organizations was a means of strengthening social cohesion among the wealthier classes. Second, that there was greater readiness to intervene medically in the home than to alleviate and suppress the ill effects of industrial working practices. Protection against tuberculosis became available in 1906, when Albert Calmette (1863–1933) and his assistant Jean Marie Guérin (1872–1961) developed the BCG vaccine from a weakened strain of tuberculosis bacteria. However, practitioners were uncertain of the efficacy of the vaccine and it was not widely used until the 1940s.

Venereal disease was another target of health policies (Figure 9.7). In the 1880s, the growing concern over syphilis was controversially raised by the Norwegian playwright Henrik Ibsen in his drama *Ghosts*, which dealt with the effects of congenital syphilis. Other writers took up the themes of marriage, prostitution, abortion and birth control – notably, in France, Emil Zola in a cycle of novels on degeneration and pathological behaviour and Eugene Brieux in his dramas *Maternity* and *Damaged Goods*. These issues were also addressed in Germany by Gerhart Hauptmann and in Britain by George Bernard Shaw. Fears about venereal disease crystallized in two international congresses held in Belgium in 1899 and 1902. In Britain, concern was further roused in 1916, when a royal commission on venereal disease found that at least 10 per cent of the population was infected with syphilis and an even greater number with gonorrhoea. Organizations were founded to help control venereal disease – in Belgium in 1899, France in 1901, Germany in 1902 and Britain in 1914. These societies brought together a wide range of people – medical practitioners (especially dermatologists), educators and feminists (Baldwin, 1999, pp.355–523; Davidson and Hall, 2001).

While all these groups acknowledged that venereal disease, especially syphilis, presented serious social and medical problems, there was a prolonged debate about how best to tackle it. The position of the various protagonists was shaped not only by medical considerations, but also by their social and religious opinions.

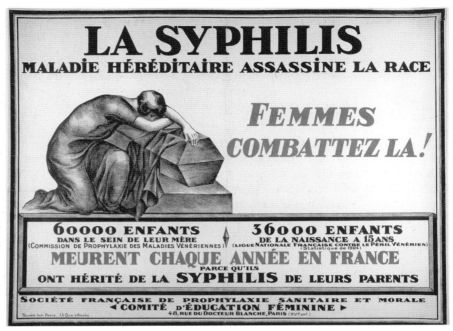

Figure 9.7   Anti-syphilis campaign, poster, Paris, *c*.1925. The caption reads: 'Syphilis, a hereditary disease kills the race. Women, fight it! 60,000 infants on their mother's breast and 36,000 children from birth to 15 years die every year in France because they have inherited syphilis from their parents.' The emotive message here is that people who contract syphilis will pay the ultimate price with the death of their children. This is both a family tragedy and a national tragedy. The call for women to act seems at odds with the image of the passive, mourning figure. Wellcome Library, London

One strategy was to regulate prostitution and make prostitutes subject to medical inspection. However, some reformers argued that police controls on prostitutes led to their ill treatment, while doing nothing to stem the demand for paid sex. Liberal-minded public health reformers in many countries supported the demands of the feminist movement. It claimed that the responsibility for the spread of sexually transmitted diseases should be shifted to all who sought paid sex, and it emphasized the need for public education on the risks of syphilis and other sexually transmitted diseases (Grossmann, 1995, pp.26–41). The views of different German groups on the content of sex education have been explored by Lutz Sauerteig.

Exercise

Read 'Sex education in Germany' (Source Book 2, Reading 9.5).

1   How do the proposals for sex education fit with other health policies of this period?

2   How do the education programmes reflect the agenda of different groups?

Discussion

1   The sex education programme set out in Germany in the 1900s required young people not to be taught about sex, but to learn 'self-control', which would, in turn, allow them to control their sexual urges. This self-control was to be acquired through exercise, and especially by avoiding alcohol. The messages about how to maintain sexual health are remarkably similar to those for maintaining good general health.

2   According to Sauerteig, attitudes to informing children and adults about sex were set by larger political agendas. In the 1920s, the Catholic church emphasized chastity and advocated telling children as little as possible about reproduction. The sex reform movement, however, with its strong feminist agenda, was eager that adults should learn how to enjoy a fulfilling sex life within marriage.

Debates on the control and prevention of sexually transmitted disease overlapped with those on birth control – if possible, an even more contentious issue. Pragmatists recognized that condoms not only served as a barrier to infection but also prevented pregnancies. Across Europe, there were furious debates as to whether the prime result of making condoms readily available to the public would be reduced rates of venereal disease or increased immorality. Conservatives demanded moral purity and restraint from sexual relations outside marriage and supported laws against the public advertising and display of birth-control devices. Generally speaking, conservative thinkers advocated large families as a means to boost the nation's strength. This principle even found its way into the world of advertising when the Michelin company mounted a campaign proclaiming that 'large families run on Michelin tyres'. Feminists advocated free choice in the use of birth control and the introduction of maternity insurance to provide financial support for expectant mothers and newborn children. In the early 1900s, French anarchists protested that having children provided fodder for factories and armies, and they advocated a *grève de ventres* ('birth strike').

Birth control soon became a political issue. Maria Sophia Quine has explored the arguments for a high birth rate that were put forward by Italy's Fascist government.

Exercise

Read 'Population and politics in Italy' (Source Book 2, Reading 9.3).

1   Why was a high birth rate seen as important by the Fascist Party?

2   Does Quine see medicine informing this policy in any way?

Discussion

1   In the late 1920s, a high birth rate was entwined with national politics in Italy. It was thought that a large population would help to boost the economy by increasing the numbers of both workers and consumers. It would also boost the

image of the Fascist Party as a radical, reforming political movement, and distinguish it from the earlier liberal regimes.

2   Quine suggests that politics was the main force driving this policy and that medical issues were of secondary importance. The Fascist Party wanted to be seen as a political movement dedicated to the improvement of the health and welfare of its people.

You saw earlier that determining the impact of bacteriological knowledge on health is complicated by the role of older ideas and practices. In a similar way, it is difficult to unpick the role of social medicine in improving health from that of other social changes. We know that rates of sexually transmitted diseases began to fall, but we do not know if this was the result of treatment becoming available, of changes in sexual behaviour prompted by education (although the organizations campaigning against venereal disease were quick to claim credit for the downturn in infection) or of some unknown factor. Tuberculosis also declined, and studies by historians have shown that the factors responsible for the fall in mortality did include diet, housing and work patterns. The extent to which there was a 'hygienization' of everyday life – with the adoption of lifestyle changes that favoured both health and the prevention of disease – is a challenging problem for social historians. Working out the impact of social medicine policies on the health of individuals and groups of people is even more complicated.

9.5   The First World War and after: moving forward, looking back

The First World War caused massive disruption to the development of health-care systems and the conflict itself generated new and serious health problems. Outbreaks of disease during the war forced governments to reinstate the type of sanitary policies that were used to combat infectious disease in the nineteenth century. This can best be seen in efforts to control typhus and its related fevers. Typhus had been a major cause of death in the mid-nineteenth century, but by the early twentieth century it had become rare. Between 1894 and 1914, the disease had disappeared from the Prussian army. In Germany, there was just one case of typhus in 1901 and seven deaths from the disease between 1901 and 1914 (most of the seven being migrant workers from Russia). Until the 1900s, typhus was thought to be caused by some environmental factor. But, just before the war, its real source, the typhus germ, was finally discovered. The louse was identified as the carrier of the germ, but the exact means of infection remained obscure. It was thought that lice picked up the germ when they sucked the blood of the sick and then injected the contagious particle when they bit a healthy host (this was the mechanism by which mosquitoes were known to transmit malaria). But experiments which aimed to transmit the disease by the direct injection of blood from individuals infected with typhus failed. This led to confusion over the transmission mechanism. There was also no conclusive evidence as to whether head lice (similar to body lice, but with a different habitat), fleas and bed bugs were culprits in spreading typhus. In 1912, however, there was a breakthrough when Charles

Nicolle (1866–1938), who worked at the Pasteur Institute in Tunis, showed that infection was passed not through louse bites but by micro-organisms in louse excreta. These micro-organisms were scratched into the flesh, where the louse had drawn blood, by the human host. This meant that to prevent transmission of the disease, not only did lice have to be killed but all excreta had to be removed by washing clothing and skin.

Despite the virtual disappearance of typhus from western Europe before 1914, the terrible conditions of war quickly led to massive outbreaks of the disease. Although the Russian advance of August 1914 was swiftly reversed by the central powers, it brought the threat of 'Asiatic' epidemics into the European heartland. When the German and Habsburg troops invaded Russian territory, they were exposed to an alien epidemiological regime. Typhus was rife in the Balkan and Turkish theatres of war, and the Austro-Hungarian and Serbian armies were soon immobilized by a raging epidemic. The Serbian typhus epidemic placed the disease on the international medical agenda. A few isolated cases quickly became a highly lethal epidemic. Within six months, more than 200,000 refugee civilians died as a result of the disease. The troops themselves were held in overcrowded and filthy conditions and mortality was as high as 70 per cent, with an estimated 150,000 deaths. Among Austrian prisoners, 70,000 died in the overcrowded camps. Sanitation was poor and the sick lay together on straw and mud in unwashed clothes that swarmed with vermin (Weindling, 2000, pp.73–87).

Bacteriological research was unable to resolve questions about a disease which did not conform to Koch's model of bacterial infection, and medical scientists could not advocate precisely targeted prevention strategies. So, policy-makers resorted to a more old-fashioned approach, tackling the environment and the infected individual. The first line of defence was to delouse clothing, uniforms and personal effects. In order to kill the parasites, clothes were doused in petrol and infested persons were scrubbed down with medicated soap and given warm baths. The pre-war delousing stations established by shipping companies were expanded and used by the military. Experiments were conducted using poison gas to kill lice. In German-occupied Poland and Lithuania, hydrocyanic acid was rapidly put into service during 1917 with the backing of the medical department of the Prussian War Ministry. Patented with a warning agent, which made anyone retch who breathed the gas in, it was marketed as Zyklon. The same gas was used by the Nazis to kill millions of people in the Holocaust on the pretext of delousing. Governments organized disinfection squadrons who went into contaminated housing in order to burn, poison or otherwise disinfect infested possessions. Anyone suffering from typhus was isolated, and no soldier recovering from typhus, typhoid or dysentery was allowed home leave. Posters that warned of the dangers of typhus were displayed in central European cities and bacteriologists portrayed themselves as defenders of European civilization against the microbial hordes. Certain groups of people – migrants, peddlers, Jews and Roma ('travellers' or 'gypsies') – were singled out as the most likely carriers of typhus. They were seen as 'human parasites' and as a menace to national hygiene. The confrontation with 'alien' disease carriers led to draconian delousing of civilians and racial stigmatization. By these means, typhus was effectively held away from the western front, although soldiers there did suffer from **relapsing fever** and another milder louse-borne disease called **trench fever**. The Germans encountered a similar fever, which they named after the localities of White Russia and Volhynia where the disease outbreaks occurred.

After the war, typhus remained endemic in areas of Poland, the Ukraine and Russia until 1921. The huge number of refugees that fled Russia during the civil war of 1919–20 exacerbated the danger of wider epidemics. Western powers and charitable organizations feared a rapid spread of typhus, particularly after the influenza epidemic of 1918–19, which had resulted in massive mortality and had exposed the limitations of infectious disease control. In the autumn of 1921, harvest failure led to famine in the normally fertile Volga region, where many refugees from the First World War German advances remained. When these Poles, White Russians, Galicians and ethnic Germans began to move westwards, the fear that they carried typhus prompted authorities to seal the borders. The Soviet authorities under Lenin invited western organizations to plan and assist in the distribution of food, medicines and delousing on a massive scale. The Norwegian explorer Fridtjof Nansen (1861–1930) (renowned for his account of survival on the polar island of Spitzbergen) coordinated this assistance, while the Americans and Germans ran independent programmes.

While typhus epidemics forced governments to fall back on policies of isolation, disinfection and quarantine, the experiences of the First World War also drove the development of new methods of delivering care. These methods laid the basis for welfare states and systems of what was variously called social medicine, social hygiene or national hygiene. This was not a simple transition and in the Soviet Union, in particular, social hygiene emerged as a distinct field, coexisting with more established forms of public health knowledge and practice. You can read about this transition in 'Social hygiene in the Soviet Union' (Source Book 2, Reading 9.4).

The post-1918 movements for democratization and national self-determination resulted in the institution of new agencies for health administration – an important step on the path to the modern welfare state. Austria established separate ministries for social welfare and public health in June 1919, and then a unitary ministry for social welfare, food and health in 1919. In Poland, a ministry of public health, welfare and labour protection was set up in 1918, under the Austrian and German occupying authorities. Prussia established a new ministry of welfare in 1919, with dual responsibilities for health and housing and with a medical officer directing the health section, as part of a concerted effort to rebuild Germany in the aftermath of defeat. This new medical bureaucracy led to a greater coordination of state medical services. Britain followed suit with the creation of the Ministry of Health in 1919. The Soviet Union instituted a commissariat for health in 1918, and established new **policlinics** and a range of socialized health measures. These clinics replaced the individual physician and provided both preventive medicine and therapy. The clinics were either attached to factories or served particular city districts; social medicine here coincided with socialist medicine. Nicolai Semashko, the first Soviet commissar for public health, was internationally minded and receptive to western medical assistance and expertise. The Soviets were interested in what the Germans called 'social hygiene', which saw disease as caused by social factors, while stressing the need for controls on fertility. Western medical observers, in their turn, had an equivocal view of the Soviet Union. Some admired its collective measures, while others disliked its authoritarian organization, which they saw as undermining the autonomy of physicians.

Governments, then, were moving towards more centralized health administration, with improved medical facilities based on the principle of welfare as a citizen's right. But the provision of health care remained divided between states, regional governments, municipalities and voluntary organizations. Most European countries had voluntary agencies which included the Red Cross, the Workers' Samaritan League and various Protestant, Catholic and Jewish welfare organizations. In some countries, different groups of workers had their own insurance schemes with enhanced benefits. While there was a perceived need for the coordination of these state and voluntary organizations, little was actually done about it. As a result, the provision of health care was an uneven patchwork of overlapping services, in which some groups were better served than others.

There were a number of distinctive features to post-1918 social medicine which grew out of wartime experience. Efforts to prevent venereal disease had intensified during the war, and after 1918 there was a pragmatic acceptance that distributing condoms was a more effective means of control than promoting sexual abstinence. There was a new interest in industrial hygiene, which advocated the elimination of health risks in the workplace and the enhancement of social security and welfare provision. The health of working women was also emphasized, in response to the increased participation of women in the labour force both during and after the war. Policies were instituted to improve hygiene in the workplace and to provide better sanitary and washing facilities. Birth control (or reproductive hygiene) also emerged as an important issue, with policies aimed at women having fewer but healthier children. Alfred Grotjahn (1869–1931), appointed as the first professor of social hygiene in Berlin in 1920, claimed that the optimum family size for the 'eugenically fit' was three children – a number which would maintain levels of population. This led to a debate with feminists, who argued for free choice in family size. The first sexual advice clinic to receive municipal funding was founded in Vienna in 1922 by Karl Kautsky Jr (1892–1978) and the anatomist Julius Tandler (1869–1936), who directed the socialized public health administration of 'Red Vienna' during the 1920s. The Austrian clinic was emulated in Germany. But there was a split between feminist and socialist advocates of sexual advice and birth control on the one side, and advocates of medically directed birth control on a **eugenic** basis on the other (Grossmann, 1995, pp.57–77). The eugenic approach was supported by state medical officers in Prussia, Saxony and Hamburg, and by 1928 there were 224 such clinics in Prussia alone.

Another feature of health services after 1918 was the rise of international initiatives that aimed to diminish the threat of disease by providing emergency food aid and other measures such as water purification. One of the first aid agencies, the Save the Children Fund, was founded in London in 1919 and, by 1921, its aid workers were active in Russia – feeding starving children. The League of Red Cross Societies, based in America, sought to extend the Red Cross principles of voluntary assistance in war and emergencies to more general welfare provision,

Eugenics is discussed fully in Chapter 10.

for example, in the care of patients suffering from tuberculosis (Figure 9.8). The League of Nations Health Organization developed from a body that was concerned with preventing epidemics to one that set standards for pharmaceutical products, including sera and the recently developed vitamin supplements. In the 1920s, cancer came to the fore as a health issue and, in 1925, the League of Nations launched a cancer commission to coordinate efforts against the disease. Epidemiological surveys attempted to isolate causal factors, laboratory research focused on the causes of tumour formation and clinics provided radiological therapy (Weindling, 1995).

The Rockefeller Foundation (funded by American oil riches) supported reform of health administration in the new states of central Europe and became a major force in the dissemination of best practice in public health. The foundation sought

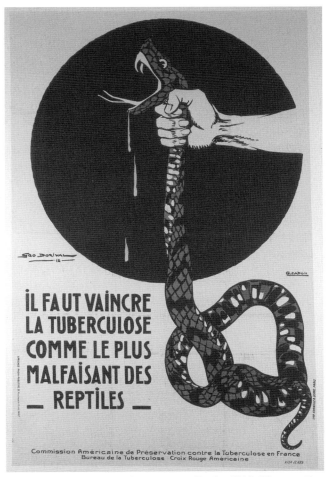

IL FAUT VAINCRE
LA TUBERCULOSE
COMME LE PLUS
MALFAISANT DES
_ REPTILES _

Commission Américaine de Préservation contre la Tuberculose en France
Bureau de la Tuberculose Croix Rouge Américaine

Figure 9.8   Anti-tuberculosis campaign, poster, Paris, 1918. The caption reads: 'We must crush tuberculosis like the most loathsome reptile.' This striking poster was issued by the American Red Cross in France as part of their campaign against tuberculosis at the end of the First World War. Wellcome Library, London

to replace the Franco-German model of health provision, with its central institute of hygiene and laboratory approach. Instead, a wide range of functions and approaches were developed, which the foundation believed to be more in tune with community interests. Each country was to have a central hygiene institute conducting research, setting policy and coordinating services. There were to be smaller provincial hygiene centres for routine monitoring, and district clinics staffed by public health nurses. By 1939, hygiene institutes financed by the foundation had been established in a belt from the Black Sea to the Baltic. One of the foundation's first European projects, however, was a campaign against tuberculosis in wartime France.

Read 'The Rockefeller campaign against tuberculosis' (Source Book 2, Reading 9.6). How did the foundation's approach to dealing with tuberculosis differ from government policies against the disease?

The foundation's approach to tuberculosis was that of a limited response to a short-term crisis. The government had to deal with the disease in the long term, and, indeed, it took over the work of the foundation in 1927. The foundation deliberately chose not to replicate services such as dispensaries and sanatoria that were already provided in France. Instead, it funded a different strategy – health education through posters and the training of nurses to care for tuberculosis sufferers in the home. Services like these had previously been provided by voluntary associations elsewhere in Europe.

The foundation's intervention was not without its critics, who saw it as interfering with existing health services. Practitioners disliked the foundation's corporate approach and science-based health care, which they felt undermined their own private practice. Historians have argued that the Rockefeller Foundation under-estimated the cultural, political and administrative differences in each country, and that this limited the effects of its intervention in the public health field. Despite the large sums of money it invested in training programmes and hygiene institutes, the foundation made little impact on the provision of medical services or on overall levels of health.

These new health policies operated alongside old initiatives. The health of children remained a priority for governments and charities. In Britain, Eglantyne Jebb (1876–1928), founder of the Save the Children Fund, championed assistance measures for starving children in central Europe. By 1924, when the threat of infectious diseases had subsided, many governments turned their attention to family welfare, with the extension of insurance benefits to family dependants and the introduction of public housing schemes. The specialist public clinics dating from before the war were extended and unified to form policlinics. In the Soviet Union, these clinics were the mainstay of health-care provision. In Croatia, Andrija

Stampar (1898–1958) developed a populist model of the clinic – *zadruga* – based on the principle that health was a citizen's right. In Germany, there was a radical socialist experiment known as the *Ambulatorien*, which was financed by health insurance. The *Ambulatorien* provided dental care, spectacles, cosmetic clinics (for patients disfigured by cancer), infant gymnastics and even access to holiday camps. In Britain, in the 1930s, a few local government authorities experimented with health centres. Inter-war health policy was characterized by pioneering schemes of health centres and modernist housing – the large-scale municipal housing blocks of Red Vienna were celebrated examples. One of these, the Karl-Marx-Hof, is more than 1.5 kilometres long and at one time had 5,000 residents. Much was done to disseminate the culture of hygiene. There were innovative efforts in health propaganda such as health weeks, health exhibitions, radio programmes, films and mothers' days. In Germany, for example, Mother's Day was instituted in 1923, and children were asked to honour and help not only their own mothers but all the nation's mothers.

Improvements in health provision during the 1920s were short-lived. Europe had barely recovered from the trauma of war when the worldwide depression of 1930 struck and disease rates and mortality began to rise. The shortfall in household incomes led to a decline in living conditions, a problem which was not addressed by politicians. And the shift to a climate of political extremism, that culminated in the Second World War, ultimately destroyed the lives and health of many millions.

9.6   Conclusion

The last decades of the nineteenth century and the opening decades of the twentieth century saw a huge shift in the role of governments in protecting the health of populations. In the 1870s, states (supported by voluntary bodies) took action against infectious diseases – especially those that occurred in epidemics. By the 1920s, their role had expanded into many new areas, and the work of governments then was similar to the role of present-day states. Governments provided services to control endemic diseases, such as tuberculosis and sexually transmitted disease. New clinics treated a wide range of conditions. Governments had also moved into the field of health education, seeking to inform the population about how to avoid disease and protect their health. All this was supported by large, modern systems of administration – the ministries of health.

Between 1880 and 1930, governments were proud of their records of declining mortality. But their claim that the expanding range of medical services was responsible for the saving of lives is hard to prove. As we have seen, long-established sanitary measures against infectious disease continued to be used alongside new 'germ eradication practices' based on bacteriological knowledge. The crisis of the First World War, and the renewed threat posed by infectious diseases such as typhus, prompted practitioners to look back and to reinstate former strategies. It is equally difficult to pinpoint the impact of social medicine on public health. Family size, diet, housing and general education were as much factors in improving health as the increased availability of medical care and the provision of treatment for tuberculosis and venereal disease. Health propaganda sought to persuade whole populations to observe the rules of hygiene in their everyday life, but it is hard to demonstrate whether this message was put into practice. Ultimately, we still lack explanations as to the interplay of the various factors affecting health, and we remain unsure of the exact reasons why mortality declined so dramatically during this period.

References

Baldwin, P. (1999) *Contagion and the State in Europe, 1830–1930*, Cambridge: Cambridge University Press.

Davidson, R. and Hall, L. (eds) (2001) *Sex, Sin and Suffering: Venereal Disease and European Society since 1870*, London: Routledge.

Dwork, D. (1987) *War is Good for Babies and Other Young Children*, London: Tavistock.

Frieden, N. (1981) *Russian Physicians in an Era of Reform and Revolution, 1865–1905*, Princeton: Princeton University Press.

Grossmann, A. (1995) *Reforming Sex: The German Movement for Birth Control and Abortion Reform, 1920–1950*, Oxford: Oxford University Press.

Hennock, E.P. (1987) *British Social Reform and German Precedents: The Case of Social Insurance 1880–1914*, Oxford: Clarendon Press.

Mitchell, B.R. (1985) *European Historical Statistics*, London: Macmillan.

Porter, D. (1999) *Health, Civilisation and the State: A History of Public Health from Ancient to Modern Times*, London: Routledge.

Smith, F.B. (1988) *The Retreat of Tuberculosis, 1850–1950*, London: Croom Helm.

Vögele, J. (1998) *Urban Mortality Change in England and Germany, 1870–1910*, Liverpool: Liverpool University Press.

Weindling, P. (1989) *Health, Race and German Politics from German Unification to Nazism*, Cambridge: Cambridge University Press.

Weindling, P. (ed.) (1995) *Epidemic and Genocide in Eastern Europe, 1890–1945*, Cambridge: Cambridge University Press.

Weindling, P. (2000) *International Health Organisations and Movements, 1918–1939*, Oxford: Oxford University Press.

Worboys, M. (2000) *Spreading Germs: Disease Theories and Medical Practice in Britain, 1865–1900*, Cambridge: Cambridge University Press.

Source Book readings

B. Latour, *The Pasteurization of France*, translated by A. Sheridan and J. Law, Cambridge: Harvard University Press, 1988, pp.116–18 (Reading 9.1).

J.A. Mendelsohn, 'Cultures of bacteriology: formation and transformation of a science in France and Germany, 1870–1914', PhD dissertation, Princeton University, 1996, vol.1, pp.589–94 (Reading 9.2).

M.S. Quine, *Population Politics in Twentieth-Century Europe*, London: Routledge, 1996, pp.34–7 (Reading 9.3).

S. Gross Solomon, 'Social hygiene in Soviet medical education', *Journal of the History of Medicine and Allied Sciences*, 1990, vol.45, pp.614–15 (Reading 9.4).

L.D.H Sauerteig, 'Sex education in Germany from the eighteenth to the twentieth centuries' in F.X. Eder, L.A. Hall and G. Hekma (eds) *Sexual Cultures in Europe: Themes in Sexuality*, Manchester: Manchester University Press, 1999, pp.16–17, 21 (Reading 9.5).

J.F. Picard and W.H. Schneider, 'The Rockefeller Foundation and the development of biomedical research in Europe' in G. Gemelli, J.F. Picard and W.H. Schneider (eds) *Managing Medical Research in Europe: The Role of the Rockefeller Foundation (1920s–1950s)*, Bologna: CLUEB, pp.19–21 (Reading 9.6).

The Fortunes of Eugenics

James Moore

Objectives

This chapter introduces the controversial new science of eugenics. Its votaries (including many medical professionals) believed that the health and welfare of any nation depended above all on the *hereditary* traits of the populace and that the task of science was to improve those traits by managing the fertility of different social groups. Here, the origins and development of eugenic policies are viewed in a comparative national perspective. When you have completed this chapter you should be able to:

- explain how eugenics originated in the work of Charles Darwin and Francis Galton;

- distinguish between theories of 'hard' and 'soft' inheritance;

- explain and illustrate methods of 'positive' and 'negative' eugenics;

- identify common factors and local contingencies in the rise of European eugenics;

- analyse characteristic features of eugenics in Germany and Great Britain;

- assess the role of medical professionals and institutions in the development of European eugenics.

10.1   Introduction: London 1912

The 'unsinkable' RMS *Titanic* was three months in her grave when on 24 July 1912 the first International Congress of Eugenics opened in London. Hundreds of doctors, professors, clergymen, social workers and activists from Europe and the United States were gathered in the majestic Hotel Cecil beside the Thames, with commanding views of the Palace of Westminster. Eager to debate the science of improving human nature, they rubbed shoulders with well-bred Britons who had lent eugenics their support. The Lord Chief Justice, the Lord Mayor of London, the president of the Royal College of Surgeons, the bishops of Ripon and Birmingham, the vice-chancellor of the University of London and the First Lord of the Admiralty, Winston Churchill, were among the congress vice-presidents. At the inaugural banquet that evening, Major Leonard Darwin (1850–1943), son of Charles, author of the *Origin of Species*, presided; beside him the former Tory prime minister, Arthur Balfour, raised a toast 'to foreign friends and invited guests'. Successive days were devoted to biological, practical, sociological and medical aspects of eugenics, and further gala events were held, including receptions by the Lord

Mayor and the US ambassador, and tea on the terrace of the House of Commons (Gillham, 2001, pp.345–6).

On 30 July, Major Darwin delivered his farewell address. As president of the London-based Eugenics Society, founded in 1907, he spoke for a growing body of intellectuals who believed that a better Britain could be bred by following the principles used to improve domestic livestock. Eugenics would 'conquer in time', he announced to hearty cheers. Already, in May, a Conservative private member's bill to prevent the 'mentally deficient' from breeding had received its second reading in the Commons, and one practical effect of the congress might be the 'hastening on' of such legislation, which would help 'stamp out feeble-mindedness from future generations'. Darwin directed all eyes to the future, to 'fields' of social policy where 'the crop' would be reaped by those as yet unborn. 'As eugenists', he urged the delegates, 'they must content themselves with feeling, each one of them, that the nation to which they belonged was, as regards its future, largely dependent upon the success of their movement.' They were their nations' 'true patriots' because they toiled on behalf of generations to come (Anon., 1912).

Yet for all the dulcet tones and lavish hospitality, the delegates left London divided about means and ends, how best to improve their peoples and the political results to expect. The congress had been inclusive; every oddball with an idea turned up. Zealots and bigots, sceptics and cranks pitched in alongside doctors and academics in a towering babble of tongues. Nor were those present untouched by international tensions and the gathering storm in Europe. Cordiality prevailed, but a competitive spirit was felt.

Take the exhibition hall and congress catalogue, where national groups showed charts and diagrams illustrating trends in human breeding. The Eugenics Society's amateurish display – typified by an 'Inheritance of Ability' pedigree of the Darwin, Wedgwood and Galton families (Figure 10.1) – was upstaged by the German exhibit, which took up more space than any other. In it, next to a family tree of degenerate peasants, stood charts showing hereditary defects among the noble Habsburgs as well as 'shocking ... inbreeding' in the family of the German head of state, Wilhelm II (Mazumdar, 1992, p.164). Britain's eugenists would never have exposed their royals in such a way (though everyone knew the Kaiser was George V's cousin). The consultants to the German exhibit were noted scholars, the majority of them medical doctors: Wilhelm Schallmayer (1857–1919), Eugen Fischer (1874–1967), Ernst Rüdin (1874–1952) and proud Alfred Ploetz (1860–1940), who boasted to the congress of the eugenics courses to be taught in the leading research universities, Berlin and Munich. Nothing of the sort was planned for Oxford and Cambridge.

Now fast-forward twenty years.

It is 1932. Schallmayer is dead, his greatest legacy a textbook, *Vererbung und Auslese* [Heredity and Selection], which has equipped generations of medical students with the technical and managerial knowledge needed to run a national eugenics programme (Weiss, 1987, pp.3–4).

Fischer, professor at Berlin University and director of the Kaiser Wilhelm Institute of Anthropology, Human Heredity and Eugenics, is about to place the organization

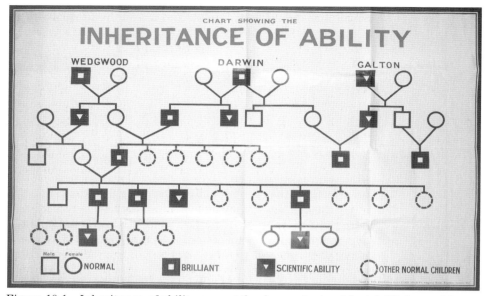

Figure 10.1   Inheritance of ability among the descendants of Josiah Wedgwood I (1730–95), Erasmus Darwin (1731–1802) and Samuel Tertius Galton (1783–1844), the model family of the eugenics movement. The pedigree, prepared for the 1912 International Eugenics Congress, shows Charles Darwin (grandson of Erasmus) married to his first cousin Emma Wedgwood and their three sons who were Fellows of the Royal Society as 'brilliant'. Of the other three, the eldest, a successful banker, is shown as a 'normal' male, Leonard as a male with 'scientific ability' (rather than 'brilliant') and the youngest son, who had a mental disability, is symbolized like 'other normal children' by a broken 'female' circle. Reproduced by permission of the Galton Institute, London

at the service of the Nazi party for training SS officers. Adolf Hitler has read his acclaimed textbook, *Menschliche Erblichkeitslehre und Rassenhygiene* [The Principles of Human Heredity and Racial Hygiene] and incorporated its teachings into his own political primer, now a best-seller, *Mein Kampf* [My Struggle] (Burleigh and Wippermann, 1991, p.52; Proctor, 1988, p.60).

Rüdin, professor at Munich University, is director of the Kaiser Wilhelm Institute for Psychiatry and newly elected (at the second, 1921, eugenics congress in New York) president of the International Federation of Eugenic Organizations. Within a year he is to become a prominent planner of Nazi race policy and an official interpreter of the government's forced sterilization law, a measure he has promoted for decades (Müller-Hill, 1988, p.5; Proctor, 1988, pp.95–6).

Ploetz has just been feted in the first issue of the Nazi journal *Nationalsozialistische Monatshefte* [National Socialist Monthly] as one of the nation's greatest heroes, a doctor who 'sought not only to preserve the health of the general population but also to maintain the higher stages of the "Nordic race"'. Later he will be honoured with a professorship at Munich University by the Führer himself (Kater, 1989, p.112; Proctor, 1988, p.27).

None of these doctors, Ploetz, Rüdin and Fischer, joined the Nazi party before 1937, by which time Hitler had been in power for four years. Each saw himself as a professional whose medical judgement stood above politics and was governed by scientific facts and the duty to promote health and prevent disease. In Britain, doctors prided themselves on the same, but the consequences for eugenics were the reverse. As German eugenics entered its most deadly phase, abetted by the nation's doctors, eugenics in Britain lost ground. Snubbed by successive governments, the Eugenics Society saw its membership turn over and decline. The motley amateurs and activists of Leonard Darwin's generation gave way to a core of cautious, medically informed biologists, geneticists, psychiatrists and sociologists. They shunned panaceas, most of all those of their German colleagues, who were aiding and abetting mass murder.

The fortunes of eugenics varied across Europe, but nowhere more tellingly than between Britain and Germany. The 1912 congress stood at a crossroads. As the delegates dispersed, Leonard Darwin's 'true patriots' marching into different national eugenic futures, little did they know that London would be a point of no return. Already those futures were being shaped and sabotaged by forces latent in the congress. Thirty years later there was a holocaust – Hitler's 'final solution' to the 'Jewish question' was implemented in 1942.

The history of eugenics involves a range of medical fields, from human genetics, to maternal and infant welfare, to public health and psychiatry. Ancillary subjects concerned with the health and fertility of populations, such as statistics and sociology, also interest historians of eugenics. This chapter touches only on those fields involved in addressing three key questions about European eugenics. What roles did medical professionals and institutions play in the development of national eugenics? How far do these roles account for differences between eugenics in democracies and under fascist or totalitarian regimes? What became of eugenics in Britain, where it all began?

10.2 Darwin family values

Eugenics is often seen as an aberration, a false science developed in Nazi Germany on the basis of ideas drawn illicitly from the great English naturalist Charles Darwin (1809–82). This 'abuse' of science under totalitarianism is contrasted with the free progress of genetics (after 1905, the study of biological inheritance) in 'open' societies like Britain's. Nothing could be farther from the truth. Fears about 'race-suicide' racked British intellectuals while Adolf Hitler was still in school; human genetics in Britain was inextricably tied up with the breeding of healthier, fitter people until at least the Second World War. Eugenics was a typical preoccupation of a nation of beef-eaters and dog-lovers, rose-growers and social climbers, long before the Germans developed it into mass murder. The only thing to be said for the conventional view of eugenics is that it *did* originate with Darwin. And the fortunes of the science, in Britain at least, were largely dependent on members of his extended family.

In an age of heroic doctors, the Darwins spawned a medical dynasty. Charles's grandfather and father were noted country physicians; his brother trained in medicine but didn't practice and Charles himself and a son followed suit. The tradition passed through the female line in the twentieth century when a granddaughter of Charles married a noted psychiatrist and another a distinguished surgeon. Three great-grandsons became physicians or physiologists, and two of them were the sixth Darwin generation to be elected Fellows of the Royal Society. The highest honour received by the family was Charles Darwin's state funeral in 1882. His interment in Westminster Abbey paid tribute not only to his science, but to an exemplary paterfamilias whose domestic life, the very 'picture of human happiness', according to the *British Medical Journal*, had been overshadowed by a strange debilitating illness (Anon., 1882; see R. Porter, 1997, pp.672–3). For forty years, Darwin presented a range of ghastly symptoms. Worse, he believed his children had inherited the condition. In the Darwin home, sickness was normal. Some of the ten developed unhealthy obsessions with preventive medicine, though their father's breeding experiments on pigeons and plants suggested that the underlying problem was, as we now say, genetic. You see, Darwin had married his first cousin Emma Wedgwood. The children were inbred.

Darwin's medical concern with hereditary weakness showed in his chief work on human evolution, *The Descent of Man* (1871). In his famous *Origin of Species* (1859), he had argued that the most important cause of life's diversity was a process called **natural selection**, analogous to the **artificial selection** practised by animal breeders. Just as in the stock-pen farmers choose the characteristics of the animals they mate, so in nature the struggle to survive and reproduce 'selects' – favours or preserves – the characteristics of organisms that succeed in leaving offspring. 'Survival of the fittest' it was called. And just as breeders, by long continued selective mating, can fix desirable characteristics and create fancy animal varieties, so nature, through the ages-long struggle for existence, has preserved a huge variety of advantageous traits in different species, adapting them to survive in different environments. That was Darwin's theory in a nutshell. Now in *The Descent of Man* he confronted a problem: 'civilized' people interfere with natural selection. They do not let nature take its course; the *unfit* – disabled, disturbed or otherwise 'inferior' individuals – are shown compassion and allowed to reproduce. How then can evolution continue to improve the human species? Surely progress must grind to a halt!

Exercise

Read the extract from Darwin's *The Descent of Man*, 'Natural selection in human populations' (Source Book 2, Reading 10.1), and mark or note down these points as you proceed:

1 Things that interfere with natural selection, which concern medical personnel.

2 Remedies for survival of the unfit, which Darwin believes will keep a nation progressing.

1   Darwin points immediately to 'asylums for the imbecile, the maimed, and the sick', 'poor-laws', life-saving treatments and 'vaccination'. These, he says, enable inferior people to do what breeders forbid in their inferior animals: 'propagate their kind'. (Being a humane gent, Darwin believes that we cannot 'neglect the weak and helpless' without damaging 'the noblest part of our nature', which is itself the product of evolution.) War keeps 'the finest young men' from marrying; early inheritance and primogeniture enable 'deficient' offspring to 'marry earlier and leave a larger number' of children, who themselves are likely to be deficient. But for Darwin these seem to be less medical than legal issues. Of more concern to doctors is the 'multiplication' of 'the reckless, degraded, and often vicious members of society', including those called 'black sheep', the 'elimination' of which in domestic herds is routine. The increase of such persons 'at a quicker rate than the provident and generally virtuous members' of society leads to a deterioration of the nation's 'intellectual' and 'moral qualities'. Medical personnel might be expected to supply a prophylactic.

2   Darwin suggests three general remedies: *selection in marriage* (the 'inferior in body or mind' should remain single and have no children; prudent men who delay marriage should choose 'women in the prime of life', capable of bearing large families); *reform of laws and customs*, including those that inhibit 'competition' arising from 'our natural rate of increase' (so Darwin implicitly opposes all artificial or unnatural forms of birth control; note also his concern about 'consanguineous marriages' like his own); and *cultural influence* ('good education during youth whilst the brain is impressible ... a high standard of excellence, inculcated by the ablest and best men, embodied in the laws, customs and traditions of the nation, and enforced by public opinion'). Note that all of these are liberal nostrums. Darwin, a rich beneficiary of Britain's laissez-faire economy, believed that the less state interference in people's lives, the better. No coercion is envisaged, though neither does he rule it out.

Like everyone in his day, Darwin was 'notoriously unsure about the mechanics' of inheritance, whether of diseased or healthy qualities (R. Porter, 1997, p.586). He simply assumed, as people had for centuries, that parents' physical and mental traits, *including those acquired as they grew to adulthood*, were transmitted to their children. (The transmission of acquired traits is known as **soft inheritance**.) Blacksmiths' sons have bigger biceps, ballerinas' daughters stronger ankles; alcoholics tend to produce drunkards, Methodists teetotallers, Quakers pacifists, professors swots, all *independently of natural selection*. Thus at the end of the extract, Darwin declares that 'the effects of habit, the reasoning powers, instruction, religion, &c.' – forms of cultural influence – are 'much more' important than natural selection for developing 'the highest part of man's nature', that is, those qualities that make for evolutionary progress. In civilized nations, the struggle for existence is muted.

But what if acquired traits are *not* inherited? What if parents' best efforts to live well do not benefit their children? What if the children's physical and mental endowment has little or nothing to do with parental investment? This was the worrying prospect raised by one of the cleverest yet strangest of Victorian gentleman, Darwin's half first cousin on his father's side, Francis Galton (1822–1911). The consequences he foresaw were radically far-reaching.

Married but childless, Galton was another family failure at medicine; he was subject to breakdowns to boot. Never mind: in the 1860s he conceived the not unflattering idea that genius runs in families, such as the Darwins. How so? In a series of gruesome blood-transfusion experiments on rabbits, he put cousin Charles's ideas about heredity to the test. The results were negative. Soft inheritance hardly occurred, if at all. Parents could *do* nothing to affect the hereditary qualities of their offspring. Geniuses were born, not made; cultural influence counted for nil. (The transmission of genetic rather than acquired traits – the view accepted today – is known as **hard inheritance**.)

On one thing Galton and Darwin agreed: civilization favoured the increase of the unfit (recall the references to Galton in the extract from *The Descent of Man*). How then – assuming only hard inheritance – could this dangerous tendency be reversed? How could Britain raise the birth rate of geniuses, 'master minds' Galton called them (1865, p.166), who would keep the nation on the up-and-up, safe from social and intellectual 'anarchy'? With cultural influence ruled out, Darwin's other two remedies remained: selection in marriage and the reforms necessary to make that possible. 'I do not for a moment contemplate coercion', Galton insisted, anticipating political flak, but he did let slip – unlike Darwin – that 'the time may come' when those who persistently 'procreate children, inferior in moral, intellectual and physical qualities ... would be considered as enemies to the state, and to have forfeited all claims to kindness' (so facing measures known as **negative eugenics**). More constructively, Galton foresaw the creation of 'some society' that would advise the state about human breeding in a 'purely scientific' way (Galton, 1873, pp.116, 120, 124, 129).

There matters stood when Darwin died in 1882. Behind the scenes, Galton manoeuvred to make political capital of Darwin's genius (and implicitly the family's), setting up the funeral and pressing for a memorial 'evolution window' to be erected in Westminster Abbey. Indeed, at this moment, in a book passing through the press, he first put a name to the science which, he hoped, would perpetuate his cousin's memory – 'a brief word to express the science of improving stock ... *eugenics*'. Eugenics, from Greek, meaning 'good in stock, hereditarily endowed with noble qualities', was 'equally applicable to men, brutes and plants', though Galton regretted that breeding was as yet unequally understood in all of its branches. 'Investigation in human eugenics ... is at present extremely hampered by the want of full family histories, both medical and general, extending over three or four generations.' No such difficulty attended the study of 'animal eugenics', which benefited from stud books and the like (Figure 10.2). But once human heredity was as well understood as that of animals, once the human equivalent of a national stud book was established, the state could begin to act. Of all eugenic policies, 'the most merciful' (known as **positive eugenics**) 'would consist in watching for the indications of superior strains or races, and in favouring them that their progeny shall outnumber and gradually replace that of the old one' (Galton, 1883, pp.24–5, 44, 307, 337).

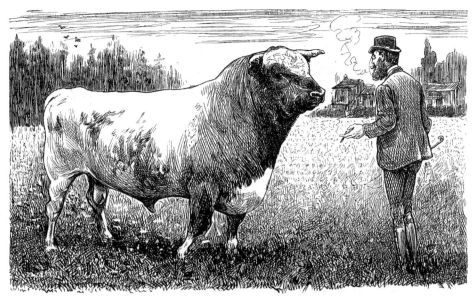

HAPPY THOUGHT! LET US ALL HAVE A VOICE IN THE MATTER.

Noble Breeder of Shorthorns. "WELL, YOU ARE A SPLENDID FELLOW, AND *NO* MISTAKE!"
Prize Bull. "SO WOULD *YOU* BE, MY LORD, IF YOU COULD ONLY HAVE CHOSEN YOUR PA AND MA AS CAREFULLY AND JUDICIOUSLY AS YOU CHOSE MINE!"

Figure 10.2   A weedy, ill-bred aristocrat (note the cigarette) reproached by his prize bull. Even in Darwin's lifetime, before Galton coined the word, eugenics was understood well enough to be satirized in *Punch*. The framed cartoon graced Galton's office for many years. From *Punch*, 20 March 1880, vol.78, p.126

Galton roped in Darwin's sons. George, a Cambridge physics professor and chronic dyspeptic, helped him with the maths for analysing differences in a population; Horace, who ran an engineering firm and was thought the family runt, built instruments for measuring those differences. A 'heredity institute' was planned for storing stud books, family trees and data about inheritance, but it fell through. When Darwin's widow died in 1896, Galton and the sons proposed to turn the family's estate into a 'biological farm' for experimental breeding. Nothing came of that either. Early in the new century, Galton bankrolled a eugenics record office at University College London to store information about 'able families', and he began talking up a 'Darwinian institute' (Pearson, 1914–30, vol.3a, pp.128–34, 311). He needed an organization – soon called the Eugenics Society – to carry out a national eugenics programme.

Exercise

Study Galton's 'The aims and scope of eugenics' (Source Book 2, Reading 10.2) and answer these questions:

1   Does Galton's programme advocate positive eugenics (encouraging superior people to breed), negative eugenics (discouraging inferior people from breeding) or both?

2   Galton often mentions 'race' and 'class'. Which concerns him more?

3   Imagine yourself an Edwardian doctor: how might you aid Galton's programme?

1   The programme is overwhelmingly positive. The only negative policy mooted is banning 'unsuitable marriages', or more subtly, via social pressure, regarding them with the 'disfavour' commonly attached to 'cousin-marriages'.

2   The word 'race' is used inconsistently. Galton first equates it with 'some one human population' (which, however, might be multi-racial); then 'our nation' and 'the race as a whole' appear synonymous; and finally eugenics enables 'the fittest races' (today's usage) to take charge of humanity. This vagueness suggests that Galton was not overly concerned about race, and in fact, he generally applied the term to any breed, variety or 'strain' of animal, including humans. Far more important to him was what a 'civilized' race *consisted of*, social classes. He regards some classes as 'useful' and others (implicitly) as less useful; some as 'upper' and others (implicitly) as lower. The crux of his lecture is that 'large and thriving families', with three or more superior children, should appear more often in the better classes than in the rest and thus 'contribute *more* than their proportion to the next generation' (Figure 10.3). In time, the whole population would improve – the ultimate aim of eugenics.

3   You should have picked up immediately on Galton's 'inborn qualities'. Doctors have an eye for birth anomalies, particularly those that hinder a person's social usefulness. Then again, the importance of men with 'more vigour' might suggest that doctors could assess levels of physical fitness, including those 'needed in a State'. 'Dissemination of a knowledge of the laws of heredity' would naturally fall to those who advise couples before marriage, and the 'systematic collecting of facts' about 'thriving families' could be part of routine medical record-keeping.

One doctor who applauded Galton's lecture was Alfred Ploetz. In 1905, with Ernst Rüdin, he founded the Deutsche Gesellschaft für Rassenhygiene [German Society for Racial Hygiene], and with Eugen Fischer he edited its journal, *Archiv für Rassen- und Gesellschaftsbiologie* [Journal of Racial and Social Biology], which continued publication until 1944. Ploetz translated Galton's lecture in the journal, boasting to him that his own term for eugenics, **Rassenhygiene**, had a good pedigree: 'I started from an English use of the word "race" and tried to investigate the conditions of preserving and developing a race' (Pearson, 1914–30, vol.3a, pp.388, 429; vol.3b, pp.546, 599, 606). 'Started from' is the operative term – Ploetz reworked the concept of 'race' considerably. He went on to offer Galton the presidency of the renamed *International* Society for Racial Hygiene, which Galton accepted, and in 1910, on a charm offensive to unite the eugenics movement under German leadership, Ploetz went to London and met Galton and his heir-apparent as president of the Eugenics Society, Leonard Darwin. The English were wary. Leonard thought the society might affiliate with its German counterpart but should never become subordinate. As he would tell the 1912 congress, eugenics was to be nationally based (Weindling, 1989a, pp.151–2).

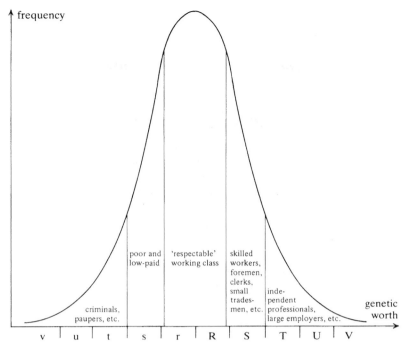

Figure 10.3   Francis Galton's view of British social structure, c.1904. To prevent the inferior classes (v, u, t, s, r) from becoming more numerous than the superior (V, U, T, S, R) – that is, to keep the whole curve from sliding to the left – Galton's programme sought to ensure that large families were more frequent in the superior or 'useful' classes, thus raising 'the average quality of our nation to that of its better moiety' – that is, shifting the whole curve to the right. Reproduced from Mackenzie (1981), p.17

10.3   Common factors and local contingencies

Darwin's theories and Galton's programme did not lead directly or inevitably to a European eugenics movement. They were only its preconditions. Three decades passed between Galton's founding of the science and the emergence of the first eugenics organizations. In this interval, additional impetus for the movement came from factors common to many countries.

The decades around 1900 have been called 'the age of the masses' (Biddiss, 1977). Birth and death rates were falling across Europe, but awareness of demographic change was on the rise, thanks to increased literacy and powerful new mass media. The effects were explosive. Mass-circulation newspapers and later the cinema and radio broadcasting opened up mass markets. News and entertainment were consumed as never before; advertising persuaded more and more people to buy cheap mass-produced goods. Mass production brought new and harsh forms of industrial organization, which led to commensurate protests – the mass picket, the mass strike. All of these in turn – mass markets, mass consumption, mass protests – were represented in the mass media for commercial and political gain. Thanks to sensational journalism, the belief became widespread that even in apparently stable societies vast forces were at work, threatening hopeful revolution or utter ruin. 'The masses', it was said, threatened 'the classes', usurping the age-old power of the mob.

Or so it seemed to noisy elites. Their fear of degeneration was another common factor in the rise of European eugenics. Anxious pundits insisted that mass culture produced mediocrity and social decay. The evidence was only too obvious. On the new mass-transit tram, in popular half-tone press photos, in the latest works on criminality – everywhere the rot could be seen in people's faces and physiques (Figure 10.4). Worse, the degraded were dragging everyone down, according to a growing alarmist literature. Reckless, thoughtless, living for the day, these people multiplied beyond their means, spreading vice and disease, their feeble offspring swamping groups with lower birth rates (Quine, 1996, p.8). Whole societies suffered; some might even die. Many thinkers assumed that the body-politic was like the human body, a functional organism greater than the sum of its parts. On this view (called the **organic analogy**), not only individuals but groups – nations, races even – could become diseased and degenerate from the growth of malignant masses within. To check the cancer, intervention was needed. Only a 'new and urgent potential science' with a strong medical component could provide the cure (Pick, 1989, p.222). Some called it **racial hygiene**, others eugenics.

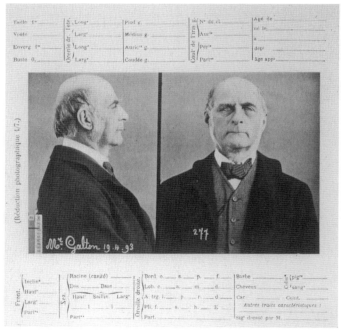

Figure 10.4   High-tech criminology in the 1890s. At the prefecture of police in Paris, Alphonse Bertillon (1853–1914) developed a system for identifying individuals from their permanent physical features and criminals from their common degenerate features. His photographs were circulated widely among law enforcement officers, enabling them to make snap arrests. Here Francis Galton was snapped on his visit to Bertillon's studio. Mary Evans Picture Library

Fear of degeneration and awareness of demographic change fed on each other, and both increased in the aftermath of war. Victorious or vanquished, nations needed to understand why. What made men fighting-fit – training, breeding or just raw guts? Did social decay lead to military defeat? If so, how could the natural defences of a body-politic be strengthened? Or perhaps the resort to war was itself a symptom of national decline. The possibilities were endless. France's humiliation by Prussia in 1870–1, Italy's futile campaigns in East Africa after 1885, Spain's loss of her last significant colonies in 1898, Britain's catastrophic clashes with Cape farmers in the Boer War of 1899–1902, Russia's retreat from Manchuria before the Japanese in 1904–5 and above all the carnage of 1914–18 touched off waves of European soul-searching. The loss of life – coupled with falling birth rates – focused minds, not just on causes, but also on the need for population renewal. What qualities were desirable in the next generation? Which women should be favoured to give birth and under what conditions? How to ensure that only healthy children are born and raised? Should these matters be left to individuals and families or may the state get involved? On the latter point, most European eugenists answered a resounding 'Yes'.

Exercise

Sometimes it is said that demographic change, national degeneration and war 'brought about', 'gave rise to' or even 'caused' the eugenics movement in Europe. Do you agree? Review the preceding paragraphs and work out a concise response.

Discussion

You may have noticed that the view expressed does not allow for the impact of Darwin and Galton. Also the factors mentioned are stated differently in the paragraphs above. The claim there is not that it was demographic change that gave a fillip to eugenics, but *awareness* of that change; not degeneration but *fear* of degeneration; not war but inferences drawn in its *aftermath*. Events per se were less influential than the spin put on them; always the question was, What do events mean?

Answers came hard. Across Europe, claims about demographic change, degeneration and war were hotly contested. For instance, 'peace' eugenists opposed military conflict because it cost the lives of able men. The war lobby countered that bloody struggle was bracing and, in effect, negative eugenics, as it tended to eliminate all but the ablest. Others insisted that war, seen as part of the Darwinian struggle leading to 'survival of the fittest' (natural selection), actually made eugenics superfluous (Crook, 1994). Most people, however, remained indifferent to eugenics or regarded it with religious and political scepticism. The controversy lasted until the Second World War. Given its depth and duration, there appears to have been nothing inevitable about the rise of European eugenics or, indeed, any national version of it. But nor could the movement have come into existence anytime, anywhere – say, in twelfth-century Turkey. Both common factors and local contingencies have to be acknowledged.

Eugenics had diverse prospects in Europe. Beyond Britain and Germany, the movement spread rapidly, acquiring a protean character. Advocates wanted to improve their nation's hereditary qualities, and there were endless ways of going about it.

As an interdisciplinary science, eugenics attracted loose federations of workers from different institutions, with different research traditions, in different national settings. While laying claim to methods and capabilities that set eugenics apart from other fields, the workers inevitably quarrelled among themselves. Party politics raised the stakes, tending to fragment the movement. What emerged after the First World War was a variety of regional, national or cultural styles of eugenics, each developing in its own historical context. Eugenics was no more monolithic than it was static. Later notorious as a racist, sexist, anti-Semitic Nazi pseudo-science, it was at first mobilized across political and class divides, by liberals as well as socialists and social democrats, often with beneficial results (Adams, 1990b).

Take France, where a eugenics society was founded in 1912, soon after the London congress. Here the emphasis fell on national regeneration through *puériculture*, an ensemble of positive eugenic methods for producing strong, healthy children. The most active eugenists were doctors – half of the founding members of the French Eugenics Society had backgrounds in medicine or physiology – and they enhanced their authority through propaganda targeted at prospective parents (Figure 10.5). Parents were seen as natural-born eugenists, able directly to improve the qualities of future generations through soft inheritance rather than any form of selection. In France, Darwin had always been overshadowed by Jean-Baptiste Lamarck (1744–1829), the zoologist whose theory of evolutionary progress stood on (and finally fell with) the hereditary transmission of acquired traits. The 'Lamarckian' belief of French eugenists, that by improving hygiene and domestic environments parents would create hereditary long-term benefits for society, displayed a nationalistic optimism 'very compatible with the political and social philosophy of the … Third Republic' (Schneider, 1990a, p.73; Schneider, 1990b). Negative eugenics through marriage restriction, immigration control and the like did not come to the fore in France until the 1930s, but even then one policy, sterilization, never gained ground.

In Italy, a eugenics society was also founded in 1912, led by an anthropologist and a demographer. Members emphasized positive policies, as in France, but here tailored for a fragile state in which political corruption, a backwards, labour-intensive economy and conflicting regional loyalties made a national programme hard to implement. Their aim was to adjust family size to maximize use of the nation's resources; optimal population growth would help increase production and cut endemic poverty. To this end, 'a distinctly Italian eugenics arose … both Catholic and Latin in outlook', with an odd oxymoronic focus on family life and sexual prowess. By playing up libidinousness as a sign of ethnic superiority, the Italian Eugenics Society tempted the working classes to 'reproduce even more prolifically', and from 1927 the ruling Fascists' programme of health and welfare

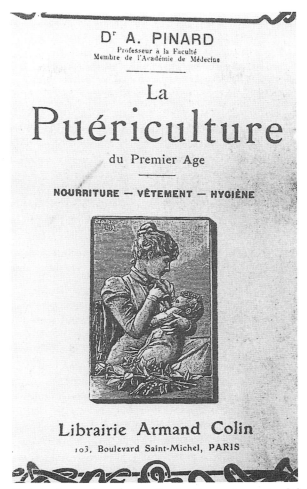

Figure 10.5 *La Puériculture du premier âge* by France's most celebrated
obstetrician, Adolphe Pinard (1844–1934), was based on talks to schoolgirls about
the feeding, clothing and bathing of infants. It became part of the school curriculum,
went through six printings by 1913 and set the tone for the nation's nascent eugenics
society, of which Pinard was a vice-president. Cover of Pinard's *La Puériculture*, 6th
edn, by permission of the Librairie Armand Colin, Paris

reforms also contributed to this end. But Mussolini's 'frantic bid' to boost the birth
rate had 'more in common with the policies introduced by successive Third
Republic governments than it did with Nazi racial hygiene' (Quine, 1996, pp.27,
132). Indeed, sterilization and abortion were never sanctioned in Catholic Italy,
while anti-Semitism under Il Duce took the comparatively mild form of political
anti-Zionism (Cassels, 1993).

Spain presents a similar case, a eugenics specialized for an undeveloped economy
in a conservative Catholic state with a strong though fractured sense of ethnic
identity. From the turn of the twentieth century, a 'clinical view' of the nation 'as
an ailing organism' gained ground among Spanish academics and politicians. In

1919, the country's first eugenics organization tackled the disorder. The Institute of Social Medicine at Madrid was founded on the premise that 'doctors, by virtue of their profession and their interest in the *patria*, should resolve to intervene energetically and actively' in Spain's 'main problem ... of poverty, of organic impoverishment'. Many high-ranking medical professionals rallied to the cause, and eugenics flourished in the ferment leading to the establishment of the Republic in 1932 (Cleminson, 2000, pp.71, 83, 84). But the nature and scope of the new science were disputed. At conferences sponsored by the prestigious *Gaceta Médica Española* [Spanish Medical Gazette], no consensus emerged; politically divided delegates could not even agree on whether there was anything distinctive about eugenics. Accepting both hard and soft inheritance, they debated selective versus environmental measures, only to opt finally for state-sponsored health reforms, with marriage restriction, rather than whole-population policies as pursued in Italy and elsewhere. A 'small but vociferous minority' supported sterilization (Cleminson, 2000, p.103), but their voices were muted after 1936 when the authoritarian Catholic Generalissimo Franco came to power.

In Tsarist Russia, eugenics attracted some public health officials but only took root after the Russian Eugenics Society, founded in 1920, made the science a 'socially responsible, socially relevant branch of the new experimental biology' (Adams, 1990a, p.159). For years, biologists had been working on Darwin's old puzzle, the mechanics of inheritance. After the 1917 Bolshevik Revolution, eugenics seemed a safe banner under which to press ahead with the research. Forward-looking and technocratic, eugenics was unlikely to raise Marxist-Leninist eyebrows, despite its class agenda, and Russian eugenists won credit for being professional and progressive. Although physicians, psychiatrists and hygienists joined the Russian Eugenics Society, geneticists were in the van, confident that their mice and fruit-fly experiments could be conducted safely alongside studies of hereditary defects in the old imperial family. Local eugenics organizations sprang up and members talked of an international movement. This was risky. In return for modest state funding, a distinctive 'Bolshevik eugenics' was expected, a synthesis of genetics and sociology geared to revolutionary ends. An activist eugenics did flourish for a time, but its negative programme – sterilization, marriage restriction and immigration control – eventually fared no better than its positive one, centrally-planned mass artificial insemination. The ideological 'great break' of 1930 proscribed all such schemes and the utopian 'biologizing' that underpinned them (Adams, 1990a, pp.171, 184). What survived was 'anthropogenetics', a clinical and laboratory-based science concerned with problems of human heredity ('medical genetics' in the west).

Eugenics fared very differently in Scandinavia. Only Sweden had a national organization, the Society for Racial Hygiene, founded in 1909 by foreign members of the German society; but in Denmark, Norway and Finland a range of welfare associations and charities took up the cause.

Scandinavia stood apart from the rest of Europe in more ways than one. Denmark and Sweden industrialized rapidly around 1900, with Norway and Finland close behind. All but Finland were spared active involvement in the Great War; afterwards Finland became an independent republic while the others remained monarchies. In each country, the state was strong and liberal, with an established Protestant (Lutheran) church, universal suffrage by 1918 and welfare systems in place or forthcoming within a decade. Everywhere, except Finland, social democratic governments were elected by 1935.

This proved fertile soil for eugenics. Individual organizations were weak, but together they saw more far-reaching legislation enacted than anywhere else in democratic Europe. Before the First World War, Scandinavians spoke openly of themselves as a superior 'Nordic' race. The notion never died; but in the 1920s experts began to place greater emphasis on improving the biological qualities and health of populations, or racial hygiene, as the key to prosperity and social progress. Sterilization laws were passed in all four countries between 1929 and 1935 with little public or parliamentary opposition. These aimed to halt the growth of crime, especially sexual offences, and to cut the number of 'mentally retarded' persons in costly institutions. The laws were meant to be persuasive rather than coercive, though in some cases surgery was carried out when an individual could not give consent. Always and everywhere, the medical professions played a 'central role' in enforcement, supplying legal and ethical guidelines, administering mental-health establishments, screening patients and carrying out the operations, the 'great majority' on females and the mentally disabled (Roll-Hansen, 1996, pp.262–3).

Exercise

Historians credit the Scandinavian management of sterilization for being 'moderate, well-organized, with loyal participation and little protest', and ascribe its success to 'the special character of the social and cultural conditions', including incipient welfare states, that existed in the Nordic countries around the Second World War. All this is contrasted favourably with the fate of sterilization in Germany and Britain during the same period (Roll-Hansen, 1996, p.268; cf. D. Porter, 1999). Such historical analysis, whatever its merits in the case of Scandinavia, can be extended. Before tackling German and British eugenics yourself, please review the paragraphs above and list (or mark) the *major* local contingencies on which the fortunes of European eugenics depended.

Discussion

It will be helpful to group the contingencies under six headings. All eugenic policies depended on *theories of inheritance*. In so far as soft inheritance was accepted, as in France and Spain, policies to improve living environments, particularly for mothers, infants and families, found favour, often at the expense of measures based on hard inheritance. But how far any policy could be implemented depended on the power of *the state* (weak in Spain and Italy, moderate in France, strongest in Scandinavia) to overcome regional and ethnic divisions, on the nature of *the economy* (poor agrarian in southern Europe and Russia; industrialized in the north) and on the character of national *politics* (volatile in Italy and Spain; stable in France and Scandinavia, with parliamentary democracy everywhere but Russia). You may have noticed other contingencies such as *religion*

(Catholics being sceptical of sexual tampering, Protestants at least tolerant, even of sterilization) and *leadership*.

The final contingency is crucial. It mattered much whether eugenics was pursued according to agendas dominated by medical professionals (France, Spain, Scandinavia), anthropologists and demographers (Italy) or biologists and geneticists (Russia). No single agenda prevailed in any country; different measures were put forward on the basis of conflicting claims to expertise (sometimes, as in Spain, frustrating concerted action). Generally, however, doctors emphasized family and public health issues, anthropologists ethnic or racial perspectives, demographers fertility and immigration, and geneticists theories of inheritance and their social implications. Much common ground could exist between any of these groups.

Outside Germany and Britain, what did European eugenists achieve before the Second World War? This cannot be measured exactly. Safe to say, hundreds of resolutions were passed by scores of organizations in a dozen or more countries. Countless journals were founded and countless meetings held, including two more international congresses, at New York City in 1921 and 1932, with declining attendance. Legislatures as well as demagogues enacted moderate eugenic measures, for the most part, hoping these would lead to favourable changes in the make-up of their populations. More people – not necessarily the 'unfit' – practised artificial birth control; more illegal abortions – not necessarily of the 'unfit' – probably took place. More mothers – not necessarily the 'fit' – raised more babies, and more families were probably healthier. More 'unfit' people were segregated in institutions to keep them from reproducing, and more were sterilized than ever before – about 5,000 Scandinavians up to 1940, according to official figures (Broberg and Roll-Hansen, 1996, pp.60, 109, 234). Eugenists were importantly but *not exclusively* active in securing these outcomes.

The greatest achievement of European eugenists was, however, pyrrhic: to qualify and complicate notions of the hereditarily unfit. For decades eugenics organizations sponsored research on human genetics, hereditary diseases and the like, only to find that much of the research made the assumptions of Darwin, Galton and their followers seem less and less tenable. By 1939, soft inheritance had been all but discredited; developments in genetics had made it extremely difficult to tell just by looking at anyone's face, physique or family tree whether their 'stock' was worthy or their children superior. Eugenists' views of inheritance, their social policies and even their aim of improving whole nations had changed irrevocably. Only in one country did the 'unfit' remain easily identifiable. A hardening of hard inheritance around assumptions about race formed the cornerstone of German eugenics.

10.4   Germany: the racial state

Everybody knows the images – torch-lit parades of jackbooted troops, huge rallies harangued by a man with a scrubby moustache; swastikas daubed, Jews arrested, synagogues burnt; the cattle wagons, the crematoria, corpses stacked like firewood. The 'banality of evil' in Germany under the National Socialist German

Workers' Party – Nazis for short – from 1933 to 1945 has itself become so familiar, so commonplace, that the appalling images may no longer shock. Some may even get a grim satisfaction from them, believing 'it could never have happened here'.

That, of course, is debatable and historians have had a field-day. Two questions have preoccupied them. Was the Third Reich the work of mad romantics or ruthless modernists, a Wagnerian opera writ large or the bleak reality satirized by Charlie Chaplin in *Modern Times*? Was it the dead end of a *Sonderweg* – separate path – of development, distinct from the normal one followed by other European democracies, or the outcome of a political catastrophe that could have occurred to any society afflicted as Germany was after its crushing defeat in the Great War?

The same pair of questions arise in the history of German eugenics. Was *Rassenhygiene* under the Nazis the product of deep Teutonic longings or of up-to-date research? Was it the terminus of a historical path separate from the development of eugenics elsewhere, or did Hitler's catastrophic rise to power force racial hygiene off the European high road of normality and into the byways of murderous pseudo-science?

The first of these questions can be answered quickly. Recent historians have argued convincingly that the Third Reich owed its existence to *both* romantic and modernistic impulses; German eugenics was the product of *both* nationalistic yearnings and advanced science. Progressive social policies and reactionary racial policies were 'different sides of the same coin' under the Nazis, a coin that fell heads or tails with appalling irregularity (Burleigh and Wippermann, 1991, p.4). For instance, Nazi doctors were the first to prove 'securely ... that smoking was the major cause of lung cancer', yet many who campaigned against tobacco blamed the Jews for promoting it and backed compulsory euthanasia (Proctor, 1999, p.10). Medical professors set up laboratories in the death camps to carry out original research alongside unspeakable human experiments. Health campaigners and environmentalists ('ecology' was coined by a German professor) established rural reserves on land where Jews and Poles had been cleared for extermination. The flip side of wiping out 'social pathogens' in the Third Reich was the cult of open-air living and physical fitness. Hence the Nazis' reputation as Europe's first 'green' party (Bowler, 1992, p.513; R. Porter, 1997, pp.632, 649).

The second question, about whether German eugenics followed a separate path of development, prompts the further question of how many paths there were. Did eugenics outside Germany stick to a single normal path? Did *Rassenhygiene* take that path until, waylaid by the Nazis, it ended up in Auschwitz? Or did the eugenics movement proceed along many national paths, Germany's *Sonderweg* being one? Political historians have studied the underlying issues in a comparative perspective and concluded, unsurprisingly, that the 'peculiarities' of German history are not half so peculiar as the horrors to which they led (Burleigh and Wippermann, 1991, p.19). In European politics there were elements of sameness and of difference, continuity with change – parallel and intersecting as well as divergent paths – and it would be extraordinary if this were not also true in the history of eugenics.

When eugenists left London in 1912 to create bright futures for their nations, they did not all set off in the same direction or even from the same place, as it were.

Within a decade or so, they had created a Europe-wide, regionally differentiated, strategically diverse and politically mixed movement committed to improving hereditary human qualities. Yet it was a movement more or less unsure or incapable of realizing its ambitious goals. Everywhere, that is, except Germany. Here the local contingencies were not unique, though their combination was exceptional. They can be summarized roughly under the headings used above.

Theories of inheritance Hard inheritance held sway thanks to the Freiburg University zoologist and medical doctor August Weismann (1834–1914), who docked the tails of breeding mice for generations without getting a short-tailed litter. He concluded that a body's 'germ plasm' – reproductive substance – cannot be affected by changes elsewhere in the body. Each individual receives and passes on a fixed set of biological characteristics. Wilhelm Schallmayer and Eugen Fischer were Weismann's students. The first issue of the German racial hygiene society's journal was dedicated to Weismann, who became an honorary chairman. In 1930, the Nazi tribute to Alfred Ploetz's medical career credited Weismann for making the 'immutability of the human genetic material' a fundamental principle of the party (Proctor, 1988, pp.30, 33; see Deichmann, 1996).

The state In 1871, Otto von Bismarck's federation of German-speaking lands under Prussian leadership created Europe's most powerful empire. Regional interests were reconciled, public administration was bureaucratized, and by the 1890s, with Wilhelm II as emperor, progressive taxation funded an extensive welfare system. None of this was achieved without conflict. To foster unity, the organic analogy was updated. Citizens and families, seen as 'cells', were urged to serve the needs of the body-politic because the health of any body depended on the proper functioning of its smallest component parts (Weindling, 1989a, pp.36–48, 291). The doctrine was backed by professors whose Reich-financed research universities led the world. They were elite civil servants who claimed to pursue science 'for its own sake' while serving the national purpose. By 1900, Germany sought a global role to match its scientific eminence.

The economy Industry forged ahead of its competitors after 1880. Huge enterprises banded together in state-sponsored cartels; exports doubled in value between 1887 and 1912. Ever-greater resources were mobilized to arm the nation, but defeat in the First World War left industry on its knees. With huge reparations payable to the allies, frantic steps were taken to regain lost ground – in vain. The economy fell into chaos, and fears grew for the Reich itself. After a brief recovery, the world banking crisis of 1929 plunged the country into turmoil once more. Mass unemployment, hardship and unrest prepared the way for a party of national salvation.

Politics The Prussian emperor and his appointed chancellor answered to federal and state parliaments elected by universal manhood suffrage. The precarious system worked until the 1890s, when demographic change and industrialization exceeded the grasp of Wilhelm II. Parties split, coalition governments were hard to achieve, and legislation often had to be justified by appeals to nationalism. Meanwhile the country's wealthiest, most technologically advanced class imbibed feudal and militaristic values through the Prussian-led education system and reserve officer corps. When a republic was proclaimed and parliamentary democracy established in 1918–19, military officers and conservative civil servants dominated the new Weimar administration. As the economic crisis deepened, coalitions disintegrated, governments collapsed, and from the wreckage a new grass-roots party of the disaffected rose to ally itself with old Prussian nationalists. Its leader laid down the terms. Under an emergency decree, in January 1933, Adolf Hitler was appointed Reichs-Chancellor.

Religion The Catholic church under Bismarck was deprived of cultural influence and forced into an enclave on the right. Protestants were an overall majority, though their proportion differed from state to state. In the absence of an established national church, the sovereign in each Protestant state was the head of the Protestant churches, the majority of which, Lutheran by confession (as in Scandinavia), believed that Christians were bound to respect the state's authority. As public welfare provision usurped traditional church prerogatives and the nation mobilized for war, loyalty could be expected from pulpit and pew. Jews formed a tiny and declining fraction of the population, wealthy on the whole, concentrated in the cities, and more responsive to their own traditions than to state demands.

Leadership Eugenics was launched by professional men committed to the nation's physical, intellectual and moral well-being. Many had trained as medical doctors and continued to practise. Some were experts in biology, others in anthropology, though neither field was yet a separate profession. The path to specialization in the life sciences led through the study of medicine. Whatever eugenists called themselves, a large proportion had medical degrees. Universities were the seedbed of *Rassenhygiene*. The planting took place at the end of the nineteenth century and after the Great War came the harvest. Courses on heredity and racial science trebled between 1919 and 1933, courses on eugenics increased five-fold. When Hitler came to power, eugenics was *already* taught in twenty-six separate lecture courses in state university medical faculties (Proctor, 1988, pp.38–9).

Why this surge of interest just as the country lurched from crisis to crisis? The history of German eugenics must not be read backwards, through Nazi-tinted lenses. Until the 1920s, *Rassenhygiene* could be fairly innocuous. 'Race' might simply refer (as Ploetz claimed) to a group of related people with similar biological characteristics. Rac*ist*, yes, eugenists shared the prejudices of other white Europeans, but this did not make them all supremacist or anti-Semitic. Nor before the First World War was *Rassenhygiene* necessarily right-wing. It was, if anything, a progressive movement, tackling perceived social problems with schemes to reverse the declining birth rate, curb mental disability and avert human suffering. Such schemes were implemented in a number of European countries. However, a flock of panacea-mongers, arch-nationalists for whom race was destiny and racial purification the cure for Germany's ills, had always hovered about the movement, and as war approached they came in to roost. Authoritarian conservatives gained control of most of the institutional centres of *Rassenhygiene*, and under their aegis in the 1920s the centres expanded. 'It was this right wing of the ... movement that was ultimately incorporated into the Nazi medical apparatus' (Proctor, 1988, p.26).

Nazi racism rested on a confusion enshrined in a myth. The confusion was about the relationship between language and race, the myth that the advanced prehistoric 'Aryan' *language*, from which scholars agreed most European vernaculars derived, had been spoken by an advanced Caucasian *race* which migrated from central Asia and conquered those parts of Europe now inhabited by groups with similar dominant traits (Poliakov, 1974, pp.255–304). According to this myth, the Aryans and their descendants were entirely separate in origin and character from the inferior Semitic race, which included the Jews. Darwin himself reinforced this distinction in *The Descent of Man*, comparing 'Europeans and Hindoos, who belong to the same Aryan stock and speak a language fundamentally the same', to 'Jews, who belong to the Semitic stock and speak quite another language' (Darwin, 1871, p.240). Impeccably scientific, this view was widely accepted in Europe before Hitler was born, though battles raged over which nations were *truly* Aryan, having mixed least with lower races.

German-speaking peoples assumed their own superiority (as did many others). The sentiment ran through their greatest literature like a Prussian blue thread long before the Aryan myth linked superiority to race and Darwin saw races struggling to survive. But, after 1871, the year of Bismarck's unification and Darwin's *Descent of Man*, it became 'scientific' to identify race with nation; and, after 1918, scientists sought out racial factors that had led to the nation's decline. Elsewhere, scholars had all but abandoned Aryanism, but in Weimar Germany the myth held sway at the highest level (Poliakov, 1974, p.327). Anthropologists studied race-anatomy, psychiatrists racial minds, and eugenists devised schemes for improving the nation's racial stock. The original Aryan type was found best preserved in the northern states, especially Prussia: tall, fair, blue-eyed people, whom Hitler labelled 'Nordic-Germanic'. In *Mein Kampf* [My Struggle], written in the 1920s, he announced his own plan to 'not only gather together and maintain the most valuable remnants of primeval racial elements' – through positive eugenics (Figure 10.6) – 'but slowly and surely lead them to a commanding position', particularly over that most dangerous and degraded racial type, 'the Jew' (quoted in Burleigh and Wippermann, 1991, pp.38, 40). A whole library has been written on the brutal development of *Rassenhygiene* under the Nazis. One of the best recent books in English is *The Racial State* by Michael Burleigh and Wolfgang Wippermann.

Read the extract from *The Racial State*, 'National socialist racial and social policy' (Source Book 2, Reading 10.3), marking or noting down evidence that enables you to answer these questions:

1   What sorts of positive and negative eugenics were practised in the Third Reich? On which does the emphasis lie?

2   How was the organic analogy developed?

3   In what sense, if at all, can German eugenics be said to have followed a separate path – *Sonderweg* – from eugenics in other countries?

1   Little is said about positive eugenics, though the words 'compelled to reproduce through a series of measures ranging from financial inducements to

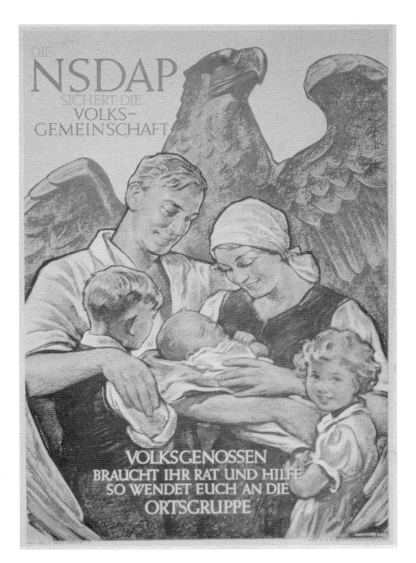

Figure 10.6   Positive eugenics in Germany: the Nazi party (NSDAP) shields the 'national community' and makes happy Aryan families. For 'help and advice, turn to your local branch'. By permission of Bundesarchiv Plak 003-002-046

criminal sanctions' cover an enormous range of activities, such as the odious *Lebensborn* ('fount of life'), a secret network of stud-farm-cum-brothels disguised as maternity homes where young people deemed racially fit (including captured Nordic women) were induced to breed for the Führer (Clay and Leapman, 1996). The emphasis in the extract is on negative eugenics, including 'compulsory sterilisation', 'murdering the sick, the "asocial", and those … of "alien" race', notably the Jews, who were considered not only alien and inferior, but a 'threat' to the Reich.

2   The key phrase is 'purification of the body of the nation', where 'the body of the nation' is equivalent to 'the regime's "national community"'. This agrees with earlier uses of the organic analogy, in which the body-politic was seen as

consisting of healthy or diseased organs, functioning or non-functioning cells. Under the Nazis, however, biomedical politics was racial. 'The "national community" ... was categorised in accordance with racial criteria', which included not only '"racial purity" but also biological health and socio-economic performance'. A body-politic with a racial identity was a refinement of – some would say a throwback to – themes and images deeply embedded in German history.

3   This is the cardinal question. You are not equipped to reply in depth, but at least you can now see how an answer might be devised. The extract says nothing about other countries until the reference in the final paragraph to 'foreign affairs and the war'. The authors explain that 'the specific and singular character of the Third Reich' lay in its determination to establish 'a hierarchical racial new order' not only for Germany, but for 'an ideal future world'. This dual objective was 'novel and *sui generis*'. The *Sonderweg* for German eugenics lay in the creation of a hierarchically organized, authoritarian racial state. Why *Rassenhygiene* diverged from the paths of eugenics elsewhere will depend on the significance you attach to the various common factors and local contingencies summarized above.

Medical doctors greeted the Nazi regime, expecting redress for hardships they had suffered for years (Figure 10.7). They were not disappointed. Opportunities opened up in the military and the civil service; top jobs fell vacant as Jewish

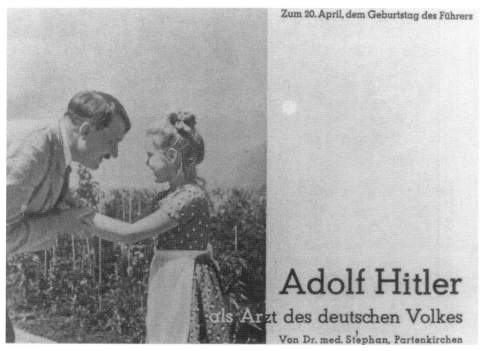

Figure 10.7   'Happy birthday Adolf Hitler, Doctor of the German People'. From *Die Volksgesundheitswacht*, Ostermond, 1935, p.3

practitioners were dismissed from universities and clinics. By 1937, doctors' average earnings were at an all-time high, and they joined the party in droves. In 1932, less than 7 per cent of physicians (excluding dentists and veterinarians) identified with the Nazis; by the end of the war the figure was 45 per cent. Doctors were over-represented in the party by a ratio of three to one compared to other sectors of the population; they were more numerous than any other academic occupation, including lawyers, teachers, civil servants and engineers. Those licensed since the 1920s signed up more often than their older colleagues, Protestants more than Catholics (Kater, 1989, pp.12–15, 56–9). Few reached high positions in the party, but all enjoyed unprecedented rising status.

In surgeries and clinics, face to face with the *volk* ('people'), doctors were the primary agents of Nazi eugenics policy. Educated in the theory and practice of racial science, they spoke with life-and-death authority. Indeed, a GP was the only 'scientist' that most Germans ever encountered, even if only in the cinema. The party used emotive propaganda and the mass media to promote *Rassenhygiene* (Figure 10.8). In the 1930s, documentary 'killing films' were produced by the Racial-Political Office under the zealous Walter Gross, MD, the party's 'racial

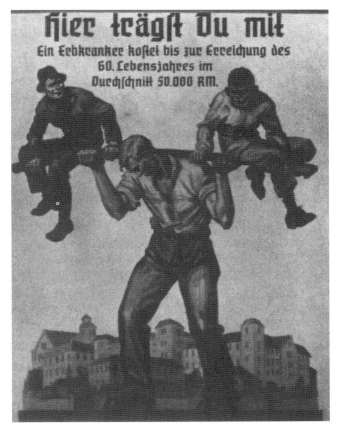

Figure 10.8   Negative eugenics in Germany: 'You are sharing the load – a genetically ill individual costs approximately 50,000 reichmarks by the age of sixty.' Taxpayers save a fortune by eliminating the unfit. From Walter Gross, 'Drei Jahre rassenpolitische Aufklärungsarbeit', *Volk und Rasse*, vol.10, 1935, p.335

warden', in collaboration with Hermann Goering's Reich Propaganda Ministry. Shown in cinemas by Hitler's order, titles such as *Erbkrank* [Hereditarily Ill], *Alles Leben ist Kampf* [All Life is a Struggle] and *Ofper der Vergangenheit* [Victims of the Past] prepared audiences for the extension of compulsory sterilization of defectives (begun in 1934) to mercy-killing and finally medicalized mass murder (Burleigh, 2002, pp.182–214; Kater, 1989, p.181; Weinreich, 1946, pp.79–80; for a description of the film 'Victims of the Past' read 'The portrayal of the fit and the unfit', Source Book 2, Reading 10.4). From the United States came calls to gas 'idiots' and sterilize the blind, but nowhere except in Germany were the Jews as a race subjected to systematic extermination.

10.5   Great Britain: a class society

Eugenics in Britain acquired its distinctive character from the same common factors and local contingencies that shaped eugenics on the Continent.

Similar *theories of inheritance* were held, but until the 1930s none gained the ascendancy of hard inheritance in Germany or soft in France. In the Eugenics Society, views were mixed. Although Galton and Leonard Darwin presided over a membership broadly committed to hard 'hereditarian' rather than soft 'environ-mentalist' explanations of social phenomena, the mechanism of inheritance remained unclear. Biologists argued bitterly over whether characteristics were passed intact from generation to generation (via what we now call genes) or blended to form intermediate traits (Mazumdar, 1992, pp.58–89). The dispute went on until the 1930s, leaving scientists at loggerheads who might otherwise have spoken with one voice about eugenics.

The state, traditionally uninvolved in society, became increasingly active in the twentieth century, providing improved schools (universities stayed private), old age pensions, national insurance and other advantages for working people. Unemployment and housing were tackled after the Great War, and during the Depression the state intervened directly in *the economy*, which nevertheless continued to decline relative to its competitors, being inefficient and over-dependent on the empire. The welfare state emerged piecemeal from decades of conflict and compromise that belied any notion of Britain as a well-functioning 'organism'.

In *politics*, parliamentary democracy was unbroken, though universal manhood suffrage came only in 1918 and equal votes for women a decade later. Coalitions governed during and just after the First World War; an emergency 'national government' held power from 1935 to 1945. There was continuous Liberal government from 1905 to 1914; Labour rose to minority administrations in 1924 and 1929–31. Between them, the Liberals and Labour (galvanized by the 1926 General Strike), pushed through most of the reforms that formed the basis of the welfare state. In *religion*, the established Church of England remained (with notable exceptions) ideologically conservative, 'the Tory party at prayer'. The increasingly affluent 'free churches' also opposed 'collectivist' state reforms, while most of the Roman Catholic laity and many Methodists supported Labour.

Leadership was concentrated in the Eugenics Society, which never had more than 800 members. Well connected and influential, they were a bourgeois mixed bag, rich rentiers, isolated intellectuals, some professionals and men with scientific training, ladies with 'bees in their bonnet' and others who cared passionately about society. (Women made up half of the membership before the First World War; 40 per cent of them were unmarried: Mazumdar, 1992, p.28; Soloway, 1990, p.128.) Like Galton, they were ultra class-conscious, preaching scientific solutions for the most pressing social problem, as they saw it, the growth of pauperism and an urban underclass. Their appeal was mainly to the comfortably well-off. People with smaller families and higher incomes, they argued, would be swamped by the rising tide of riff-raff unless laws were passed to alter the birth rate *selectively*, skewing population-growth towards those at the upper end of the social scale (see Figure 10.3). For British eugenists, a population made up of classes *was* 'the race'. An excess of dull, dependent and diseased lower-class persons was the root of the nation's ills, not some hypothetical non-Aryan enemy within. The Eugenics Society enrolled many prominent Jews (MacDougall, 1982, pp.127–30; Searle, 1976, p.41) and emphasized voluntary rather than compulsory solutions to 'hereditary' social problems (Figure 10.9).

But leading academics refused to join. Most churchmen, journalists and reformers held aloof, and politicians, with few exceptions, steered clear. Frustrated, eugenists slated most of the reforms sponsored by the pre-war Liberal and post-war Labour governments. The 1913 Mental Deficiency Act (which Leonard Darwin anticipated at the congress the year before) did provide for segregation of the 'feeble-minded' to prevent their breeding, but all reference in it to eugenics was expunged. Taxes soared as welfare provision grew and politicians persisted in treating individual hardship without regard for its hereditary causes or the interests of 'the race'. Eugenists attacked them bitterly 'not simply as Radical mischief-makers working to set class against class, but as ignorant men attempting to set the laws of biology at nought ... as "bad stockmasters"' (Searle, 1976, p.113). As early as 1912, one activist could foresee a great irony unfolding: while 'modern eugenics are the work of an Englishman' (meaning Galton), it would be 'the German, with his accustomed painstaking capacity, [who] will probably be the first to turn them to advantage. He shows the wisdom. He looks to other people to pioneer the way, and once the path is open he gallops merrily along the road' (quoted in Larson, 1991, p.56).

Exercise

It has been suggested that 'comparison of British and German ... eugenics would provide a valuable test for the *Sonderweg* thesis' (Weindling, 1989b, p.323). You have evidence to conduct such a comparison, and there is more in 'An alternative programme' (Source Book 2, Reading 10.5) by Dorothy Porter. Read the extract now to discover one local contingency, at least, that stood in the way of British eugenics, effectively keeping it off the German 'path'.

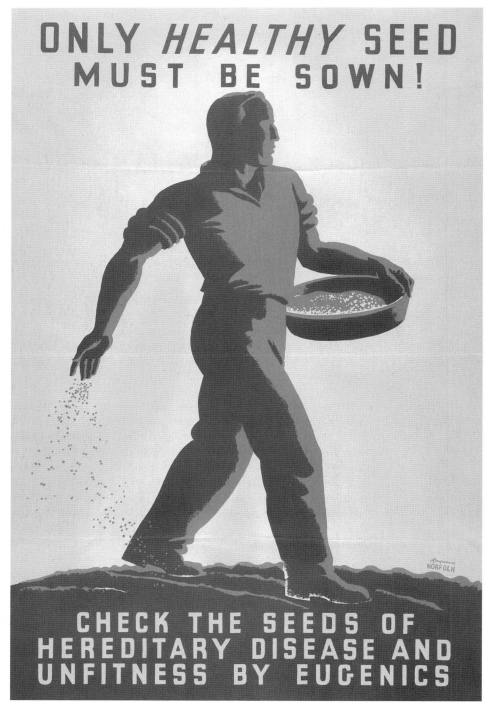

Figure 10.9   Negative eugenics in Britain: 'Only healthy seed must be sown!'
Individuals are urged to avoid spreading hereditary disease. Reproduced by
permission of the Galton Institute, London

In a word, you could call it 'doctors'. Far from spearheading eugenics, as in Germany, they were a stumbling-block. According to Porter, the opposition of the public health movement and health-service professionals to hard hereditarian – 'social Darwinist' or 'biologistic' – approaches to social problems explains the 'extremely limited success' of eugenics in Britain. Public-funded and powerfully entrenched doctors emphasized the *environmental* causes of pauperism, and *preventive* medicine as 'the panoptic overseer of communal life'. Permanent social improvements were to come 'through nurture rather than nature', by town planning, housing renewal, free school meals, medical inspection of pupils, antenatal care, health visitors and so on – not via state-sponsored selective breeding. The focus was still on the individual. Governments held out against collectivist 'planning and eugenic health policies', although their reforms proved to be the first steps towards a *national* health service. The founding of the National Health Service (NHS) in 1945 marked the final triumph of state-funded environmentalism over the state-sponsored Darwinism of Galton's dreams and of Nazi reality. Today, every NHS hospital, every NHS trust, is a monument to the death of classical eugenics.

10.6 Conclusion: London 1939

Disappointments piled up for British eugenists. The Great War was a dysgenic disaster: mass rationing favoured the unfit; the fittest fell in battle, leaving 'cowards' and 'cripples' to replenish the population. Voting reforms empowered those who cared only for 'cigarettes, chocolates and cinemas' (one professor quipped): what good was a gardener 'if his tenure of office depended on the consent of the weeds' (quoted in Searle, 1976, pp.68–9). The battle against birth control was lost; the 'better' classes continued to limit their families, the tax-supported poor did not. Larger family allowances for those with higher incomes might have upped the bourgeois birth rate, but in the impoverished 1930s eugenists failed to agree on a policy and flat-rate allowances remained in place. The biggest setback was over sterilization. Leonard Darwin drafted a law in 1927 permitting operations to be conducted on medical grounds, thus passing the buck to doctors (Thomson, 1998, p.182). When the Sterilization Bill of 1931 was defeated, the Eugenics Society lobbied for measures based on the 1934 Brock Report, which proposed to allow surgery for certain categories of person who gave informed consent. The opposition was fierce. Geneticists attacked the science, lawyers raised legal objections and the Catholic church moral ones; medical professionals insisted on the social and environmental causes of many disabilities. When Labour condemned sterilization for being anti-working class, the charge stuck. With Nazi horrors making headlines, it practically ensured 'the failure of eugenics in inter-war Britain' (Macnicol, 1989, p.147).

Successive medical authorities presided over the Eugenics Society after Leonard Darwin's retirement in 1928. But it was the general secretary elected three years later, C.P. Blacker, a Catholic physician and psychiatrist, who transformed the organization. Under his guidance, the old fearful class-conscious membership gave way to men (for the most part) with broader, more moderate and inclusive views, bona fide professionals who accepted hard inheritance and sought the roots of social problems *not either* in defective biology *or* in defective environments, but in their interplay. The society set up and funded groups to front its campaigns, such as the Family Planning Association and the Marriage Guidance Council. Anxious to escape association with the Nazis, Blacker even proposed in 1935 to change the society's name to 'The Institute for Family Relations' (Soloway, 1990, p.72; Thomson, 1998, p.192).

One sign of Blacker's success was a manifesto published in London in September 1939. 'Social biology and population improvement' (Source Book 2, Reading 10.6) appeared in *Nature*, the world's leading science weekly, a fortnight after Churchill declared war on Germany and a month after Albert Einstein wrote to the US president, warning of the threat of atomic weapons. Signed by twenty-two leading biologists, including British eugenists, it called for the creation of social conditions such as 'equal opportunities' that would aid the 'genetic improvement of mankind'. Under these conditions, the state, by 'estimating and comparing the intrinsic worth of different individuals', and then selecting those with 'better genetic equipment', could adopt a 'rational' policy for the attainment of 'health', 'intelligence', and those 'temperamental qualities which favour fellow-feeling and social behaviour'.

For all its success with animals and plants, eugenics had failed as a method of improving a nation committed to laissez-faire and individual rights. But in 1939, as war began against a state practising racist eugenics in the extreme, here was scientific authority for believing in the old eugenics ideal (Figure 10.10). Except for the word 'genetic', the manifesto could have been written by Blacker's hero, Francis Galton. Leonard Darwin might have signed. Only time would tell whether that ideal could be achieved.

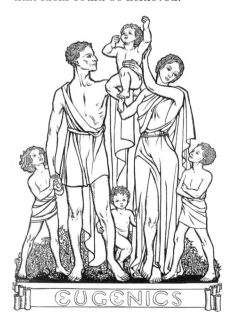

Figure 10.10   Positive eugenics in Britain: a big happy family groomed after the classical ideal. Note the frequency of birth. Reproduced by permission of the Galton Institute, London

References

Adams, M.B. (1990a) 'Eugenics in Russia, 1900–1940' in Adams (ed.) *The Well-Born Science: Eugenics in Germany, France, Brazil and Russia*, New York: Oxford University Press, pp.153–216.

Adams, M.B. (1990b) 'Toward a comparative history of eugenics' in Adams (ed.) *The Well-Born Science: Eugenics in Germany, France, Brazil and Russia*, New York: Oxford University Press, pp.217–31.

Anon. (1882) 'Charles Darwin', *British Medical Journal*, 29 April, pp.634–5.

Anon. (1912) 'A survey of the work of the Congress', *The Times*, 31 July, London.

Biddiss, M. (1977) *The Age of the Masses: Ideas and Society in Europe since 1870*, Harmondsworth: Penguin.

Bowler, P. (1992) *The Fontana History of the Environmental Sciences*, London: Fontana.

Broberg, G. and Roll-Hansen, N. (eds) (1996) *Eugenics and the Welfare State: Sterilization Policy in Denmark, Sweden, Norway and Finland*, East Lansing: Michigan State University Press.

Burleigh, M. (2002) *Death and Deliverance: 'Euthanasia' in Germany, c.1900–1945*, new edn, London: Pan Books.

Burleigh, M. and Wipperman, W. (1991) *The Racial State: Germany, 1933–1945*, Cambridge: Cambridge University Press.

Cassels, A. (1993) 'Italy and the Holocaust' in S.S. Friedman (ed.) *Holocaust Literature: A Handbook of Critical, Historical and Literary Writings*, Westport: Greenwood, pp.380–407.

Clay, C. and Leapman, M. (1996) *Master Race: The Lebensborn Experiment in Nazi Germany*, London: Hodder & Stoughton.

Cleminson, R. (2000) *Anarchism, Science and Sex: Eugenics in Eastern Spain, 1900–1937*, Oxford: Peter Lang.

Crook, D.P. (1994) *Darwinism, War and History: The Debate over the Biology of War from the 'Origin of Species' to the First World War*, Cambridge: Cambridge University Press.

Darwin, C. (1871) *The Descent of Man, and Selection in Relation to Sex*, vol.1, London: John Murray.

Deichmann, U. (1996) *Biologists Under Hitler*, translated by T. Dunlap, Cambridge: Harvard University Press.

Galton, F. (1865) 'Hereditary talent and character', *Macmillan's Magazine*, vol.12, pp.157–66, 318–27.

Galton, F. (1873) 'Hereditary improvement', *Macmillan's Magazine*, new series, vol.7, pp.116–30.

Galton, F. (1883) *Inquiries into Human Faculty and Its Development*, London: Macmillan.

Gillham, N.W. (2001) *Sir Francis Galton: From African Exploration to the Birth of Eugenics*, Oxford: Oxford University Press.

Kater, M.H. (1989) *Doctors under Hitler*, Chapel Hill: University of North Carolina Press.

Larson, E.J. (1991) 'The rhetoric of eugenics: expert authority and the Mental Deficiency Bill', *British Journal for the History of Science*, vol.24, pp.45–60.

MacDougall, H.A. (1982) *Racial Myth in English History: Trojans, Teutons and Anglo-Saxons*, Montreal: Harvest House.

Mackenzie, D.A. (1981) *Statistics in Britain, 1865–1930: The Social Construction of Scientific Knowledge*, Edinburgh: Edinburgh University Press.

Macnicol, J. (1989) 'Eugenics and the campaign for voluntary sterilization in Britain between the wars', *Social History of Medicine*, vol.2, pp.147–69.

Mazumdar, P. (1992) *Eugenics, Human Genetics and Human Failings: The Eugenics Society, Its Sources and Its Critics in Britain*, London: Routledge.

Müller-Hill, B. (1988) *Murderous Science: Elimination by Scientific Selection of Jews, Gypsies and Others, Germany, 1933–1945*, translated by G.R. Fraser, Oxford: Oxford University Press.

Pearson, K. (1914–30) *The Life, Letters and Labours of Francis Galton*, 3 vols in 4, Cambridge: Cambridge University Press.

Pick, D. (1989) *Faces of Degeneration: A European Disorder, c.1848– c.1918*, Cambridge: Cambridge University Press.

Poliakov, L. (1974) *The Aryan Myth: A History of Racist and Nationalist Ideas in Europe*, New York: Basic Books.

Porter, D. (1999) 'Eugenics and the sterilization debate in Sweden and Britain before World War II', *Scandinavian Journal of History*, vol.24, pp.145–62.

Porter, R. (1997) *The Greatest Benefit to Mankind: A Medical History of Humanity from Antiquity to the Present*, London: HarperCollins.

Proctor, R.N. (1988) *Racial Hygiene: Medicine under the Nazis*, Cambridge: Harvard University Press.

Proctor, R.N. (1999) *The Nazi War on Cancer*, Princeton: Princeton University Press.

Quine, M.S. (1996) *Population Politics in Twentieth-Century Europe*, London: Routledge.

Roll-Hansen, N. (1996) 'Conclusion: Scandinavian eugenics in the international context' in Broberg and Roll-Hansen (eds), *Eugenics and the Welfare State: Sterilization Policy in Denmark, Sweden, Norway and Finland*, East Lansing: Michigan State University Press, pp.259–71.

Schneider, W.H. (1990a) 'The eugenics movement in France, 1890–1940' in Adams (ed.) *The Well-Born Science: Eugenics in Germany, France, Brazil and Russia*, New York: Oxford University Press, pp.69–109.

Schneider, W.H. (1990b) *Quality and Quantity: The Quest for Biological Regeneration in Twentieth-Century France*, Cambridge: Cambridge University Press.

Searle, G.R. (1976) *Eugenics and Politics in Britain, 1900–1914*, Leyden: Noordhoff.

Soloway, R.A. (1990) *Demography and Degeneration: Eugenics and the Declining Birthrate in Twentieth-Century Britain*, Chapel Hill: University of North Carolina Press.

Thomson, M. (1998) *The Problem of Mental Deficiency: Eugenics and Social Policy in Britain, c.1870–1959*, Oxford: Clarendon Press.

Weindling, P. (1989a) *Health, Race and German Politics between National Unification and Nazism, 1870–1945*, Cambridge: Cambridge University Press.

Weindling, P. (1989b) 'The "Sonderweg" of German eugenics: nationalism and scientific internationalism', *British Journal for the History of Science*, vol.22, pp.321–33.

Weinreich, M. (1946) *Hitler's Professors: The Part of Scholarship in Germany's Crimes against the Jewish People*, New York: Yiddish Scientific Institute – YIVO.

Weiss, S.F. (1987) *Race, Hygiene and National Efficiency: The Eugenics of Wilhelm Schallmayer*, Berkeley: University of California Press.

Source Book readings

C. Darwin, *The Descent of Man, and Selection in Relation to Sex*, London: John Murray, [1874] 1883, pp.133–43, 617–18 (Reading 10.1).

F. Galton, 'Eugenics: its definition, scope and aims' in his *Essays in Eugenics*, London: Eugenics Education Society, 1909, pp.35–43 (Reading 10.2).

M. Burleigh and W. Wippermann, *The Racial State: Germany, 1933–1945*, Cambridge: Cambridge University Press, 1991, pp.304–7 (Reading 10.3).

M. Burleigh, *Death and Deliverance: 'Euthanasia' in Germany, c.1900–1945*, London: Pan Books, [1994] 2002, pp.183–5 (Reading 10.4).

D. Porter, 'Enemies of the race: biologism, environmentalism, and public health in Edwardian England', *Victorian Studies*, 1991, vol.34, pp.164–74 (Reading 10.5).

F.A.E. Crew *et al.*, 'Social biology and population improvement', *Nature*, 1939, vol.14, 16 September, pp.521–2 (Reading 10.6).

11

The Rise of the Asylum in Britain

Jonathan Andrews

Objectives

When you have completed this chapter you should be able to:

* describe some of the major developments in the history of psychiatry in Britain, especially the growth of asylums for dealing with the mentally ill;

* comprehend different historiographical and methodological approaches to the history of psychiatry;

* appreciate the ways in which the growth of British psychiatric institutions was influenced by wider social, economic, political and cultural contexts;

* understand the range of different source materials used by historians in writing the history of psychiatry.

11.1 Introduction

In the nineteenth century, the asylum became – as never before – the accepted place for the care and treatment of insanity. Until that time, people suffering from mental disorders were mostly cared for at home. Of the few institutions that offered care, most were rather small. They were funded by a combination of fees charged to patients and charitable donations or subscriptions. From the early nineteenth century, the number of asylums increased all over Europe as governments accepted a responsibility to care for the mentally ill via various (but strikingly consistent) means and timescales. Most importantly, by the 1840s and 1850s, most European governments required local authorities to build asylums. Yet this shift was not directed solely by central government. From the later eighteenth century, local Poor Law boards, regional departments, townships and other local authorities, as well as a range of private benefactors, individual social reformers and charitable agencies, were agitating for the establishment of larger-scale, purpose-built asylum accommodation. While significant opposition to asylum-building persisted at national and local levels, there was an increase in both the number and the size of such institutions. British Victorian asylums were massive complexes of buildings. County and borough asylums were catering, on average, for over 800 patients by 1890, and some were accommodating over 1,000 inmates, with growing (but often inadequate) numbers of staff to see to their needs. The rise of the asylum was not just about bricks and mortar: governments created regulatory bodies to oversee the care offered by institutions, and comprehensive bodies of lunacy legislation. (This complex of institutions, laws and agencies is referred to as **asylumdom**.)

But why (and to what extent) did the asylum become the accepted way of dealing with lunacy during the nineteenth century? In this chapter, I look at a range of arguments put forward by historians to explain (as well as to question the comprehensiveness of) this change. These accounts fall into two categories. First, there are analyses that set the growth of asylums in the context of wider social changes, including the rise of capitalism, urbanization and increasing 'social control'. Second, there are analyses that relate the growth of asylums to medical factors: reforms in the conditions of asylum life, claims for the role of the asylum in curing patients, and the rise of the power of medical practitioners. Clearly, the rise of the asylum is a complex issue. To simplify the task a little, I focus on asylums in Britain, with some limited comparative reference to France and elsewhere in Europe. The objective of looking at a number of historical analyses of the same problem is not to decide which is the 'correct' answer (although I examine which arguments have stood up best to the scrutiny of other researchers). Instead, this chapter is designed to give you a feel for how historians approach broad questions from a range of perspectives through detailed historical researches.

11.2 From Bedlam to asylumdom

Before looking at the different explanations for the growth of asylums in the nineteenth century, I offer here a brief overview of how insanity was treated before 1800, and some sense of the extent of the growth in institutional care.

It is important to remember that until the nineteenth century few insane people were confined in institutions. The vast majority were cared for within their local communities, by families, assisted by various forms of outdoor relief from their local parish. This relief might take the form of nursing care, medicine, material goods (food, clothing, etc.), regular pensions or occasional doles. While institutional care was the exception, not the rule, over the course of the eighteenth century, new institutions appeared to confine the mad and other social undesirables – prisons, Bridewells (or houses of correction), workhouses and poorhouses in Britain, *maisons de force*, *hôpitaux-généraux* and *dépôts de mendicité* in France. In Britain and much of Protestant Europe, institutional provision for the insane was a predominantly secular affair. In Catholic countries, a range of religious orders offered institutional care for the insane, from the Franciscans, Cordeliers and the Christian Brothers, to the Charitains or Brothers of Charity. In France, for example, seven of the twenty-three hospitals run by the Charitains specialized in caring for the insane, including the famous Charenton Hospital in Paris. Despite the existence of such specialist institutions, in France most of the institutionalized insane wound up in mixed institutions, alongside the unruly, the criminal and the poor. Even in monastically administered houses, a majority of lunatics mingled with a minority of *correctionnaires* – moral reprobates placed there by their families or local authorities for correction of their vices (Jones, 1990). In Britain, a smattering of lunatics found their way into workhouses and houses of correction. Only a handful of institutions dealt specifically with the insane. Separate institutional provision for the poor insane had been offered by Bethlehem (or Bethlem – proverbially, Bedlam) Hospital in London since at least the fifteenth century and, since the early eighteenth century, by Bethel Hospital in Norwich and by Guy's Hospital in London, which had a few beds for incurable lunatics (Andrews *et al.*, 1997). Nonetheless, as late as 1750, fewer than 250 lunatics were confined in these specialist institutions.

After 1750, a second generation of lunatic hospitals appeared in Britain, paralleling the growth in the number of voluntary hospitals established to care for the sick poor. As with the voluntary hospital movement, the government took little part in such initiatives. Asylums were founded and run on subscriptions from local benefactors. There was also a proliferation of private mad-houses in England and Wales that offered care to individuals from wealthy families. As late as 1800, however, the British and European insane had not yet been systematically separated as a class from other types of deviant, such as criminals, vagrants and sturdy beggars (individuals thought to be capable of work who 'preferred' to beg). Similarly, psychiatry was only just beginning to define itself as a medical specialty. 'Mad-doctors' did not receive a specialist training, and many worked in general practice while at the same time holding posts at hospitals for the insane or attending private mad-houses: medical attendance at lunatic hospitals and asylums took the form of honorary, visiting appointments, rather than full-time employment. Mad-doctors had no professional associations or journals of their own. The treatment provided was little different from that used for physical ailments – patients were bled, purged and blistered in an effort to rebalance the body's fluids or energies.

The funding and running of voluntary hospitals is described in detail in Chapter 2.

In his hugely influential book *Madness and Civilization*, first published in 1961, Michel Foucault has famously argued that the period between 1660 and 1760 saw a *grand renfermement* (great confinement) of the insane. The mad, along with the idle, immoral, dangerous and deviant, were segregated and confined in new forms of institution (Foucault, 1965). While Foucault is right to see something different in perceptions of insanity at that time, Roy Porter has shown that in numerical terms there was no 'great confinement' of the insane, either in Britain or in France (Porter, 1987). The nineteenth and early twentieth centuries saw by far the greatest increase in the numbers of those segregated and confined in various institutions, and it is this later period that might more accurately be described as being a time of 'great confinement'.

The basis of this transformation was a whole host of new, specialist institutions for the confinement and treatment of madness, and for the increasing numbers of individuals identified as insane. From the 1750s, a generation of public asylums had been established, funded predominantly by private means, by legacies, public subscriptions and patients' fees. All over Europe during the nineteenth century, central state legislation to regulate the entry of patients and the care they received was one of the driving forces behind the building of more and larger asylums. In England and Wales, for example, (Wynn's) Lunacy Act 1808 saw the start of the building of publicly funded asylums, paid for by taxes rather than by charitable giving. It granted powers to local authorities to erect asylums financed out of the rates. In fact, only nine counties actually built asylums during the following twenty years. Fundamental machinery for the certification of patients and the local overseeing of asylums was established via the amendment acts of 1811–19. The County Asylums Act 1828 required counties to erect asylums. Traditionally, the

Lunacy Act of 1845 has been seen as the major piece of Victorian lunacy legislation for England, providing comprehensive procedures for the certification of all lunatics and the inspection of all asylums. Yet more recently, historians have concluded that this Act simply codified existing patterns of practice, and have argued that the essential apparatus had already been developed via the lunacy and Poor Law Acts which preceded this (Bartlett, 1999a, b; Wright, 1998). The English 1845 Act was followed in 1857 by parallel legislation in Scotland. Attempts at comprehensive legislation in Scotland had largely foundered (including an 1818 bill to erect district asylums). The three Scottish Lunacy Acts of 1815, 1828 and 1841 were mostly concerned with the regulation of private licensed mad-houses and with certification.

By 1844, according to the annual report of the English Metropolitan Commissioners in Lunacy, in England and Wales there were seventeen publicly funded county asylums servicing mainly the poor and lower middling sort, paid for by local rates, and eleven asylums of a mixed character for private and pauper cases, funded by both rates and private fees or donations. There were also 139 private licensed houses for insane members of better-off families. By the beginning of the twentieth century, the number of public asylums alone had risen to over 70, with an average patient population of almost 1,000 each. In 1827, just over 1,000 patients were confined in English and Welsh county and city asylums (see Table 11.1). By 1890, the number of inmates had risen to somewhere around 53,000. Although a similar growth can be seen across Europe, the development of institutions took slightly different forms. In Scotland, for example, there were very few private mad-houses – only twenty-three in 1857. The timing of the growth in asylum populations also varied from place to place. In Britain, the highest rates of increase occurred between c.1827 and 1850, when the number of local authority asylums more than quadrupled and their average populations more than trebled. And the dramatic rise abated only slightly after this date, with yearly admissions more than doubling, and average numbers of (mainly 'chronic') patients more than trebling once again by 1890 (Scull, 1993). By contrast, in Prussia, for example, the major increase in asylum populations occurred much later, rising by 429 per cent during 1880–1910 (Goldberg, 1999).

It was not just that the place of care for the insane had changed; the whole perception of madness and the way it was dealt with had also been transformed. Andrew Scull, one of the most prolific writers on asylums and the care of the insane, sums up the situation:

> By the mid-nineteenth century ... [i]nsanity had been transformed ... into a condition which could be authoritatively diagnosed, certified, and dealt with by a group of legally recognized experts ... the asylum was endorsed as the sole, officially approved response to the problems posed by mental illness.
>
> (Scull, 1980, p.38)

I look at these changes in more detail later in the chapter.

Table 11.1 The growth of asylums in England and Wales, 1827–1900

Year	No. of county and city asylums	Total no. of patients	Average no. per asylum
1827	9	1,046	116
1850	24	7,140	297
1860	41	15,845	386
1870	50	27,109	542
1880	61	40,088	657
1890	66	52,937	802
1900	77	74,004	961

(Jones, 1993, p.116)

It is easy to see legislation that required local authorities to build asylums as a motor driving the growth of asylums. But this simply begs the question of why this legislation was passed. It is better to think of legislation as a response to a perceived need for more asylums. So why did governments and local authorities decide to build asylums in the nineteenth century?

11.3 Contemporary views on the growth of asylums

The most obvious explanation for the increase in the number of asylums and asylum patients is simply that the general population was increasing, and with it the number of persons suffering from some form of mental illness. However, if you look at the statistics, it becomes clear that the increase in the number of people in asylums was greater, proportionally, than the growth in population (see the figures for England and Wales in Table 11.2). The same pattern holds true for much of Europe, although there were some regional variations.

Table 11.2 Growth in the number of cases of mental illness as a proportion of the whole population of England and Wales, 1859–99

Year	Known persons of unsound mind	Increase on previous year	Number per 1,000 population
1859	31,400	–	1.60
1864	38,700	+7.3	1.93
1869	46,700	+8.0	2.17
1874	54,300	+7.6	2.36
1879	61,600	+7.3	2.44
1884	69,900	+8.3	2.77
1889	75,600	+5.7	2.66
1894	83,000	+7.4	2.79
1899	95,600	+12.6	3.03

(Jones, 1993, p.116)

Was it really the case that mental illness was becoming more common? This is an extremely difficult question to answer, since modern definitions of mental illness are not the same as nineteenth-century diagnoses of 'insanity'. However, this question was frequently discussed by contemporary commentators and the extracts that form the first reading for this chapter look at some of their conclusions.

Exercise

Read extracts (i)–(iii) of 'Contemporary accounts of the increase of insanity' (Source Book 2, Reading 11.1). Who do the three authors identify as the main social group suffering from mental illness? What explanation do they put forward for the alleged increase? Are these explanations social or medical?

Discussion

None of the commentators sees the growth in the number of asylum inmates as a direct consequence of a general epidemic of mental illness. While an increasing number of asylum patients are coming from the poorer classes, there is no such increase among the middle classes. All three authors are particularly concerned with the growth in the number of pauper lunatics, who end up in local authority asylums, paid for through local rates. Coxe argues that there may not be an absolute increase in the number of the insane. Rather, patients who were dealt with in the home, and were unknown to the authorities, are now in asylums. Hawden, by contrast, points out a greater increase in the number of pauper insane than the increase in the total number of people claiming poor relief. Her figures suggest that there is a greater prevalence of mental disease. The commentators suggest that this may be linked to urban living and working conditions. They associate urban life with the consumption of alcohol. Also, the greater cost of housing in cities means that families cannot afford to accommodate an insane relation. As this modern lifestyle spreads to rural areas, it may produce more cases of insanity. Hawden also suggests that many cases of insanity are inherited.

However, they conclude that the main causes of the growth in the numbers of asylum inmates are the simple availability of institutional care coupled with a greater willingness on the part of the public to send members of their families to asylums. This in turn is linked to an inability (or unwillingness) to tolerate strange behaviour within the home. Carswell suggests that this may reflect a more general willingness to turn to the state for help with all sorts of social difficulty. The increasing number of inmates also reflects the fact that patients are steadily accumulating within the asylums; while many inmates do recover and are discharged, there are more admissions than discharges.

Thus far, these reasons are all social. However, Carswell sets the problem at the doors of certifying medical practitioners, who are more willing, partly through pressure from relations, to diagnose patients as mentally disordered and in need of asylum care.

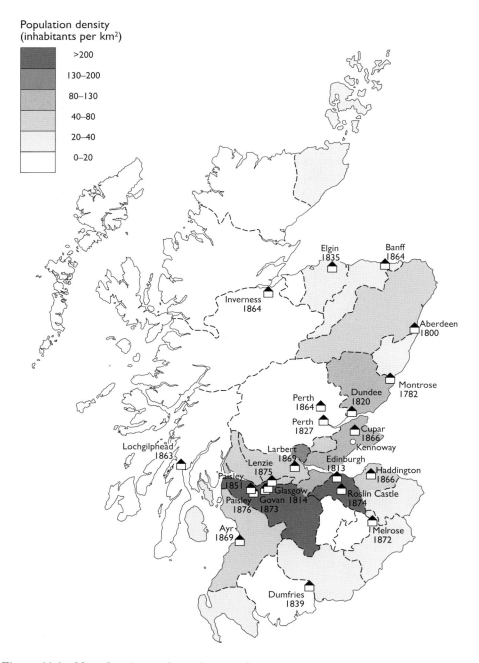

Figure 11.1   Map showing early asylums in Scotland and population densities of counties. This map shows the location of public, pauper, district and 'idiot' asylums built before 1880, and Kennoway, Scotland's most famous village centre for the boarding-out of lunatics. The map reveals the difficulty of relating asylum-building to industrialization and urbanization. While the concentration of asylums around Scotland's populous central belt is quite clear, a significant number of institutions were located in thinly populated areas

11.4   Social factors in the growth of the asylum

Industrialization, urbanization and migration

How do historians' interpretations of the growth of asylums compare with these contemporary accounts? Many historians link the rise of the asylum with the huge social changes of the nineteenth century. Some link the rise to industrialization and urbanization, pointing to the fact that asylums grew up in industrial regions and large cities. Frank Rice, for example, argues that in Scotland the great majority of asylums grew up if not within urban centres, then at least servicing urbanized communities, in the central belt of Scotland (Figure 11.1). Only two of twenty-three Scottish private mad-houses identified as being in existence in 1855 'were situated outside the central belt', and demographic research suggests that after 1811 there was never less than 81 per cent of the Scottish population concentrated within the urbanized central regions (Rice, 1985, p.44). Rice emphasizes (but fails to offer specific statistics on) the chronological correlation between the size of Scottish towns and the number of institutions erected within them. Many cities appear to have embarked on new and enlarged asylum programmes out of a recognition of the inadequacy of existing, mainly urban-sited, provision for the insane in hospitals and poorhouses. Furthermore, Rice argues, these new asylums were built just as urban communities were attaining the peak of their industrial and demographic growth rates.

However, other historians have questioned the simplicity of the link between the new cities and the asylum. They point out that asylums were in many cases sited in rural areas that had little, or limited, industrial and urban growth. The first Victorian asylums were characteristically sited at some distance from towns and cities. The archetypal model of the nineteenth-century asylum, the Quaker York Retreat, opened in 1796, was a 'retreat' offering 'asylum' from the strains and stresses of everyday life (Figure 11.2). Early prints emphasized the idyllic situation of asylums, in expansive grounds with sheep and cattle grazing nearby (Figure 11.3). Many asylums' physician-superintendents emphasized the rural nature of their catchment areas, and the easy recruitment of staff from among the servants and farmworkers of the surrounding country. In England, as Scull argues, while rural communities enthusiastically built public asylums from the 1780s onwards, few of the counties in England's most industrial, urban Midlands and northern regions built asylums until obliged to do so by the 1845 Lunacy Act (Scull, 1979, p.29). Even in Scotland, it would be stretching the point to characterize Montrose (1781–2) and Dumfries (1839), the sites of two of the earliest asylums in Scotland, as highly urbanized and industrialized regions. Elgin, the site of Scotland's first district asylum for paupers only (1835), was even further distant from the central belt. The industrialization–urbanization theory also fails to explain why poor-houses with lunatic wards attached grew up in rural areas like Stranraer or Irvine. My own studies of the catchment area for Glasgow Asylum (later Glasgow Royal Asylum) during the first decades of the nineteenth century show how broadly the institution spread its net outside Glasgow and the more industrialized regions of Lanarkshire and Renfrewshire, with significant numbers of patients coming from the more rural regions of Argyllshire, Ayrshire and Fifeshire. Unfortunately, we

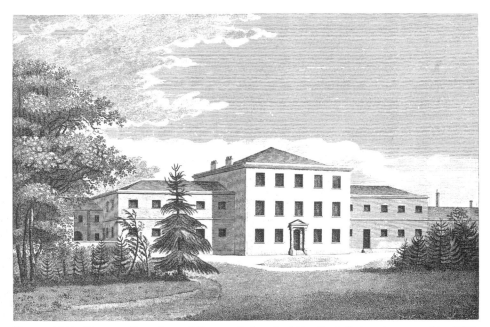

Figure 11.2   Perspective view of the north front of the York Retreat, opened in 1796 and run by William Tuke (1732–1822), a retired tea merchant, and his family. It was intended primarily for members of the Society of Friends (Quakers), although as time went on it became increasingly multi-denominational. The engraving shows the plain edifice of the Retreat, and its leafy site, removed from the bustle of York. The inspiration for the foundation of the Retreat was the Tukes' disgust at the ill treatment and death of a Leeds Quaker, Hannah Mills, in the York Asylum. This image is taken from the frontispiece of *Description of the York Retreat* (1813), written by William's grandson Samuel, which did more than any single publication to broadcast and popularize the virtues of the Tukes' distinctive approach to madness, known as 'moral therapy'

still lack enough detailed surveys of the origins of Scottish asylums and their demographic profiles to attempt an overall model.

Another issue in question is whether or not the growth of asylums occurred at the same time as the growth of cities. Andrew Scull argues that the main growth of asylums took place before Britain was truly urbanized. While more than half of the populations of England and Wales lived in cities or towns by the middle of the nineteenth century, most of these communities were small. Only around one-third of the population lived in cities of 20,000 or more people. By this time, the asylum movement was well established, with all the major pieces of legislation in place and large numbers of asylums founded.

However, recent historical research has produced new evidence in two areas that challenges Scull's assertion that asylum-building preceded urbanization and industrialization. This work has shown that there was a significant phase of proto-industrialization which preceded and laid the foundations for larger-scale industrial, urban and commercial growth. There was no radical divide between

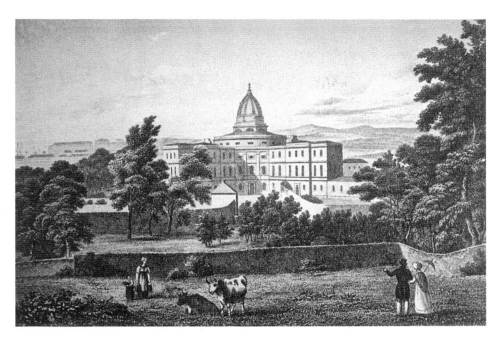

Figure 11.3   The first Glasgow Asylum for Lunatics, at Parliamentary Road, Dobbie's Loan, opened in 1814 and renamed the Glasgow Royal Asylum after it acquired a royal charter in 1824. This engraving underlines the representation of the asylum as a rural retreat. Clearly, the site was selected because of its appreciable remove from the urban sprawl of Scotland's rapidly expanding second city. The architect, William Stark, and its directors and staff, certainly claimed common ground with the ethos of the Retreat. This engraving was reproduced repeatedly to publicize the asylum, even after it had been rebuilt in Tudor-Gothic style on a new site at Gartnavel, Glasgow (where it remains to this day)

urban and rural areas in terms of industrial development, with many factories (especially textile works) and proto-industrialized crafts growing up within urban networks but closely linked to rural economies. Recent surveys of English urbanization have emphasized the dramatic nature of the shift away from rural dwelling-places into townships and cities in the period c.1780–1850, and suggest that towns of 5,000 ought to be ranked as urbanized in contemporary terms (King and Timmins, 2001).

Scull and other historians have pointed to capitalism and the rise of an economy based on the payment of wages, rather than urbanization or industrialization, as important factors in the growth of institutional care for the insane. The next reading, from Scull's book *The Most Solitary of Afflictions: Madness and Society in Britain, 1700–1900*, reviews the debate over whether urbanization or capitalism drove the increase in asylum populations.

Read 'The impact of industrialisation' (Source Book 2, Reading 11.2).

1   What aspects of capitalism does Scull believe contributed to the rise of the asylum?

2   How does his analysis compare with the contemporary accounts you read earlier?

1   Scull argues that capitalism and the emergence of a commercial society in the late eighteenth and early nineteenth centuries, which occurred *before* large-scale industrialization, destroyed the old ways of dealing with insanity within a domestic setting. A money-based, highly competitive economy broke the old social bonds between upper and lower classes that had helped poorer families to care for a mentally disordered person. In cities, where housing costs were high, families were unable to support an unproductive member, or to care for them, especially as their wages rose and fell dramatically during periods of boom and bust.

2   Scull is broadly in agreement with the contemporary accounts in seeing social change as the key factor in asylum growth. However, he has the benefit of standing back and using earlier historians' interpretations of broad social change in the nineteenth century. The contemporary accounts are much more impressionistic, relying on personal observations.

This is a very appealing argument. However, recent work by a number of historians suggests that we need to treat it with a certain degree of caution. This new research is built on a different approach: rather than trying to link a broad asylum movement with major social change, it focuses on particular institutions and the experience of individual patients, and forms part of the movement to study 'history from below'. It uses hitherto neglected sources such as medical certificates, family members' descriptions of patients' behaviour prior to admission, and patient records from asylums. This provides a quite different perspective on the asylum, one that highlights issues of demand and need as well as supply. You will encounter a number of such studies in the rest of this chapter. On the question of why patients were admitted to asylums, studies of accounts provided by the friends and families of the mentally disordered lend only qualified support to Scull's view that economic strain was the main trigger for seeking admission. Families and friends occasionally spoke of loss of income to the household through the expenses associated with nursing and managing a mentally disordered individual, through their own, or that individual's, inability to get employment. But there is little evidence yet from these sources that such rationales for committal figured any more prominently than they had done in previous times (Adair *et al.*, 1998; Walton, 1981, 1985; Wright, 1998).

Similarly, detailed work on the geographical origins of asylum patients has also questioned the portrayal of the link between urban migration, social dislocation and the asylum. We might assume that the migration of families into towns in search of work would have loosened networks of support, and ultimately led to families placing members in asylums. The story is not that simple, however. My research on Glasgow Royal Asylum shows that although there were recent migrants to the city among the inmates, they were not a conspicuously large group. An extensive survey of the route to the asylum in the Devon region during the second half of the nineteenth century by Adair *et al.* (1997) has argued that the relationship of migration to asylum admission was actually the reverse – at least in some areas. They find that it was not the migrants who were more prone to end up in the region's asylums. On the contrary, it was 'from the deeply rooted, physically less mobile and more socially entrenched families that the bulk of ... patients came', and thus from those sectors of society where kinship and household ties would be expected to be more resilient (Adair *et al.*, 1997, p.393). Longer distance migration in Devon was actually associated with *lower* admission rates. The key factor here seems to be that insanity (like other forms of illness) prevented families from being mobile and moving into the cities.

Social control, the family and the asylum

Both contemporary commentators and historians have argued that the pressures of capitalism resulted in families being not only less capable of supporting family members but also less tolerant of unruly behaviour. In Scull's phrase, the asylum became a dumping ground for 'inconvenient people'. It is clear from contemporary admission documents, including private correspondence and diaries, that caring for a mentally ill relative put all sorts of emotional strains on families. Many strove in vain to keep the problem within doors. They struggled to cope with the verbal incongruities and indiscretions of people with florid delusions, or with the often frightening and wearing behavioural anomalies of those who were destructive, violent, despondent and self-harming. Most felt the strain of dealing with the associated problems of compromised working lives and interrupted sleep. Most admission records dwell on the troublesome, bizarre and traumatic nature of the behaviour of the mentally disordered. Such behaviour was likely to bring the insane into contact with the police and other authorities engaged in maintaining good social order. This is the basis of another explanation for the growth of asylums: that these institutions were used for the social control of deviancy. This thesis sees the asylum as an instrument for the (bourgeois) establishment of norms and social order, via the incarceration of those defined as socially, morally, politico-religiously and physically deviant and dangerous (Doerner, [1969] 1981; Goffman, [1961] 1990; Rothman, 1971). Ireland, where the insane and mentally disabled were confined (and conflated with the criminal) in accordance with the Dangerous Lunatics Act 1838, seems to provide particular evidence for the intensification of representations of insanity as 'dangerous in this period' (Walsh, 1999).

So were asylums geared to dealing with Scull's 'inconvenient people' or were they about confining disorderly persons who threatened bourgeois property and livelihoods? John Walton has made a detailed study of admissions to Lancaster County Asylum which presents some useful evidence for deciding between these two viewpoints.

Read 'Getting rid of "inconvenient people"?' (Source Book 2, Reading 11.3).

1   What does Walton conclude about the reasons for admission of persons to the Lancaster Asylum?

2   How does his work challenge the claims made by Scull?

1   Walton dismisses the idea that the asylum is used in any systematic way to deal with the 'disorderly poor' – although a small number of asylum admissions did come through the law courts. He also finds little substantial evidence that asylums served the function of quelling political or religious dissent: only a handful of patients seem to have been admitted on such grounds without other signs of mental disorder. He suggests that the machinery of asylum admission was simply too complex to make it an effective method of social control.

2   Walton argues that people admitted to the asylum were not the 'inconvenient people' of the Scull thesis but were, rather, 'impossible people'. Drink and violence, especially violence towards other family members, as well as deep depression and suicidal behaviour figured in over half of the admissions. There is little evidence that any failure to contribute to family income was a reason for incarceration. Walton argues that families did not dump their relatives in the asylum: institutional care was a last, not a first, resort. Family bonds and social networks were resilient under the pressures of hardship and destitution.

Other studies back up Walton's conclusions by showing that the police were rarely involved in committing lunatics. My study of Gartnavel Royal Hospital (Glasgow Lunatic Asylum) reveals that as many as 10 per cent of committals had some kind of police involvement, but that a large proportion of these patients came voluntarily to police stations, or exhibited highly delusive, dangerous or disruptive forms of behaviour. Others were sent to asylums at the behest of their families after getting into trouble (often repeatedly) with the police. Such findings do not entirely fit with the idea of close social control through intensified policing of Victorian societies.

There seems no doubt that, as Walton puts it, 'the roots of most asylum committals clearly lay in domestic troubles, as families at the end of their tether sought succour even though it meant the Poor Law and the asylum' (Walton, 1985, p.139). Does this mean that we should accept the views of contemporary commentators that families' increased willingness to confine individuals was the result of the availability of asylum accommodation? Was the growth of the asylum a result of the supply of places, or a real demand for such care? Given Walton's argument that families did look after mentally ill relations until the situation became difficult or even dangerous, and the way in which asylums were constantly forced either to expand, to rebuild or to refuse large numbers of applicants, the answer seems to be that there was a genuine demand for places, and not that working-class families were cynically exploiting a resource to deal with awkward family members. Almost invariably, the number of applicants exceeded the available accommodation, and the mounting waiting lists for admission suggest that the demand increased ahead of supply.

11.5 Medical factors in the growth of the asylum

Apart from the social factors I have discussed, historians have also pointed to developments in medicine as a cause of the growth in the asylum: that the definitions of madness expanded, that the asylum became a more attractive option for the care of the insane, and that through the development of psychiatry as a specialism and claims to be able to treat insanity, doctors acquired greater powers to commit and confine the mentally disordered.

Redefining madness

The idea that the boundaries of what constituted madness expanded during the nineteenth century was articulated by many Victorian medical practitioners who dealt with madness (or **alienists**, the term widely employed in Europe until around the 1930s). The Scottish Lunacy Commissioner James Coxe (1811–78) declared in 1872, 'the definition of lunacy has expanded, and many a one is accordingly treated as a lunatic who formerly would not have been regarded as coming within the meaning of the term' (quoted in Renvoize, 1991, p.61). From the mid-eighteenth to the early nineteenth centuries, insanity was as much a moral (and mental) as a physiological disorder. Bad behaviour, vitiated judgement and inordinate passions or emotions – from excessive joy or pride to excessive dolour, and from drunkenness, sexual licence and extrovert religious fervour to rudeness towards parents and masters – were often key signs of madness. During the early 1800s, such perceptions culminated in the articulation of novel diagnostic concepts such as 'moral insanity' (coined by the alienist James Cowles Prichard (1786–1848)) and 'monomania', whereby certain types of insanity might be manifested and understood solely in terms of disordered or perverted moral sensibilities, or as a partial delirium affecting a single subject, idea or mental faculty. The asylum was advocated by many as a kind of moral reformatory, where patients could be taught to re-establish their own internal controls over their behaviour and distorted morals or faculties.

After the 1840s, however, while traditional moral and behavioural aetiologies continued to have a place in mental diagnostics and in committal papers, the Victorian asylum movement was more pervasively grounded on new definitions of madness. In accounts of madness written in the later nineteenth century, organic and physical causes took precedence over external behaviour. Increasingly, as insights from phrenology and research into the localization of mental faculties (described in Chapter 4) took hold, mind and brain began to be seen as coterminous, and insanity was regarded as rooted fundamentally and primarily in the brain. Nineteenth-century notions of insanity emphasized physiological causes, and stressed in particular the damaging effects on the body and brain of vice, dissipation and overindulgence. Later in the century, influenced by anthropological and evolutionary theory and **Social Darwinism**, and by models of defect such as those proposed by Francis Galton and B.A. Morel (1809–73), alienists stressed the role of heredity and racial degeneration as underlying causes of insanity, although the disease might still be triggered by circumstances or behaviour (Pick, 1989). Yet even though alienists became more convinced as to the underlying organic root to most mental disorders, relatives continued to conceive of insanity in multi-causal terms, specifying a wide range of factors in their explanations of the mental derangement of a family member and in the process of a committal. James Coxe, like many commentators, stressed the multiplicity of 'different influences' and causes that might lead to people being certified as insane, among them 'temper, disease, vice, intemperance, or old age' (quoted in Renvoize, 1991, p.61). In around 20 per cent of patients admitted to asylums like Glasgow Royal in the 1870s and 1880s, the cause of their problems was ascribed (primarily) by their relations in admission documents to alcohol, yet in as many as 44 per cent of cases their problems were attributed to moral, emotional and environmental causes such as love and grief, with over 52 per cent of patients having some such constituent as an ingredient of their aetiologies. When alienists sought to categorize different forms of mental condition, they too marked the emotional behaviour of patients as well as attempting to identify characteristic physical appearance and facial expressions (Figures 11.4 and 11.5).

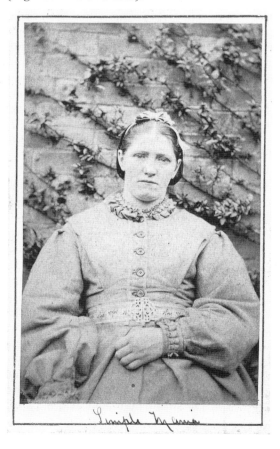

Figure 11.4   Simple mania. Photograph of a female patient at the West Riding Lunatic Asylum. Photography, which initially promised to provide alienists with the means of fixing more accurately the physical and facial characteristics of a diagnosis and, via multiple photographs, charting progress or decline in a case, soon became a more limited undertaking exploited primarily to identify individual patients rather than for diagnostic purposes. Wellcome Library, London

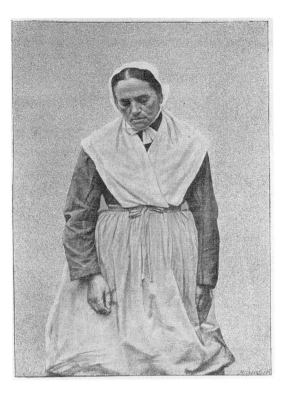

Figure 11.5 *Mélancolie anxieuse* (anxious melancholy), from Henri Dagonet, *Nouveau traité elementaire* (New Elementary Treatise), 1876. Another photograph attempting to fix the diagnosis scientifically. The representation is intended to show the downcast head, eyes and facial expression, along with the 'continual moaning' and 'imaginary guilt' that are deemed characteristic of the condition. Wellcome Library, London

New guidelines for committal devised in the nineteenth century may also have expanded the boundaries of what constituted insanity. Eighteenth-century lunacy law focused on those lunatics adjudged 'dangerous to themselves or others', placing the onus on families and communities to keep them within doors. Nineteenth-century lunacy legislation widened this brief to include not only those who were dangerous, but also those adjudged unable to take proper care of themselves. In Britain by the 1810s, certifying medical officers were completing detailed questionnaires as to patients' behavioural anomalies as derived (mainly) from relatives' testimonies. By the middle of the nineteenth century, reception orders became more medically authoritative, distinguishing between facts observed by medical men and those observed by others. Eighteenth-century institutions like London's Bethlem had attempted to prioritize the admission of acute, dangerous and violent cases, although it is debatable what proportion of patients had genuinely threatened or committed violent acts prior to admission, while 'incurables' or chronic cases became a substantial proportion of such hospitals' provision from the second third of the century (Andrews *et al.*, 1997). Buoyed up by enthusiastic conviction in the philosophy of moral management (see below), and with traditional moral explanations reinforced by more organic understandings of insanity, nineteenth-century institutions and alienists may well have widened definitions of certifiable impairment. Certainly, as you have seen, contemporary commentators believed that medical men were willing to diagnose an increasing range of symptoms as forms of madness. Whatever the case, it seems indubitable that alienists were increasingly accepting of chronicity and incurability as inherent in asylum populations (Ray, 1981, esp. pp.252–9).

Moralizing the insane: the 'reformed' and 'domesticated' asylum

A further argument to explain the growth of asylums in the nineteenth century is that the asylum was itself reformed, making it a more attractive option for families seeking to care for the mentally disordered. Early nineteenth-century asylums, such as the York Retreat, pioneered the use of moral therapy or moral management. There was an increased stress on appealing to patients to employ their own inner self-control instead of relying on outer, mechanical forms of restraint. Patients were classified and segregated more effectively to ensure social and sexual decorum, and asylum administrators stressed the need to recruit and train staff of a high moral and professional calibre who would show kindness towards patients. Mad-doctors and medical specialists after 1750 emphasized as never before the benefits of confinement in asylums and the need for patients to be removed from their families and from the context of their disturbance. Asylum clinicians and lunacy administrators alike argued that confinement was absolutely necessary for the cure of most forms of insanity.

The later nineteenth century saw further profound changes in the way madness was managed – changes that have been described as the 'domestication of madness' (Scull, 1989a). Efforts were made to render the asylum more 'homely' and comfortable, and to bring its accommodation into line with the surroundings that its inmates and their families might expect to find at home. On the one hand, many asylums became huge 'museum-like' structures, ever-expanding agglomerations of buildings covering huge areas the size of a village, in which patients must have felt overawed (Figure 11.6). On the other hand, concerted efforts were made to improve the range of comforts and amenities offered, in an attempt to mimic the situations from which patients had sprung. This meant not only improving the furnishings of asylums, but making them fit the particular purchasing powers of patients and their relations, so that accommodation was available on a series of scales. Asylums supported an increasingly wide-ranging programme of activities and pastimes, from board games, magic lantern shows, bowling, cricket, dancing and music, to literary clubs and patient magazines. In accordance with dominant social strictures and market-oriented philosophies, many of the more genteel of these recreations were reserved exclusively for the better class of patient. The large-scale provision of manual occupations in asylums for paupers – including digging, farming and gardening (for males), and housework, sewing and laundry (for females) – brought the physical and psychological benefits of vigorous work for patients and substantial economic benefits for the institution. The fatiguing or soporific effects of such work can also be seen as an effective means of quelling and diverting the potential unrest and excitement of large captive populations – and some historians have perceived nineteenth-century carceral institutions as putting the deviant, as never before, to work. Bullying, coercion and exploitation of 'drudge' patients by staff, alongside clear employment-mediated pecking orders, plainly occurred at some asylums. However, the punishment, restraint or withdrawal of privileges for patients refusing to work was increasingly seen as an abuse of the system. Occupational and recreational provision also served to some degree as a means of convincing the public of the productivity and reformatory nature of asylum care. The nineteenth-century asylum was just one of a range of institutions, including the almshouse, the workhouse, the penitentiary and the factory, that aimed to instil 'habits of industry' in 'unproductive' inmates, although the accumulation of chronic cases dulled early hopes of turning most asylum patients into 'productive members of society'.

This period also witnessed a transformation of the relationship of the wider community to the asylum. Until the late eighteenth century, families and friends had enjoyed considerable influence over when, in what circumstances and for how long the mentally disordered were incarcerated. In the nineteenth century, these powers passed to the medical profession and to official watchdogs like the Lunacy Commission. Visitors to early nineteenth-century asylums found themselves subject to increasingly restrictive rules. The first generation of nineteenth-century asylums exerted tight controls over contact between patients, families and friends. Indeed, asylum doctors of the 1820s and 1830s seem to have been more prone than earlier alienists to barring friends whose interaction they saw as harmful or risky from further contact with patients, while patients' correspondence was withheld or censored. Many patients were not even allowed pen and ink at these early asylums. From the 1840s, restrictions began to be eased, although throughout the late eighteenth and nineteenth centuries patients' mail was subject to being

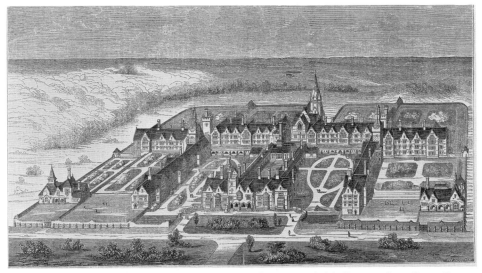

Figure 11.6   Essex County Lunatic Asylum, Brentwood, bird's-eye view, from the *Builder*, 16 May 1857. A typical village-like asylum on a grand scale, this encapsulates what Scull means in his evocative phrase 'museums of madness'. It was one of the asylums in which the famous Victorian alienist Sir Henry Maudsley (1835–1918) cut his teeth as a medical officer. Opened on 23 September 1853, its initial population of 300 patients had expanded to 450 by 1858. It offered a model of contemporary segregative and proportional design: large airing court expanses to the side and behind the main building ensured separate exercise for each sex, and the administrative block was placed hierarchically at the centre front, with the chapel at centre back. Wellcome Library, London

withheld in most asylums. Only in the late nineteenth century did patient letterboxes appear in some asylums. The later part of the century saw increasing freedoms being made available to patients, for example the wider granting of leaves of absence, the removal of locks from many wards and the demolition of the imposing asylum walls.

But are historians right to argue that the asylum became more acceptable to the public? There is evidence for a continuing stigma of committal, not least in the vocal opposition one finds in patients' correspondence, admission documents and case notes. Fears of false confinement and of abuse of patients within asylums remained rife, as evidenced in the work of contemporary bodies like the Alleged Lunatics' Friend Society (Hervey, 1986). However, the psychiatric profession worked hard to combat such stigma, and a steady effort to reform and transform the physical and therapeutic environment of the asylum did placate some of society's concerns.

Medical men as 'moral entrepreneurs'

Alongside his thesis concerning the social consequences of capitalism as a cause of the increase of confinement, Scull argues that the expanding use of asylums was closely linked to the acceptance that medical practitioners alone possessed the expert knowledge required to treat and cure insanity. They exploited an adaptation of moral therapy and non-restraint – forms of treatment that were only partially reliant on medical theory – in Scull's evocative term, becoming 'moral entrepreneurs' (Scull, 1989b). While many historians would not accept Scull's argument *in toto*, most do associate the rise of asylumdom with the emergence of a cadre of specialist practitioners.

Closer examination casts doubt on this argument. Undoubtedly, medical men did press the case for the use of moral therapy to treat madness. The establishment of the Quaker York Retreat in 1796 and the work and writing of Philippe Pinel (1745–1826), medical director of the Salpêtrière Asylum in Paris, mark the rise of an innovative approach to the treatment of the insane known as 'moral treatment' or 'moral therapy'. The system was characterized by techniques of resocializing patients through the disciplines and diversions of work and entertainment, and through rewards, privileges and punishments, applied according to good or bad behaviour. This had a far-reaching impact on the mental medicine of nineteenth-century Europe. Moral treatment was publicized in the *Description of the York Retreat*, 1813, by Samuel Tuke (1784–1857), grandson and successor of the York Retreat's founder, William. Pinel, credited rather inaccurately by subsequent generations with having spectacularly struck off the chains from the Salpêtrière's female inmates, was to achieve similar fame to the Tukes for his own brand of moral therapeutics detailed in his *Treatise of Insanity* (1806). Alienists undoubtedly succeeded in bolstering their reputations through their adoption of non-restraint, as popularized during the 1830s and 1840s, especially by Drs Charlesworth and Robert Gardiner Hill (1811–78) at Lincoln, and John Conolly (1794–1866) at Hanwell Asylum. From the 1860s, policies such as 'open-doors' (or unlocked wards) and voluntary admissions in asylums, pioneered in Britain by

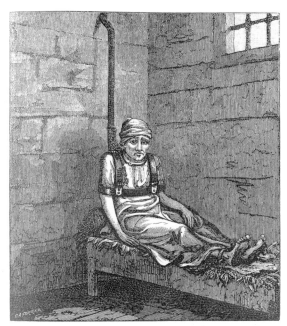

Figure 11.7   James Norris (wrongly called William in official reports and newspapers), an 'insane American' sailor, under restraint in his Bethlem cell. Norris became a *cause célèbre* for reformers during the 1815–16 House of Commons Enquiry into Madhouses. He was found in 1814 in an elaborate, highly constrictive and shocking iron harness contraption of mechanical restraint, in which he had been kept confined for more than ten years. His case was the most conspicuous of the patient abuses uncovered by the Quaker Edward Wakefield and his co-reformers. This engraving was just one of many produced at the time and in the years that followed the enquiry to dramatize Norris's plight. More than any other image, it came to be seen as emblematic of the former excesses of restraint and old Bedlam mad-doctoring. Wellcome Library, London

Scottish asylums, further eroded the old images of the physically restrained madman (Figure 11.7).

Around this time, alienists made new claims for the power of the asylum to cure insanity. The prevalence of new notions of insanity as a disorder rooted in the brain but amenable to re-education meant that the asylum could be designed as an agent of cure that would help rationally to remodel the minds of the insane. The wide appeal of moral therapy helped to foster the founding of a whole host of such purpose-built asylums. Foundations of model asylums, from the York Retreat to the Crichton Royal in Dumfries, and the promotional publications of asylum doctors and officials, such as Tuke's *Description of the York Retreat* (1813) and W.A.F. Browne's *What Asylums Were, Are and Ought To Be* (1834) helped to legitimate the role of the reformed asylum. Early utopian notions of asylum construction, like the panopticon Glasgow Asylum of 1814 (Figure 11.8), presented a complex building in which patients were rigidly classified according to sex, class and type of disorder, and where carefully controlled social intercourse would help to restore reason.

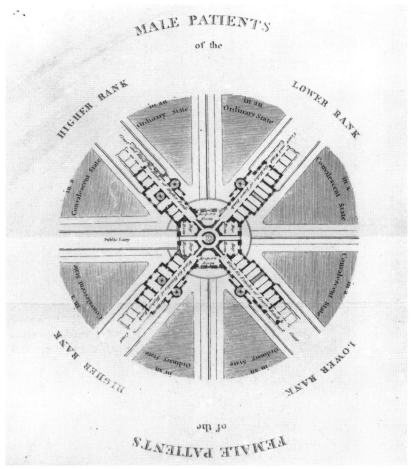

Figure 11.8   William Stark's (1770–1813) plan of the panopticon-like Glasgow Asylum, published in the 2nd edition of his *Remarks on the Construction of Public Hospitals for the Cure of Mental Derangement*, 1810 (first published 1807). There are clear similarities between Stark's plan and panopticon prisons, hospitals and asylums built on the Continent. Using this institutional plan, staff numbers were minimized and observational efficiency maximized by the use of radiating wings fanning spoke-like from a central circular corridor and tower. The plan emphasizes the concerns with segregation, classification and surveillance, patients being separated not only by class and sex but by degree of illness (i.e. whether 'frantic', 'incurable', convalescent' or 'in an ordinary state'). Patients' recovery was to be facilitated by the fact that they were unable to catch even a glimpse of inmates from other classes, either from the wards or from the asylum's four enclosed airing courts. This idealized classificatory system was never really implemented at Glasgow, since it proved impractical. Instead, the evacuative treatments, mechanical restraints and intimidatory tactics of old were applied, at least initially. The rigid and rather forbidding characteristics of this plan may be contrasted with the idealized version of the asylum in Figure 11.3. And significantly, though Stark's asylum was initially praised by native and foreign observers alike as ultra-modern, it was roundly censured by Samuel Tuke as 'prison-like'. By permission of the British Library, shelfmark 7306.b.13(1)

How successful were alienists in developing new and effective therapies? Although we would now dismiss them as useless or even harmful, physical remedies – purges and vomits, regimen, exercise and diet – were the mainstays of practice until the 1840s. In the early nineteenth century, the new sciences of hydraulics and hydrotherapy developed during the scientific and industrial revolutions were applied by means of new restraining chairs, whirling chairs or douche bathing contraptions (Figures 11.9 and 11.10). The use of 'shock' tactics was a pretty staple part of eighteenth- and early nineteenth-century mad-doctoring. Such recourses were sanctioned on a variety of theoretical grounds. The body might be loaded with corrupted matter, which required violent intervention and evacuation in order to expel it. Literally jolting the system might be required to raise patients out of their torpor. Finally, lunatics were seen as often stubborn, and therefore as requiring 'terrific', if not punitive, tactics to break down their wills and intimidate them into good behaviour. Such theories were also justified by classical medical models that had long countenanced the use of fear and of opposites (stimulation for torpor and calm for excitation) in treating lunatics, and had also recommended supplanting one prevailing impression with another, stronger impression. The next reading is a series of extracts from case notes on the use of the rotary chair at Glasgow Asylum, 1820–1.

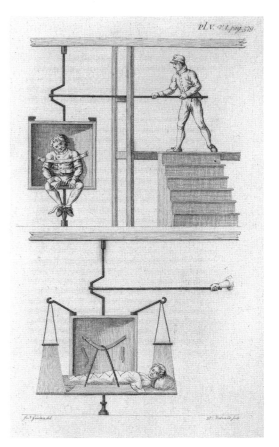

Figure 11.9   Rotary machine, or whirling chair, from Joseph Guislain, *Traité sur l'aliénation mentale*, 1826. This contraption was designed to revolve patients in order to induce dizziness and vomiting (without the use of artificial chemicals). Vomiting was, according to the dominant theories of medicine, a salutary aid in the voiding of corrupt matter from the body. The machine was adapted by a number of different alienists and institutions in Europe, and calibrated by some to be able to procure a particular number or speed of revolutions. The popularity of this device was, however, short-lived at most asylums. Wellcome Library, London

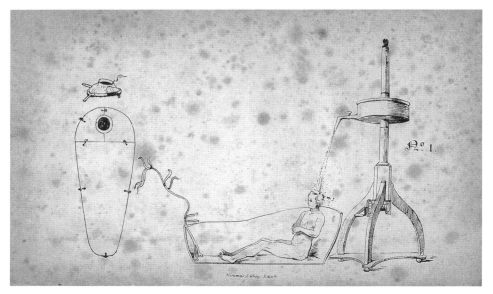

Figure 11.10   Douche, or shower-bath, from Alexander Morison (physician-superintendent at Bethlem Hospital), *Cases of Mental Disease*, 1828. Another form of 'shock' therapy employed at a wide range of asylums from the eighteenth century and through the nineteenth century. The apparatus was designed (and was increasingly intricately calibrated) to allow for the fall of variable amounts of water on the bare or shaven head of the patient. Morison's design for this machine was somewhat primitive, being basically 'a bucket ... regulated by a rope and pully – by the cock inserted into the lower part of the bucket'. This image also depicts the warm bath apparatus to which patients were often simultaneously or separately subjected, as well as straps which were used to restrain patients if necessary. The combined apparatus allowed for total and forcible immersion, and a stark contrast of temperatures and effects. This form of treatment was deemed to have both a cooling or soothing and a shocking impact on patients (maniacs were formerly conceptualized as 'hot-headed', while many early nineteenth-century alienists continued to see insanity as an inflammation of the brain). Wellcome Library, London

Exercise

Read 'The effects of the whirling chair' (Source Book 2, Reading 11.4). What are the reasons for advocating use of the whirling chair? What effects does it appear to have, and can you think of any reason why these might be thought to be beneficial? Do you think the chair was used as punishment or therapy?

Discussion

Unruly behaviour seems to be the main reason for prescribing the use of the chair. Male and female, private and pauper patients were subjected to this treatment. One patient was evidently whirled due to masturbation ('self-pollution'), and others because they were unruly, or obstinate. The physical effects of nausea and vomiting were seen as efficacious in that they might evacuate purulent or noxious matter from the body. Meanwhile, the powerful impact the treatment exerted on the senses, and its strong psychological effects, might help to alter the patient's behaviour – and staff noted that after time in the chair some patients became docile, obedient and tractable. Such treatments were also a form of threat and intimidation, the mere mention of the chair often sufficient on its own to subdue patients. Such techniques must have been physically exhausting, and so can be seen as a form of sedation prior to the development of more effective chemical tranquillizers. Although it is easy to think that the whirling chair was used to punish patients – sometimes to the point of torture – we must remember that contemporary medical theories justified the salutary use of fear in managing the insane.

Few of these technologies endured or brought genuine kudos to the special competence of alienists. The development and wider use after 1850 of new tranquillizers or hypnotics such as chloral hydrate and sulphonal, and the hypodermic injection of morphia, rendered asylums more ordered and quiet, but also did little to bolster their therapeutic image. Even by the 1910s, mental medicine had nothing to compare with antisepsis or inoculation, and alienists themselves sometimes bemoaned the lack of a therapeutic breakthrough.

Medical 'imperialism' and the making of psychiatry

Most historians link the rise of institutional care for the insane with the development of psychiatry itself as a specialism. Scull has often spoken of such developments as professional 'imperialism' and the product of alienists' self-interest. While this has raised the hackles of some historians (especially those who are clinically trained), most historians would at least accept that Victorian asylum doctors succeeded in promoting their position as arbiters of mental illness, just as other practitioners enjoyed status as experts on a wide range of medical matters by the end of the century.

Before the late eighteenth century, few medical practitioners specialized in the treatment of insanity. Those that did so had little sense of a common professional identity, their rather ambiguous status being encapsulated in their popular title 'mad-doctor'. This situation was not helped by the scandals of the private 'trade in lunacy' (Parry-Jones, 1972). Since the early eighteenth century, the pages of British magazines, periodicals and broadsheets had been peppered with a litany of reports of false confinements and ill treatment of patients in private mad-houses, from the case of Sarah Clerke in 1718, to that of the prime minister Spencer Perceval's son, John, in the 1830s (Andrews, 1990; Peterson, 1982). A number of such patients penned long narratives of their experiences, berating the iniquities of mad-houses and those who ran them. Parliamentary enquiries such as those of 1763 and 1815, and the associated legislation that followed, provided for only limited inspectorial oversight over the operations of this business prior to 1845. Mad-doctoring by its very nature, and by virtue of the social unpalatability of the patients it dealt with, seemed to attract the distrust and stigma of the public at large. As late as 1864, alienists still complained of the low status of mental medicine in the eyes of the public. Things were apparently little better on the

Continent. The verdict of the renowned visiting German alienist Baron Mundy (1822–94) was that 'our science does not exist at all ... every snob has now become accustomed to sneer at mad-doctors' (quoted in Turner, 1991, p.6).

By the end of the nineteenth century, alienists had accumulated an impressive body of literature and experience on the basic pathology of mental disease and its various manifestations. In 1841, practitioners formed the Association of Medical Officers of Asylums and Hospitals for the Insane. By the 1860s, it had become a truly national association, renamed in 1865 the Medico-Psychological Association (MPA), with subordinate divisional organizations for Scotland and Ireland. The association had its own journal (the *Asylum Journal* [*of Mental Science*], later the *Journal of Mental Science*), which furthered the formation of a cohesive professional identity among alienists. Just as in general medicine, where hospital training and practice became vital to a successful medical career, the specialty of mental medicine became steadily associated with the public asylum.

The specialism was further developed through the growth of formal medical education and training in psychiatry. From the 1830s to the 1840s, some renowned asylum superintendents and private practitioners gave public lectures on mental diseases, and institutions increasingly conducted informal training for their medical assistants and attendants. In the last decades of the century, however, the MPA began to supervise the format of examinations for medical students in mental diseases and inaugurated a formal training programme for asylum attendants. Towards the end of the century, insanity also began to be taught as a separate subject within the university medical curriculum. Alienists gained university chairs; Thomas Clouston, for example, succeeded to the first Scottish university lectureship in mental diseases at Edinburgh in 1879, followed the next year by David Yellowlees, of Glasgow Royal Asylum, who was appointed to a lectureship in insanity at Glasgow University. Others sought and garnered a substantial degree of social status, profession kudos and financial success in work beyond the asylum sector, in private consulting practice, tending to the nervous and deranged among the well-heeled classes. Quite a few leading Victorian alienists chose to abandon their asylum posts to become society physicians, including Sir John Charles Bucknill (1817–97), Sir James Crichton-Browne (1840–1938) and Sir George Henry Savage (1842–1921) (Figure 11.11), one-time doctor to Virginia Woolf.

The growing influence of alienists was also apparent in the area of legislation. For decades, practitioners had given testimony before government enquiries into lunacy, only to have their recommendations and their drafts of bills rejected. Gradually, however, and partly through the MPA and other professional organizations, they began to exert themselves in a more concerted way as a pressure group. Politicians began to consult with practitioners during the framing of new lunacy law. Disputes over definitions of insanity, particularly in law courts, were a prominent feature of the profession's activities throughout the nineteenth and twentieth centuries. By 1900, the authority of the psychiatrist's testimony was firmly established.

However, medical men did not have total authority over all matters connected with mental illness. Lawyers, politicians and local government officials also enjoyed a good deal of influence over the lunacy law and its administration. Throughout the

There is a clear parallel between the processes by which alienists acquired respectability within medicine and the professionalization of medicine described in Chapter 5. Both groups based their claim to status on possession of a body of highly specialized knowledge and skills in treating illness.

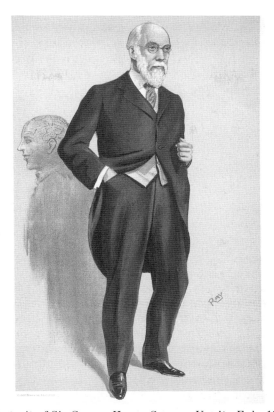

Figure 11.11   Portrait of Sir George Henry Savage, *Vanity Fair*, 1912. Savage's inclusion in the gentle caricatures of *Vanity Fair* (as with that of his contemporary, James Crichton-Browne) is a sign of his status as a society physician. Following appointments as medical officer (1872–9) and physician-superintendent (1879–88) at Bethlem Hospital, like many of his prominent alienist colleagues, Savage gravitated towards a career in private consultative practice. In this capacity, he treated Virginia Woolf. His prescription of a 'rest-cure' was little appreciated, however, by the independent-minded author, who deeply resented being banned from writing and banished to the boredom of country life. She got her own back in her novel *Mrs Dalloway* (1925), when she used him as one of her models for the character of the socially unpolished psychiatrist Sir William Bradshaw. Not only a physician, Savage was also a clubbable socialite, a keen sportsman and a proponent of physical fitness as a way to mental health and hygiene. He made a record ascent of the Matterhorn and gave his name to the 'Savage Shield' for fencing. In this image, Savage is shown with a phrenological head, being an enthusiastic and early proponent of phrenology (as he was of hypnotism and psychology). He retained an interest in the 'science' long after it had been substantially discredited as a legitimate professional preoccupation for other serious, career-minded alienists

late eighteenth and the nineteenth centuries, practitioners complained of being hampered in the removal of individuals to asylums by sentimental families, legalistic minds and penny-pinching officials. The activities of the Lunacy Commission reveal an often uncomfortable compromise between lay and medical interests. The commission was composed not only of specialists in mental medicine, but also of general practitioners, lawyers and legalistically inclined politicians. The English commission was headed by a politician, Lord Shaftesbury, whose powerful personality was stamped very firmly on its operations. Evidently then, medical specialists remained only one significant group of actors in contemporary management and arbitration of lunacy matters. The final reading for the chapter, from an article by David Wright, looks in some detail at the role of medical practitioners in the crucial process of certification of the insane in nineteenth-century England and Wales.

Exercise

Read 'The power of medical men?' (Source Book 2, Reading 11.5). In the light of this research, do we need to modify Scull's claim that medical men had gained authority to pronounce on matters connected with mental medicine?

Discussion

Wright shows that various lunacy acts gave medical men an important role in certifying lunatics, and thus controlling admissions to asylums, but that, contrary to Scull's thesis, they gained no new powers as the century progressed. If anything, medical men lost some authority as the role of medical superintendents in certification was constrained to guard against abuses. Families and lay people continued to play a role in providing vital information in the certification process. Wright's research gives the impression that medical practitioners worked within a complex legal framework, with strictly defined roles, often subordinate to magistrates, who held a good deal more power over certification and inspections.

11.6   Asylumdom as a local affair: the Poor Law, parochial administration and the family

A growing number of historians now argue that earlier studies have overestimated the influence of medicine and medical men in the identification and management of lunacy. Wright has gone so far as to assert that asylum specialists 'were peripheral agents in the great confinement of the insane', the 'social forces' at the heart of most confinements being a family and local affair 'beyond their control' (Wright, 1997, p.154). Historians of medicine and psychiatry have also begun to re-examine the role of Poor Law authorities – the guardians, relieving officers and Poor Law commissioners – in the committal and care of the insane.

The structure and operation of the Poor Law is described briefly in Chapter 2.

Poor Law authorities had since the late seventeenth century overseen the confinement of poor lunatics in workhouses, prisons and private mad-houses, and so to some extent the nineteenth-century use of public asylums may be seen as an extension of this long tradition. The late eighteenth century saw a move away from supporting lunatics through outdoor relief towards sending the poor to large-scale institutional establishments. After the passing of the Poor Law Act 1834 and the subsequent lunacy acts, the role of the Poor Law authorities was greatly expanded.

Parochial authorities funded and to some extent oversaw the huge Victorian pauper lunatic asylums.

Historians now emphasize the important role of Poor Law workhouses in identifying paupers as insane and thus suitable for the asylum. Rather than asylum medical officers, it was magistrates, guardians and union personnel who tended to determine the route to the asylum for paupers (Adair *et al.*, 1998). Peter Bartlett has shown that there was considerable cooperation between Poor Law and asylum officials working within a network of lunacy administration. He emphasizes how asylums acted in a complementary way to workhouses, receiving their more difficult and acute cases. Similar relationships existed between Scottish asylums and poorhouses (Bartlett, 1999a, b).

In the past, both of these perspectives – the supremacy of medical or of Poor Law authorities – encouraged the view that families and friends of the insane were impotent onlookers to the process of institutionalization. Yet it was they who initiated confinement and who also often curtailed it. Historians have begun to investigate the important role of households and relations at the local level in certification, and have shown that the process consisted of 'a complex pattern of negotiations with families and friends of ... pauper lunatics' (Adair *et al.*, 1998, p.3). Indeed, however much the role of patients' relations in institutionalization was eroded by the heightened powers of medical and other authorities, patients' families continued regularly and successfully to demand the discharge of the mentally ill via applications to the boards of Poor Law guardians and directly to asylums. Such interactions, by their very nature less likely to be recorded in asylum records, too often remain a dimension hidden from the initial investigations of psychiatric historians.

11.7   Outside the asylum walls: limits to the primacy of the asylum as a solution

Although historians have written about the asylum as the only response to insanity, there was in fact a widely used alternative. **Boarding-out**, or 'family care' of the insane, offered a genuine alternative to asylumdom. The exact form of boarding-out differed from one national and regional context to another, but basically it supported patients within domestic and often rural settings, generally with guardians or relatives in single dwellings and cottages. The practice had long been used by local authorities, but after the middle of the nineteenth century it was subject to much wider centralization and official oversight. Boarding-out was widely used, from Gheel and Liemeux in Belgium to Dun-sur-Auron in France, and to Massachusetts in the USA. In Scotland, the Fifeshire village of Kennoway, where children had been long boarded by local parishes, was the best known and most touted of the Scottish initiatives (see Figure 11.1).

The practice was not without its critics. It was alleged that boarding-out was only practicable for a minority of the harmless, chronic insane and demented, and that patients were sometimes exposed to ill treatment. Yet there is evidence that by the 1870s many patients faired well in such settings (Parry-Jones, 1981; Sturdy and Parry-Jones, 1999). In Belgium and Scotland, and in some areas of France, boarding-out can be characterized as a mainstream solution to the problem of harmless chronic and imbecile patients who accumulated in asylums. While strong and growing fears about the propagation of the unfit meant that women were often boarded-out only post-menopause, and harmless female patients might be retained in asylums until past the age of fertility, the embracing of boarding-out as a policy under centralized supervision by the Scottish Lunacy Commissioners, in collaboration with local authorities, won plaudits and esteem from a wide range of international commentators and observers. In this context, a British approach to lunacy significantly influenced other contemporary international initiatives with family care of the insane, lunatic colonies and cottage asylums.

In addition, we know that a whole host of alternatives to asylums were tried for the convalescent, the nervous and even the more seriously mentally troubled among the middle and monied classes. Such alternatives ranged from home-based regimen and exercise routines, to visits to spas and hydropathic establishments, and to travel at home and abroad. These options were increasingly available to the lower middling classes by the end of the nineteenth century (Andrews, 2000; Oppenheim, 1991; Wright and Bartlett, 1999).

11.8   Conclusion

This chapter gives some of the sense of how historians work – by developing explanations of historical events, which are in turn challenged by new research that re-examines these ideas. In the case of the nineteenth-century asylum, much of the research carried out since the 1980s is based on new sources and detailed case studies which test old explanations for the timing and causes of the growth of asylums. In part, this reflects a trend in other areas of medical history and in the broader field of social history.

The result has been to challenge the nature of the link between the growth of asylums and the forces of broader social change – urbanization, industrialization and capitalism. Detailed work suggests that links between urbanization and asylums are not straightforward: asylums did not grow up in large cities (which were thought to be inappropriate sites for such institutions), and their patients came from both urban and rural areas. Urban life did not necessarily undermine the social bonds within the family that helped to support a mentally disordered family member – families facing such a strain tended to stay put. Admission to the asylum was not merely, and often not directly, a response to economic difficulty, but was also closely bound up with the longer-term emotional strain of dealing with violent and difficult family members. Its meanings were wider and more variable than has formerly been postulated in terms of the socio-economic and life-cycle pressures on families in variously configured industrializing, commercializing regions and societies. Such findings suggest the need to recognize and explore personal experiences of dealing with insanity in different regions before patterns of resort to the asylum in the Victorian age can be explained.

It is difficult to pin down how changes in the treatment of the insane and the rising status of doctors specializing in mental disorder may have fed into the growth of asylums. While reforms within asylums – the replacement of physical restraint with moral therapy, and the domestication of asylum architecture, amenities and furnishings – undoubtedly made the asylum seem a more pleasant place to the families of the insane, these reforms seem to come too late to explain the growth in asylum numbers. Similarly, improvements in the status of doctors dealing with asylum patients (which owed little to their ability to cure patients) came in the second half of the century, when the asylum had already achieved its place as an important (although as we have seen, not the only) means of dealing with the insane. New research on the roles of the legal and welfare authorities also suggests that we should not place too much weight on the role of medical men in driving change.

References

Adair, R., Forsythe, B. and Melling, J. (1997) 'Migration, family structure and pauper lunacy in Victorian England: admissions to the Devon County Pauper Lunatic Asylum, 1845–1900', *Continuity and Change*, vol.12, no.3, pp.373–401.

Adair, R., Forsythe, B. and Melling, J. (1998) 'A danger to the public? Disposing of pauper lunatics in late-Victorian and Edwardian England: Plympton St Mary Union and the Devon County Asylum, 1867–1914', *Medical History*, vol.42, no.1, pp.1–25.

Andrews, J. (1990) '"In her vapours: ... [or] indeed in her madness?" Ms Clerke's case: an early eighteenth-century psychiatric controversy', *History of Psychiatry*, vol.1, pp.125–44.

Andrews, J. (2000) 'Letting madness range: travel and madness, *c.*1700–1900' in R. Wrigley and G. Revill (eds) *Pathologies of Travel*, Amsterdam: Rodopi, pp.25–88.

Andrews, J., Briggs, A., Porter, R., Tucker, P. and Waddington, K. (1997) *The History of Bethlem*, London: Routledge.

Bartlett, P. (1999a) 'The asylum and the Poor Law' in J. Melling and B. Forsythe (eds) *Insanity, Institutions and Society, 1800–1914: A Social History of Madness in Comparative Perspective*, London: Routledge, pp.48–67.

Bartlett, P. (1999b) *The Poor Law of Lunacy: The Administration of Pauper Lunatics in Mid-Nineteenth Century England*, London: Leicester University Press.

Doerner, K. [1969] (1981) *Madmen and the Bourgeoisie: A Social History of Insanity and Psychiatry*, translated by J. Neugroschel and J. Steinberg, Oxford: Basil Blackwell.

Foucault, M. (1965) *Madness and Civilization: A History of Insanity in the Age of Reason*, translated and abridged by R. Howard, New York: Random House.

Goffman, E. [1961] (1990) *Asylums: Essays on the Social Situation of Mental Patients and Other Inmates*, New York: Doubleday.

Goldberg, A. (1999) *Sex, Religion, and the Making of Modern Madness: The Eberbach Asylum and German Society, 1815–1849*, Oxford: Oxford University Press.

Hervey, N. (1986) 'Advocacy or folly: the Alleged Lunatics' Friend Society', *Medical History*, vol.30, pp.245–77.

Jones, C. (1990) 'Medicine, madness and mayhem from the "Roi Soleil" to the Golden Age of Hysteria (seventeenth to late nineteenth centuries)', *French History*, vol.4, pp.378–88.

Jones, K. (1993) *Asylums and After: A Revised History of the Mental Health Services, from the Early Eighteenth Century to the 1990s*, London: Athlone.

King, S.A. and Timmins, J.G. (2001) *Making Sense of the Industrial Revolution: English Economy and Society, 1700–1850*, Manchester: Manchester University Press.

Oppenheim, J. (1991) *'Shattered Nerves': Doctors, Patients and Depression in Victorian England*, Oxford: Oxford University Press.

Parry-Jones, W. (1972) *The Trade in Lunacy: A Study of Private Madhouses in England in the Eighteenth and Nineteenth Centuries*, London: Routledge & Kegan Paul.

Parry-Jones, W. (1981) 'The model of the Geel lunatic colony and its influence on the nineteenth-century asylum system in Britain' in A.T. Scull (ed.) *Madhouses, Mad-doctors, and Madmen: The Social History of Psychiatry in the Victorian Era*, London: Athlone, pp.201–17.

Peterson, D. (1982) *A Mad People's History of Madness*, Pittsburg: University of Pittsburg Press.

Pick, D. (1989) *Faces of Degeneration, a European Disorder, c.1848–c.1918*, Cambridge: Cambridge University Press.

Porter, R. (1987) *Mind-Forg'd Manacles: A History of Madness in England from the Restoration to the Regency*, London: Athlone.

Ray, L.J. (1981) 'Models of madness in Victorian asylum practice', *Archives of European Sociology*, vol.22, pp.229–64.

Renvoize, E. (1991) 'The Association of Medical Officers of Asylums and Hospitals for the Insane, the Medico-Psychological Association, and their presidents' in G. Berrios and H. Freeman (eds) *150 Years of Psychiatry*, London: Gaskell, pp.17–28.

Rice, F.J. (1985) 'The origin of an organisation of insanity in Scotland', *Scottish Economic and Social History*, vol.5, pp.41–55.

Rothman, D.J. (1971) *The Discovery of the Asylum*, Boston: Little, Brown.

Scull, A.T. (1979) *Museums of Madness: The Social Organisation of Insanity in Nineteenth-Century England*, London: Allen Lane.

Scull, A.T. (1980) 'A convenient place to get rid of inconvenient people: the Victorian lunatic asylum' in A.D. King (ed.) *Buildings and Society*, London: Routledge & Kegan Paul, pp.37–60.

Scull, A.T. (1989a) 'The domestication of madness' in A.T. Scull, *Social Order/ Mental Disorder: Anglo-American Psychiatry in Historical Perspective*, London: Routledge pp.54–79.

Scull, A.T. (1989b) 'Medical men as moral entrepreneurs' in A.T. Scull, *Social Order/Mental Disorder: Anglo-American Psychiatry in Historical Perspective*, London: Routledge, pp.118–61.

Scull, A.T. (1993) *The Most Solitary of Afflictions. Madness and Society in Britain, 1700–1900*, New Haven and London: Yale University Press.

Sturdy, H. and Parry-Jones, W. (1999) 'Boarding-out insane patients: the significance of the Scottish system' in D. Wright and P. Bartlett (eds) *Outside the Walls of the Asylum*, London: Athlone, pp.86–114.

Turner, T. (1991) '"Not worth powder or shot": the public profile of the Medico-Psychological Association, *c*.1851–1914' in G. Berrios and H. Freeman (eds) *150 Years of Psychiatry*, London: Gaskell, pp.3–16.

Walsh, O. (1999) '"The designs of providence": race, religion and Irish insanity' in J. Melling and B. Forsythe (eds) *Insanity, Institutions and Society, 1800–1914: A Social History of Madness in Comparative Perspective*, London: Routledge, pp.223–42.

Walton, J.K. (1981) 'The treatment of pauper lunatics in Victorian England: the case of Lancaster Asylum, 1816–1870' in A.T. Scull (ed.) *Madhouses, Mad-Doctors and Madmen: The Social History of Psychiatry in the Victorian Era*, London: Athlone, pp.166–97.

Walton, J.K. (1985) 'Casting out and bringing back in Victorian England' in W.F. Bynum, R. Porter and M. Shepherd (eds) *The Anatomy of Madness: Essays in the History of Psychiatry*, vol.2 *Institutions and Society*, London: Tavistock, pp.132–46.

Wright, D. (1997) 'Getting out of the asylum: understanding the confinement of the insane in the nineteenth century', *Social History of Medicine*, vol.10, no.1, pp.137–55.

Wright, D. (1998) 'The certification of insanity in nineteenth-century England and Wales', *History of Psychiatry*, vol.9, pp.267–90.

Wright, D. and Bartlett, P. (eds) (1999) *Outside the Walls of the Asylum: The History of Care in the Community*, London: Athlone.

Source Book readings

J. Coxe, 'On the causes of insanity, and the means of checking its growth', *Journal of Mental Science*, 1872, vol.18, pp.311–33 (Reading 11.1i).

J. Carswell, 'Contribution to the inquiry into the increase in pauper lunacy in Scotland', *Glasgow Medical Journal*, 1892, vol.5, pp.262–70 (Reading 11.1ii).

E. Hawden, 'On the supposed increase in insanity: a plea for prevention', *Poor Law Magazine and Local Government Journal*, 1901, vol.11, pp.349–59 (Reading 11.1iii).

A. Scull, *The Most Solitary of Afflictions: Madness and Society in Britain, 1700–1900*, New Haven and London: Yale University Press, 1993, pp.26–33 (Reading 11.2).

J.K. Walton, 'Casting out and bringing back in Victorian England: pauper lunatics, 1840–70' in W.F. Bynum, R. Porter and M. Shepherd (eds) *The Anatomy of Madness: Essays in the History of Psychiatry*, vol.2 *Institutions and Society*, London: Tavistock, 1985, pp.137–41 (Reading 11.3).

Case notes of the use of the rotary chair at Glasgow Asylum, 1820–1, Greater Glasgow Health Board Archives, 13/5/2–6 (Reading 11.4).

D. Wright, 'The certification of insanity in nineteenth-century England and Wales', *History of Psychiatry*, 1998, vol.9, pp.271–6, 288 (Reading 11.5).

12

Medicine in War

------------------ R o g e r C o o t e r ------------------

Objectives

When you have completed this chapter you should be able to:

- describe some of the main medical problems associated with war;

- understand historical approaches to the subject and how these have changed in recent years;

- provide both supporting and opposing evidence for the proposition that 'war is good for medicine', and appreciate the interpretative limitations of this proposition;

- appreciate the difficulty of generalizing on the practice of medicine in wartime, and the need to attend to the socio-economic forces involved in shaping the relations between war and medicine.

12.1 Introduction: war in the history of medicine – from poverty to promise

The relations between war and medicine have only recently come in for serious historical discussion. Hitherto, neither military nor medical historians thought much about them. Medicine's place in war and war's place in the history of medicine were assumed to be straightforward, obvious and rather boring. In military history, it was only after the publication of John Keegan's *The Face of Battle* (1976), with its fresh insights into military history and the central place of health and medicine in war, that some attention came to be given to the wartime experiences of soldiers and doctors. In the history of medicine, with few exceptions, the interest in military matters came later. As in other branches of history, war was regarded as something separate from the rest of society and culture. Worse, it was often regarded as a disastrous deviation from the 'march of civilization', of which medicine was perceived as both stunning exemplar and handmaiden.

Early historians of medicine were more interested in public health, mental care, hospitals and other features within what they perceived as the expanding social domain of medicine. In these accounts, warfare might be seen as a fillip to medical welfare and professionalization (especially specialization), but it could not become a primary focus for fear of endorsing militarism. For similar reasons, war was unfashionable among historians of medicine in the 1970s and 1980s. In their view, warfare was inimical to welfare; moreover, it was a politically incorrect topic of study in the shadow of the war in Vietnam. Its prospects were not improved in subsequent years when historians focused on social and cultural representations of the body and disease. War's mundane practicalities, its unsubtle 'politics by other means', its emphasis on great men and great battles, and its general machismo image marked it a distinctly 'unsexy' subject.

Only in the 1990s did some historians of medicine begin to crack it open. Attracted in particular to path-breaking cultural studies of the First World War as a crucible of modernity, they began to focus on subjects such as the history and meaning of shell shock, medicine's role in the reshaping of military command, and military medicine's place in the surveillance and discipline of populations. Many historians became interested in Nazi medicine during the Second World War, either from the perspective of the history of medical ethics, or in terms of the relations between medicine, ideology and politics. Gradually, war-focused (or at least war-attentive) endeavours in the history of medicine expanded to include, in one way or another, virtually every aspect of health and welfare discourse and practice. This is reflected in recent specialist studies such as those on disablement and rehabilitation, professionalization, epidemiology and nursing. These have spilled over to inform myriad undertakings across the sweep of history and historical sociology which, in their turn, have structured books and inspired chapters devoted to war in new general surveys of the social history of medicine (e.g. Hardy, 2001; Lane, 2001).

My own work in this area emerged from the study of a particular medical specialty – orthopaedics, the 'modern' version of which (concerned with the repair of musculo-skeletal injury) is usually thought to have been forged during the First World War (Cooter, 1993). One of the obvious questions for me to ask was how exactly was the modern specialty made during the Great War – if 'made' it was? On the face of it, the answer was as simple and straightforward as the question, for the war had clearly placed urgent demands upon medical experts in the treatment of fractures and the rehabilitation of the disabled. The surgeons who came together at the end of the war to form the British Orthopaedic Association had doubtless taken advantage of the professionalizing opportunities the war afforded. This was true, but it only begged the question of why these surgeons chose to professionalize in this particular manner, since 'orthopaedics' up to this point was about the treatment of crippled children (a medical backwater) and had little to do with fracture treatment or rehabilitation. (Fracture treatment was then still primarily a part of general surgery, while rehabilitation was associated with various cranky branches of massage and manipulation.) Other questions intruded, such as what exactly constitutes 'the making' of a specialty, and what precisely is 'modernity' in medicine? The former, it emerged, was integral to the latter; modernity in medicine consisted in large measure of the adoption of certain idealizations of efficiency. These were drawn from 'progressive' management practices in contemporary business and industry, such as coordinated divisions of labour, and the standardization and routinization of procedures. Modernity in medicine embraced a view of the body which incorporated these aspects of 'scientific management'. Thus, perfect health or musculo-skeletal function was seen as the result of the body working at maximum efficiency through an appropriate division of labour between the different parts – yet with all working within an integrated physiological system. During the First World War, the organization of orthopaedic services under the command of certain medical reformers followed a model of such efficient organization, while the orthopaedic image of the body's dynamic locomotor system served to legitimize it to the wider world. But, as might be expected, 'modernity' did not arrive in medicine without a struggle, or without putting up the backs of traditionalists opposed to specialization and its rationales.

This is not the place to unpack the politics of modernity in medicine; I only need to say here that my orthopaedic pathway into the relations between war and medicine added to the difficulty of subscribing to the conventional views of civilian and military medical spheres as more or less autonomous. Nor, on the basis of this and similar historical examples, was it possible to sustain the common distinction between wartime and peacetime. 'War' and 'medicine', hitherto all too readily separated and compartmentalized, came to appear more entwined, both being equally bound to the rest of society, culture and economy. Medicine, far from something merely wheeled out in war, began to look like something that was intimately a part of it.

Since this chapter addresses developments in medicine within a specific context, it explores many issues that have been discussed in earlier chapters – surgery, laboratories, the medical profession and public health.

You will have a chance to reflect on this recasting of the relations between war and medicine towards the end of this chapter. The following sections are intended to lead you there by reviewing some of the contrasting ways in which the relationship has been conceptualized in the past. Because these conceptualizations stand at odds with the *integrative* view of war and medicine suggested above, the case for the latter can be made partly through reference to the former.

12.2   The positive audit of war and medicine

Conventional commentary on war and medicine typically highlights a relationship that is deemed to be one of the great ironies of medical history – the notion that war, with all its horrors and sufferings, has nevertheless brought lasting medical benefit to mankind. According to this view, medicine may even be war's redemption – 'the good that cometh out of evil' (Watson, 1950, p.130). What is usually meant is that war has operated as a positive external influence on medicine, providing unique learning opportunities, which have resulted in better curative and humanitarian therapies. For example, from the medical literature of the early nineteenth century, it seems that young practitioners who entered the army or navy during the Napoleonic wars acquired a great deal of knowledge and experience in the treatment of wounds, the contagiousness (or otherwise) of diseases, the amputation of limbs and, above all, in anatomy and pathology (as a result of unrestricted access to corpses for dissection). It is also apparent that the urgent medical demands of wartime encouraged valuable therapeutic techniques and procedures. Thus, Napoleon's famous army surgeon Dominique-Jean Larrey (1766–1842) is celebrated for his pioneering hip amputations, and for the 'flying ambulance' he devised for the rapid transport of injured troops. Similarly, the Prussian military surgeon Johannes Freidrich August von Esmarch (1823–1908) is fondly remembered for devising, during the Schleswig-Holstein wars of the 1860s, the 'first field dressing' and the rubber bandage that renders a limb bloodless before amputation. Best known of all, perhaps, are the nursing achievements of Florence Nightingale during the Crimean War of 1854–6, in response to the sufferings she witnessed at Scutari, discussed in Chapter 6.

Story-telling

Such stories are not innocent; to put it bluntly, we know of them only because it has been in someone's interest to tell them. The heroic story of Nightingale – 'the lady with the lamp' – for instance, has served the interests of those who wished to cultivate national pride, to celebrate women's achievements, or to seek support for the nursing profession (Plate 13). It is revealing that the work of another Crimean nurse, the black woman Mary Seacole (1805–81), was lost to posterity until the civil rights and black culture movement of the mid- to late twentieth century.

While the interests of military medicine are served by rhetoric that insists that 'for the medical profession ... war [is] a very efficient schoolmaster', as the Surgeon-General of the United States army put it (Ireland, 1921, p.763), the medical profession's recounting of the achievements of Larrey, Esmarch and others serves a self-celebratory function. These stories, often truncated, frequently misinform. For example, the French doctors who served in Napoleon's foreign campaigns may have been enriched by their experiences but they were also closed off to new knowledge. Only upon their return home did they learn about the spectacular discovery of vaccination, introduced into France in 1800, and find 'a widespread interest in hygiene and public health, owing partly to a voluminous literature stimulated by the war' (Weiner, 1993, p.281).

The two world wars did much to cement the view of war as something that advanced medicine and health care, and encouraged the idea of medicine as an inherently progressive force. The First World War, besides introducing blood transfusions and hastening developments in plastic surgery and the design of artificial limbs, propelled research into vitamins, wound shock, shell shock and gas asphyxia, among much else. In Britain, the war consolidated the Medical Research Council. This had been mandated in 1911 for the study of tuberculosis, but by the war's end in 1918 it had become a clearing-house for almost all the country's biomedical research.

Such post-world-war stories of medical progress mask the fact that prior to the First World War almost all wartime medicine was concerned not with technological and therapeutic innovations but overwhelmingly with infectious diseases (above all, typhus, typhoid, smallpox and yellow fever). Battles were often won or lost on the virulence of such epidemics, and whole territories gained or forfeited. The First World War was really the first war to break that mould, as can be seen from the comparison of deaths from disease with deaths from wounds in different major wars presented in Table 12.1.

Table 12.1   Major wars and medical problems, 1793–1918

War	Date	Combatants (000s)	Killed	Wounded	Casualties (000s) (a) Deaths from disease	(b) Deaths from wounds	Ratio of (a) to (b)	Particular problems
French Revolutionary and Napoleonic (British army only)	1793–1815	198	16	70	194.0	8.0	24:1	fevers, diarrhoea, typhus, dysentery
Peninsular War (British under Wellington)	1808–14	64	7	32.0	30.0	4.0	7.5:1	typhus, yellow fever
Mexico-American	1846–8	100	1.5 (incl. wounded)	–	11 (1.5%)	–	7:1	yellow fever
Crimean War (French, British and Russian)	1854–6	730	34	–	130.0	26.0	5:1	cholera, typhus, scurvy
American Civil War (North only)	1861–6	2,000–3,000	118 3.3%	–	344.0 6.5%	63.0	5:1 66%	typhoid, malaria, typhus, smallpox, dysentery
Franco-Prussian (Prussians only)	1870–1	1,100	17	–	15.0	11.0	1.36:1	typhoid
Russo-Turkish (Russians only)	1877–8	100	30	–	81.0	5.0	16:1	typhus, typhoid
Spanish–American (USA only)	1898–1902	172	–	–	3.0	0.8	3.75:1	malaria, typhoid, yellow fever
South African (British only)	1899–1902	500	–	–	14.0	7.5	1.9:1	typhoid
Russo-Japanese (Japanese only)	1904–5	1,350 650 (mean ave.)	76 43	– 153	36.0 13.0	17.0 8.0	2:1 1.6:1	typhoid, enteric fever, smallpox, cholera, diphtheria
First World War	1914–18	61,140	7,848 (+6,778 missing)	19,669	included	in	'killed'	fractures, tetanus, trench fever, gas asphyxia, shell shock
(British and empire only)		11,096	418 (+ 362 missing)	2,004 (8,040 'sick or injured')	113.0	167.0	0.67:1	

(Adapted from Dumas and Vedel-Petersen, 1923; Duncan, 1914, p.160; Garrison, [1922] 1970; Mitchell and Smith, 1931; Prinzing, 1916)

Although infectious diseases could still seriously affect military manoeuvres (as during the influenza pandemic of 1918), the sheer quantity of the battle casualties during the First World War and the relatively puny numbers of deaths from disease rendered the long-standing distinction between 'killed by disease' and 'killed by enemy action' seem rather bizarre and virtually superfluous (Cooter, 2003, p.298). This is reflected in the third column of Table 12.2, which merges deaths from disease with deaths from battle wounds.

Table 12.2   Estimated military losses during the First World War

Nation	Mobilized	Killed and died from wounds or disease	Wounded	Missing or prisoners	Total
British empire	8,654,467	929,812	2,097,994	32,391	3,063,664
France	8,407,000	1,109,000	3,025,613	252,900	4,387,513
Russia	12,000,000	1,700,000	4,950,000	2,500,000	9,150,000
United States	4,175,367	112,855	224,089	14,363	351,207
Italy	5,550,000	460,000	947,000	1,393,000	2,800,000
Belgium	267,000	104,779	77,422	10,000	192,201
Romania	750,000	200,000	120,000	80,000	400,000
Serbia	707,343	322,000	28,000	100,000	450,000
Montenegro	50,000	3,000	10,000	7,000	20,000
Greece	230,000	15,000	40,000	45,000	100,000
Portugal	100,000	4,000	15,000	200	19,200
Japan	850,000	300	907	3	1,210
Germany	11,000,000	1,686,061	4,211,469	991,341	6,888,871
Austro-Hungary	6,500,000	800,000	3,200,000	1,211,000	5,211,000
Bulgaria	400,000	101,224	152,399	10,825	264,448
Turkey	1,600,000	300,000	570,000	130,000	1,000,000
Totals:					
Allied powers	41,640,177	4,960,746	11,535,718	4,434,857	20,934,995
Central powers	19,500,000	2,887,285	8,133,868	2,343,166	13,364,319
Grand total	**61,140,177**	**7,848,031**	**19,669,586**	**6,778,023**	**34,299,314**

(From Garrison, 1970, p.199)

In reading statistics such as those in Tables 12.1 and 12.2, it is important to bear in mind the observation of the early nineteenth-century military theorist Carl von Clausewitz that 'the returns made up on each side of losses in killed and wounded

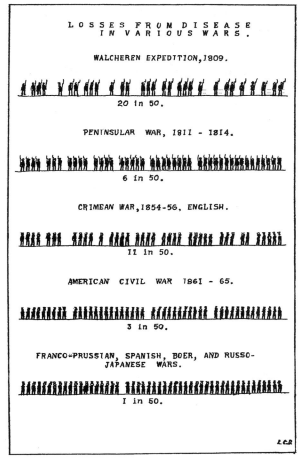

Figure 12.1   Operating on the assumption based on past experience that microbes are more deadly than bullets in warfare, doctors entered the First World War confident that the decline in deaths from disease would continue in proportion to the maintenance of sanitary and preventive measures. They were right, but failed to anticipate the nature and extent of the injuries of industrial warfare, which greatly dwarfed the lethal significance of the microbe. Reproduced from Duncan (1914), p.160

are never exact, seldom truthful, and in most cases, full of intentional misrepresentation' (from *On War* (1832), quoted in Winter, 1985, p.67). In other words, such statistics constitute yet further stories. Jay Winter cites thirty-three different sources on 'total British war dead, 1914–18', the estimates of which range from 550,000 to 1,184,000 (Winter, 1985, pp.68–9).

The conventional distinction between the two different main causes of death among combatants was further blurred by new understandings of disease causation and prevention. During the First World War, typhus still raged in Serbia and other parts of eastern Europe (stirred by the movement of refugees); however, as you read in Chapter 9, for the first time the disease came to have both its bacterial cause and its louse-borne mode of transmission understood. By 1914, typhoid fever was revealed by epidemiologists and bacteriologists to be borne by contaminated water or food, and 'bacteriologic research had provided a remedy in inoculation' (Hardy, 2000, p.282). Delighting in such achievements, military doctors before the First World War scripted a happy story of ever diminishing deaths from disease in military conflicts, as can be seen in Figure 12.1. The story was self-empowering for military doctors, for the diminution of deaths from disease could be credited to their sanitary achievements. The First World War undermined that particular boost to the profession, however, not because it disproved the pattern of decreasing mortality for diseases during war but because it rendered the story irrelevant in the face of the massive carnage on the battlefield.

It is important to note this fundamental difference between military medical realities before and after the First World War, for it helps explain why, before 1914, it was difficult for anyone to entertain the notion of 'war-as-good-for-medicine'. Most often, the medical profession was impotent in the face of battle injuries and infectious diseases. Thus, few writers on war and medicine before 1914 ever thought to suggest that war was good for medicine; at most they spoke of the medical 'lessons' of war, though even that not much before the late nineteenth century. This is illustrated in the first two readings for the chapter, by Edward M. Wrench (published 1899) and Mary Seacole (published 1857).

Exercise

Read 'Military medicine in the Crimea' (Source Book 2, Reading 12.1) and 'Nursing in the Crimea' (Source Book 2, Reading 12.2). Is war presented as being good for medicine? Do these authors attempt to find 'lessons' in the Crimea for future conflicts?

Discussion

Neither author suggests that war is in any way good for medicine – rather, that the medical services in the Crimea were sadly inadequate. Wrench's account – published in a medical journal and aimed at a medical audience – clearly fits into the genre of 'lessons of war'. He portrays the chaos and inadequacy of the medical services in the Crimea and, as he clearly states at the beginning of the article, his object is to provide one of the last eye-witness accounts that might teach 'lessons of progress' for future conflicts. However, he does not blame the medical staff – the problems arise from misfortune (the hurricane and the sinking of ships) and inefficient organization. Mary Seacole writes for a rather different purpose and a different audience. Her book was for a general audience to present herself as a heroic individual performing unforgettable acts of kindness that transcend rank and nationality. She does not overtly criticize the medical services or suggest reforms – indeed she speaks highly of the doctors – but emphasizes that she occupies a particular 'niche' – standing in for the domestic care soldiers would have received from family and servants at home, and cooperating, not competing, with army doctors.

It was not until after the Second World War that the further step was taken of estimating retrospectively the relative worth of medicine to different wars in the past. This hitherto bizarre type of backward audit is to be found in an article entitled 'The medical balance sheet of war' composed by one of the editors of the official medical history of the Second World War, Zachary Cope (1881–1974), a London hospital consultant (Cope, 1961, pp.169–83). In this, little if any real value to medicine is seen as having emerged from wars before the twentieth century. Cope's article, focused on the medical achievements of the victors of the Second World War, predictably reads these as the 'fulfilment' of the medical advances 'anticipated' mainly during the First World War.

Professional opportunities

Academic historians of medicine, no less than doctors and popular writers, have contributed to the notion of war-as-good-for-medicine, especially in connection with the First World War, and with regard to medical specialization. The Anglo-American studies of the historian Rosemary Stevens, for example, are emphatic that medical specialization thrived during the war, with the army acting as a 'filtering system for quality' (Stevens, 1971, p.127). Recent studies of cardiology, psychiatry and rehabilitation medicine have elaborated this process, revealing how at least three of the four requirements seen as necessary for specialty development were fulfilled: large groups of patients (Figure 12.2), specialized facilities and financial resources from the state to support specialization.

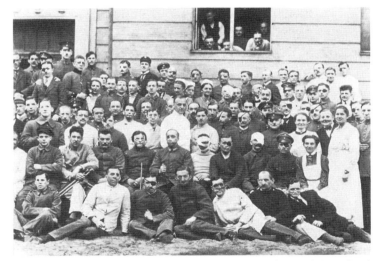

Figure 12.2   A group of soldiers in Berlin in the early 1920s awaiting plastic surgery. One of the requirements for medical specialization is the high incidence of a specific medical problem. Yet, vast numbers of the same type of medical problem do not necessarily compel the creation of occupational divisions of labour. The size of the problem can, however, create the opportunities for professional engagement and allow doctors to carve out new territories. The First World War provided this opportunity for plastic surgery, as it did for the 'new cardiology' and for 'modern orthopaedics'. Reproduced from de Moulin (1988), p.327, Kluwer Academic Publishers

Only the fourth postulate for the making of a medical specialty, a technological innovation (like the ophthalmoscope for ophthalmology), has come to be seen as unnecessary. After all, medical specialties such as orthopaedics and plastic surgery did not require these kinds of tools to become professionally coherent. Technologies of organization and hard-nosed professionalizing politics counted for more.

The impact of the First World War on the careers of medical women is discussed in Chapter 6.

It is not only in relation to specialization and the professionalization of specialists that the 'Great War' has been perceived as medically great. For medical women, among others, it has been regarded as presenting unique opportunities. As increasing numbers of male doctors were called to arms, women doctors got their first real chance to prove themselves in spheres other than far-flung colonies or, at home, exclusively women's hospitals or low-status public health services.

For many, there was now work in general practice on the home front, as well as recruitment opportunities abroad with the Red Cross and other affiliated voluntary units. In Britain, the numbers of female medical graduates rose from a handful in 1914 to 3,000 by the end of the war, by which time women made up 31 per cent of all medical students. Female nurses, of course, had been employed in military service long before Nightingale's involvement in the Crimea, and they were involved in even greater numbers thereafter. During the First World War, many more women entered the nursing profession, if only on a temporary basis. The Voluntary Aid Detachment movement, begun in 1909, comprised nearly 2,000 branches by 1914, with dozens of women (VADs) attached to each branch (Leneman, 1994; Summers, 1988).

Public health

Nor is it only in relation to the self-interested advancement of the caring professions that war has been regarded as benefiting medicine. Medical provision for civilian populations during wartime, and for their health and nutrition, have also been brought within the audit. In one of the few monographs specifically to address the question of the effects of war on public health, the historical demographer Jay Winter has argued on the basis of life-expectancy figures that the health of the poorest sections of British society was in fact much improved during the First World War (Winter, 1985). The paradox of the war for Britain, he concludes, was that victory was not at the expense of the civilian population. In the next reading, taken from his *The Great War and the British People*, published in 1985, you can see his observations on female mortality rates during the First World War.

Exercise

Read 'Civilian health in the First World War' (Source Book 2, Reading 12.3) and then summarize Winter's argument by answering the following questions.

1 What diseases does he claim declined during this period, and why?

2 Why does tuberculosis not decline?

3 What sources does he use to construct his argument?

1   Winter traces a pattern of mortality decline from a number of diseases – degenerative diseases, complications of pregnancy and childbirth, diarrhoeal diseases and (for most age groups) respiratory diseases. He hints at several causes and notes that maternal mortality was diminished partly through fewer pregnancies. However, the main cause of diminished mortality was better nutrition – a factor affecting all ages and classes.

2   He attributes the persistently high death rate from tuberculosis to the movement of people, poor housing, 'stress' and long working hours, and argues that improved nutrition had little impact on the disease.

3   He constructs his argument almost entirely from statistics, and the extract gives very little evidence to support his claims about social factors such as nutrition and housing.

In general, Winter's thesis harmonizes with the story of how programmes in maternal and child health and welfare, described in Chapter 9, were encouraged by startling revelations of the physical unfitness of Britain's slum denizens during recruitment for the Boer War (Cooter, 1991; Dwork, 1987; Searle, 1971). Parallel arguments for similar reforms, as well as for eugenics and industrial research into health and economic production, were bolstered by the lurid light cast on people's health during the call-up for the First World War. These revelations also abetted campaigns and legislation against the spread of venereal disease, and did more besides: while soldiers and sailors were familiarized with the uses of condoms, the medical profession, in their treatment of venereal disease, were led for the first time to an appreciation of chemotherapy. The anti-syphilitic drug Salvarsan, which came into wide usage during the war, was the first ever 'magic bullet'.

Science and technology

Few historians of medicine today would wholly endorse the bold claim made immediately after the First World War, in 1919, by the distinguished physician Sir Thomas Clifford Allbutt (1836–1925) that the war transformed medicine from 'an observational and empirical craft to a scientific calling' (Allbutt, 1921, p.542). But several studies provide support for the view that the war hastened the movement of science and technology to the bedside (discussed in Chapter 4). One means to this end was the development of the pharmaceutical industry, especially in America. Becoming more intent on research around this time, the industry's commercialization of new and pirated products (such as the German-patented Salvarsan, and Bayer's aspirin) were greatly accelerated as much by the economic dislocations of the war as by its medical demands. Another means to the 'scientization' of medicine was the exposure of the profession to new or unfamiliar medical technologies, such as X-ray equipment and laboratories for bacteriology and pathology.

The First World War also exposed doctors to new surgical techniques, which were soon applied to civilian hospitals. In Britain, this had the effect of both increasing the scale and intensity of hospital workloads and enhancing public demand for services operating beyond the scope and provision of general practice. At the same time, the old Poor Law hospitals, which had been commandeered for the war-injured, were exposed to modern medical treatments (surgery in particular), and thereafter undertook programmes of improvement in their medical and convalescent facilities. In some cases the War Office bequeathed them the operating theatres they had installed during the war, and many acquired new surgical equipment from the cheap surpluses that flooded the market after the war (Lawrence, 1992, p.305).

Also extending from the war was the application to medical practice of the principles of modern management – technologies of organization driven by the compulsion for efficiency. The laboratory provided one model of coordinated working (described in Chapter 4). Although these innovations were not born of war so much as imposed upon it from the world of business and industry that was acutely concerned with productivity and profit, war facilitated their application – not least through the view of it as a 'giant industrial accident' requiring the application of industrial medicine to 'soldier-workers' (Lerner, 2000, p.16). Many of the basics of 'scientific management', such as record-keeping, became routine parts of everyday medical practice in the war's aftermath. Other wartime organizational arrangements were hastened, such as team-work, and continuity in patient care between different sets of specialist practitioners. The management of injured soldiers during the war, from casualty clearing stations at the front, through to base hospitals and convalescent camps at the rear, proved to be a model for the integration of medical services in civilian practice when the war was over. It informed, for instance, the much celebrated 'Dawson Plan', first outlined in 1918, for the organization of **primary** and **secondary care**. Such war-inspired schemes are historically important, not because they had significant clinical impact during the inter-war period (the Dawson Plan was never implemented), but rather because they reveal how those who were keen to reform the structure and function of medicine used their wartime experience. Whether such idealizations were good or bad for medicine is another matter. Suffice to say here that they were a part of the process by which medicine was fitted to the mass society it was increasingly intended to serve.

12.3   The negative audit of war and medicine

It has never been proposed that war was *universally* good for medicine and health care. Even medical authors have expressed some doubt, especially in relation to supposed advances in medical technology. The American military historian and bibliographer Fielding Garrison, for example, reflected in 1929 that, in contrast to the remarkable administrative achievements of the world war, the 'medical innovations and inventions ... seem clever, respectable, but not particularly brilliant' (Garrison, 1929, p.790). In 1946, in the flush of media enthusiasm for 'the miracles of modern military medicine', a writer on 'wartime influences on health and welfare institutions in the United States' submitted:

The melancholy truth seems to be that wars generally have contributed but little to the progress of medical science. War undoubtedly does spread skills in medical practice as a result of the opportunities it gives doctors for operating on men in masses. It produces more surgeons, and improves their skills by practice ... Yet, in spite of the ballyhoo, I fail to recall a single medical discovery of primary importance that has come out of this or any war.

(Deutsch, 1946, p.318)

Even the clinical study of 'shell shock' (the equivalent of today's post-traumatic stress syndrome), which has often been regarded as a good example of a development born during the First World War, fails to pass muster in view of the growing medical literature from the 1860s on the same subject, albeit called 'railway spine' (shock resulting from railway accidents) and 'traumatic neurasthenia' (acute nervousness). As with so many other medical pursuits, war can be seen as accelerating medical interest in older problems, although in this case it also contributed to a clinical redefinition. Railway spine had been construed as an organic problem of mind: that is, a physical rather than a mental condition, whereas the discussion of shell shock marked a move toward conceiving disturbed minds in purely psychological terms (Leese, 2002; Lerner, 2003; Shephard, 2000). The next reading is made up of extracts from the evidence of Drs W.J. Adie and W.H.R. Rivers presented to the War Office Committee of Enquiry into 'Shell-Shock', which reported in 1922.

Exercise

Read 'The causes of shell-shock' (Source Book 2, Reading 12.4). How does Adie's account of the causes of shell shock differ from that of Rivers? What do the two accounts suggest about the men who succumb to shell shock?

Discussion

Adie expresses a militarist 'stiff upper lip' view of shell shock. He argues that it is a consequence of fear, and that all soldiers to some extent suffer from 'nerves' but the brave soldier, or one in a platoon with good morale, will survive. Cowardly or badly led soldiers will go through an unmanly emotional breakdown. He hints that by claiming shell shock many soldiers have evaded their duty.

Rivers seeks to de-moralize the condition. He argues that shell shock, far from being the result of shirking duty or poor morale, stems from men trying to persevere in the performance of their duty under conditions of extreme duress – sleeplessness, fatigue, etc. Whether or not soldiers develop shell shock depends on their personality, their duties (if they are able to control their own situation, they are less likely to be stressed) and their training (better trained regular soldiers are better able to deal with frontline conditions). In direct contrast to Adie, Rivers believes that notions of morale can add to stress by intensifying feelings of guilt and shame.

Worthless lessons

For the most part, the wars between 1800 and 1939 encouraged research only into problems of direct concern to the military. Like shell shock, the treatment of gunshot and shrapnel wounds, gas asphyxia, gas gangrene and trench foot, for instance, are rarely called for in peacetime. Moreover, wartime research priorities with civilian applications, such as the treatment of fractures, flat foot and venereal disease, have normally reverted to low status in peacetime medicine because of the poor remuneration they have offered in private practice. Thus, while war might cause new light to be cast on hitherto neglected patient populations (e.g. the physically disabled individuals revealed at recruiting stations) and on neglected problems (e.g. the best treatment of fractures), sustaining that illumination after the war has been another matter.

Often, too, in relation to the treatment of acute injuries, wartime conditions are so different as to render the military experience virtually irrelevant to peacetime. The need for urgency in wound treatment and amputations, for instance – well appreciated since the Napoleonic wars, and a major impetus to the development of ambulances and front-line dressing stations – was less essential in the controlled and eventually aseptic hospital environment with its anaesthetized patients. Vice versa, the medicine of peacetime was often out of place on the battlefield. Wounds encountered in civilian medicine rarely displayed the massive destruction of the surrounding tissue in the manner of battlefield wounds. Partly as a result of such differences, 'errors may be committed by being too exclusively guided by the experience gained in civil hospitals', a doctor noted during the Franco-Prussian War (MacCormac, 1871, p.viii). A specific example is the discovery by neurologists during the First World War that their rule of thumb in civilian practice for assessing the gravity of head injuries – loss of consciousness – was misleading with regard to gunshot wounds of the head (Sargent and Holmes, 1915).

Because each war between 1800 and 1939 was, technologically and environmentally, substantially different from its predecessor, and because civilian medicine changed rapidly in the intervals between, the lessons of one conflict were often of little value to the next. For instance, injuries from high-velocity jacketed bullets, explosive shells, hand grenades, aerial bombing and chemical gassing were hardly known before the First World War. The experience of previous wars could seriously deceive. A well-known example is the discovery by surgeons at the beginning of the First World War of their misplaced confidence in the power of antiseptics to disinfect wounds as a result of their experience in the Boer War. In the bacteria-infested battlefields of Europe and Mesopotamia, unlike the Transvaal, nearly all wounds resulting from explosions were septic. Conventional treatment methods failed to check infections and amputation rates rose steeply, to as high as 80 per cent of all cases of wounded limbs. Until new methods of wound treatment could be devised, the practice of 'conservative surgery' – based on the principle of cutting the least to save the most – was lost.

Professionalization revisited

It might be expected that the fate of those areas of medicine that were extensively professionalized through war must be different. Surely, the gains made by specialties during wartime could not be lost simply by war's end. Yet this is very much the case with some of the specialties that were placed on the medical map during the First World War. While neurosurgery, plastic surgery and rehabilitation, for instance, had to wait until the Second World War to find a demand for such specialized skills, orthopaedics found its progress checked even before the First World War had ended. In July 1918, 'traditional' authority structures in medicine were reasserting themselves, and a special committee of the Royal College of Surgeons viewed with 'mistrust and disapprobation the movement in progress to remove the treatment of conditions always properly regarded as the main portion of the general surgeon's work from his hands, and place it in those of "Orthopaedic specialists"' (quoted in Cooter, 1993, p.133). Consequently, the desire among orthopaedic surgeons for the post-war control of fracture treatments in civilian hospitals was frustrated. After the war, most of the members of the new British Orthopaedic Association were compelled to retreat to the poorly remunerated therapeutic territory that had been 'orthopaedics' before the war – that is, hospital outpatient departments for the treatment of the crippled children of the poor. Other would-be specialists were equally frustrated when they endeavoured to carve a niche for themselves in post-war civilian practice. Not only was the market glutted by demobilized medical men, but it was difficult to re-establish the informal patient referral networks with general practitioners (GPs) upon which private specialist practice relied.

The case for the war improving the lot of GPs (male or female) is even less convincing. For women doctors, the advantages conferred were lost with the war's ending. They were forced into retirement or back into the traditional areas of work accorded to women doctors. Moreover, they found that their war experience raised uncomfortable tensions and ambiguities. Many now felt caught between two equally unsatisfactory poles: on the one hand, the professional demands placed upon them within the military's 'culture of expertise and efficiency', while on the other, 'older idealizations of spiritual womanhood' and codes of 'woman as healer' (More, 1989, pp.645, 637).

As for male GPs, when conscripted, they had far less reason than either women doctors or specialists to regard modern war as enhancing their professional interests. Especially in countries where military service was not compulsory, or where, as in Britain before the First World War, the medical profession had been exempt from military service, the enforced discipline, routine and red tape of medicine in the military were frequently regarded with disdain. Whereas consultant specialists might delight in the greater clinical autonomy they obtained in military hospitals than in civilian voluntary ones (where their activities were still partially controlled by lay managers), GPs were compelled to remain in the lowest classes within the medical hierarchy.

Many GPs, under-employed for the most part during the war, found the whole experience a colossal bore. 'I had joined the Royal Army Medical Corps in July 1916,' wrote one medical officer to his Member of Parliament, '[but] I had at the most about two hours' work a day until the battle of Arras, which, as you know took place in April 1917 ... Since then I have ... no medical work to do at all. My case is not an exceptional one' (quoted in *Hansard*, 14 August 1917, col.1084). Others recalled medical experiences that were anything but the 'instructive [ones] of a lifetime' remembered by the hospital consultant and future Cambridge (and then Oxford) don, Captain John A. Ryle. Ryle enthused about:

> the good comradeship, the complete absence of the competitive evil, the living and working at close quarters of friendly teams, the direction of unanimous effort to the one object of doing the best possible both for the Service and for the individual sick or wounded soldier, sailor, or airman – all these provide[d] an atmosphere which might with advantage, but does not yet, exist in our less united and less whole-hearted civilian organizations.
>
> (Ryle, 1939, p.1202)

Richard Clarke, on the other hand, recollected experiences that were probably far more typical. He was posted to No. 19 Casualty Clearing Station on the western front in November 1915, where he dealt with wounded soldiers brought from the battlefield dressing stations. He reported:

> The surgery, such as it was, was being done by the general practitioner from South Africa and the Edinburgh graduate. As the consulting surgeon of the army hardly ever appeared – and when he did was as ignorant as we were – the science of war surgery did not get very far in our unit. Looking back on that period in the light of further knowledge, our ignorance was deplorable.
>
> (Clarke, 1937, p.4)

While some impecunious practitioners may have welcomed the security of military service, most resented the loss of their civilian income and were incensed by the 'stay-at-homes' who (allegedly) 'materially improved their financial positions ... especially if they sympathetically supported the [ill-health] pleas of some of their patients who were of military age [that is, aided them in avoiding being conscripted into the services]' (Bayly, 1934, p.189). For many rank-and-file doctors, the consequences of experiencing salaried servant status and loss of their autonomy cemented a distaste for all forms of medical provision involving the state.

Public health

Public health and welfare, when looked at more closely, also fail to offer up much to the war-as-good-for-medicine thesis. It is generally agreed among historians that one of the consequences of the First World War throughout the western world was a dampening down, rather than an intensification, of pre-war social welfare movements. As in Britain, the promised 'land fit for heroes' soon fell to the axe of post-war austerity (Abrams, 1963; Davis, 1967; Johnson, 1968). In general, during wartime states cut back on funding for socio-medical projects other than those deemed essential to the military. And this *demedicalization* of civilian-directed initiatives could have profound consequences. In the short term it might mean that medical infrastructures become ill-equipped to handle outbreaks of disease, such as occurred during the influenza pandemic at the end of the First World War. Long term, it might mean that ideologically and politically informed initiatives, such as those for combating insalubrious housing and environmental dangers to health, would succumb to cheaper, short-term wartime-like 'quick-fixes' (Murard and Zylbermann, 1996).

You read earlier about Winter's thesis on the improved life expectancy of the poor as a result of altered conditions during the First World War. This position has been seriously challenged by Linda Bryder, and the next reading is an extract from her critique of Winter's argument in an article entitled 'The First World War: healthy or hungry?', published in 1987.

Exercise

Read 'Civilian health re-examined' (Source Book 2, Reading 12.5).

1   How does Bryder challenge Winter's conclusions?

2   What sources does she use, and how do these differ from those used by Winter?

Discussion

1   Bryder casts doubt on Winter's assumption that mortality and nutrition are linked in any clear and direct way. She questions Winter's reliance on mortality statistics, arguing that they do not necessarily reflect the health of a population. She argues that better nutrition may result not simply from *more* food (as Winter implies) but from a better quality of food.

2   Whereas Winter draws on aggregated mortality statistics, Bryder relies on epidemiological statistics on morbidity and draws on the insights of social historians of medicine. However, she does not use these uncritically – she regards certain contemporary statistics as 'rhetoric', rather than accepting them at face value.

Others have noted that the high pre-war incidence of complications in pregnancy and childbirth (such as puerperal fever) continued unchanged during the war, and that standards of hospital care for civilians in fact seriously declined (Abel-Smith, 1964; Berridge, 1990, p.222). Weak and vulnerable social groups, such as elderly people and those with mental and physical disabilities, lost out in the reallocation of scarce medical resources. So severe was the effect on elderly people in Britain during the early years of the First World War, that the rules for claiming old-age pensions had to be relaxed. And so harsh was the financial effect on children's hospitals (normally an obvious target for charity) that Mr Punch was moved on more than one occasion to help out (Figure 12.3).

The competition for sympathy and alms was such that, as physically disabled non-war veterans soon discovered, without a military uniform their begging bowls stayed empty. Historian of tuberculosis F.B. Smith has shown that the Great War was anything but 'great' for sufferers of that disease. Indeed, TB was 'probably the largest single cause of civilian casualties in all the belligerent nations' (Smith,

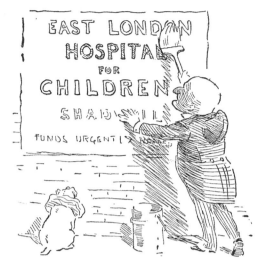

IN A GOOD CAUSE.

Mr. Punch ventures to appeal once more in a cause that has always been nearest his heart—the cause of suffering children. The East London Hospital for Children at Shadwell stands in urgent need of help. The economy of its management has been commended by those who control the King Edward's Hospital Fund, and further reduction in current expenses is impossible. Therefore if no help comes it will have to close its doors. This is unthinkable in these times when the care of the children of our fighting men is an obligation laid upon us all, and the health of the new generation is more than ever of vital importance to the nation. Mr. Punch begs his generous readers to help this Children's Hospital that serves the needs of a very poor district, isolated from the natural sources of charity. Gifts of money, great or small, will be gratefully received by The Secretary of " Punch," 10, Bouverie Street, E.C.

Figure 12.3   Hard-hit financially by the reallocation of charitable funds to wartime causes, the East London Hospital for Children receives a special appeal from Mr Punch. Note the caption's eugenic and militaristic overtones with reference to the health of future generations. Reproduced from *Punch*, 29 November 1916, p.384

1988, pp.171–3). While in Britain the mortality from this cause among young women jumped from 1.3 per 1,000 in 1914 to 1.65 per 1,000 in 1918, in Germany, 1 person for every 10 military casualties died of it (Smith, 1988, p.222). Those in mental institutions suffered most, although TB was not the only reason for their shockingly high mortality. In Germany, over 140,000 such patients died as a result of a more or less deliberate mass starvation policy and other 'mistreatments' (Schmiedebach, 1997, p.115).

In other European countries, too, the nutritional and other effects of the 1914–18 war on civilian populations were far from benign. In Germany, gout is said to have disappeared because of the leaner diet, but there was an eight-fold increase in rickets, hunger-induced tissue damage and other problems. In Russia, obesity, alcoholism, gout, gastritis, appendicitis and biliary disorders are said to have declined, but there was a marked increase in bowel, stomach and heart conditions (Bennett, 1990). Also, the tendency to racialize certain diseases accelerated in situations where military conditions deteriorated. In Germany, Jews were increasingly represented as a lethal sanitary threat; as a result, they were deloused and herded into concentration camps. Bacteriology itself became racialized as the need to control typhus led to attempts to seal borders against 'ethnic undesirables' from the east (Weindling, 1999, p.231). Whether from an ethical or a practical point of view, then, it is hard fully to endorse the idea of the beneficence of war on public health; the opposite is rather more apparent.

Furthermore ... the view from the trenches

War appears still less medically beneficent when attention is directed to the ostensible objects of military medicine: the troops. To ask what medicine in war did for them is to bring to light the paradox of medicine in war − the fact that its primary goal is not to preserve health for the sake of it, but rather to provide it purely in order to allow combatants to incapacitate one another. Since participation in such acts of violence is often not the preferred choice of conscripts, their interests and those of the medical profession in war are in this respect (as in others) fundamentally opposed.

One by one, recruits were stripped for examination, measured, weighed, tapped and interrogated (Figures 12.4 and 12.5). During the First World War, as physical fitness categories were refined over the bodies of recruits, the search for 'officer material' led to the development of IQ testing. Robert Yerkes (1876–1956) and a group of American psychologists devised the first scales for measuring intelligence (Figure 12.6). Aware of psychology's tenuous status in the military, Yerkes and his team made every effort to make their work 'more military in appearance', as Yerkes confessed in his diary, 25 June 1918: 'The psychological ratings have proved valuable not so much because they make a better classification than would come about in the course of time through natural selection but chiefly because they greatly abbreviate this process by indicating immediately the groups in which suitable office material will be found, and at the same time those men whose mental inferiority warrants their elimination from regular units in order to prevent the retardation of training. Speed counts in a war that costs fifty million dollars per day' (Carson, 1993, p.300).

From the reluctant combatant's point of view, the more the medicine of war is technically and therapeutically efficacious, the worse it is as a tool of exploitation. For the war-weary soldier, as Figure 12.7 suggests, a comfortable wound has often been a desirable passport off the battlefield. Hence a medical service that could quickly restore a soldier or sailor to fighting fitness was by no means admired by combatants. From their perspective, war is not good for medicine so much as medicine is good for war.

Wars such as the American Civil War and the First World War exposed large numbers of men to modern medicine for the first time. Along with the soldiers and sailors whose lives and limbs may have been spared by the skills of military surgeons, some combatants may have returned home from war with higher demands and expectations of orthodox medicine than when they left. If so, here

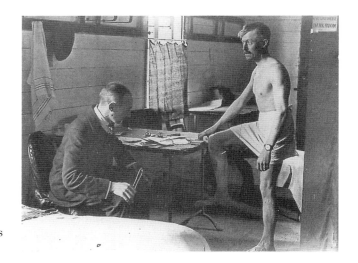

Figure 12.4   A medical officer examining a recruit. Crown Copyright, reproduced by permission of the Controller of Her Majesty's Stationery Office (IWM Q30062)

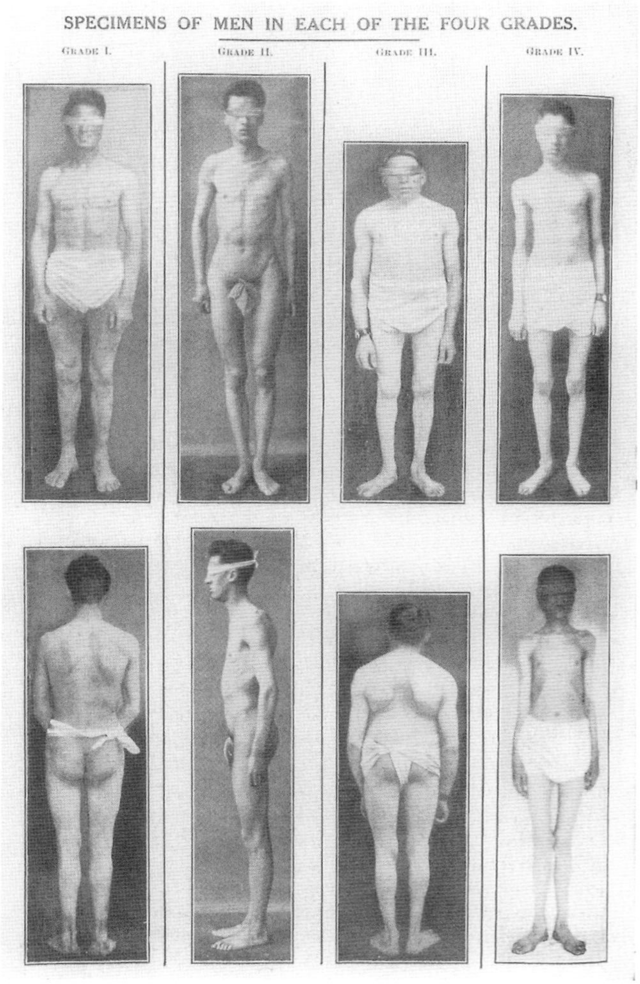

SPECIMENS OF MEN IN EACH OF THE FOUR GRADES.

GRADE I.   GRADE II.   GRADE III.   GRADE IV.

Figure 12.5   Specimens of the four grades of British recruits as adopted in 1917 when the medical examination of recruits was taken out of the hands of the War Office and placed under civilian authority. The photographs were published in the British parliamentary papers to indicate to politicians the dramatic differences between men in each of the four different grades. This classification replaced the old 'A', 'B', 'C' typing and enabled more men to be recruited to the front. The old class 'A' became Grade I; Grade II absorbed the old designations 'B-1' and 'C-1', which consisted of men who had some disability but sufficient fitness for garrison service abroad or at home. Grade III was drawn from the rest of the 'B' and 'C' categories: men unfit in varying degrees and ways but still able to serve as auxiliary troops, sanitary inspectors, batmen, cooks, storekeepers, butchers, clerks and in a wide variety of non-combatant labouring capacities. From *Parliamentary Papers*, 1919, vol.26, 308. Reproduced from Bourke (1996), Figure 45

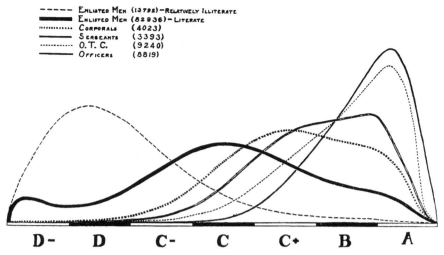

Figure 12.6   The distribution of intelligence ratings in typical army groups, showing the value of the tests in the identification of officer material. The illiterate group was given Beta; other groups were given Alpha. Reproduced from Carson (1993), p.300. © 1993 by the History of Science Society

was a further wartime gain to the medical profession. But equally noteworthy are the bases for the troops' distrust of the agents of the enforced medicalization of military life. Not least was the fear of being made the subject of a medical experiment. Like slaves, prisoners and orphans, soldiers and sailors were easy prey for medical experimenters. As early as 1587, Barnaby Rich (*c*.1540–1617) in his *Pathway to Military Practice* felt the need to advise surgeons to 'work according to arte, not practisinge newe experiments upon a poore soulder' (quoted in Firth, 1902, p.253). However, given the number of healthy male bodies available in the military, and the authoritarian conditions, the temptation to do otherwise was irresistible. For Zachary Cope, two of the plus factors of medicine in modern war were, first, that the discipline among the troops rendered it 'more easy to test any method or drug on a sufficiently large scale to endure a definite result', and second, '[that] it is possible to introduce compulsion and in this way confirm by large-scale experiment that which had been previously proved on a smaller scale' (Cope, 1961, p.169). Conventional ethical behaviour in medicine could be put aside in the interest, ostensibly, of ultimately greater military might, although often it was in the more immediate interest of professionalizing groups. For instance, in Germany during the First World War, army pathologists were permitted to conduct post-mortems on soldiers without the consent of relatives in order to further their expertise. However, the very fact that these pathologists felt the need to argue that offering up one's body for autopsy was 'definitely the pinnacle in comradeship and Christian love for one's neighbour even in death', suggests that there was considerable resistance to overcome (Prüll and Sinn, 2002, p.79).

Another reason for combatants to be on their guard against the medical profession was in connection with malingering and the self-infliction of wounds. Both practices, when undertaken to contrive honourable discharges, were punishable

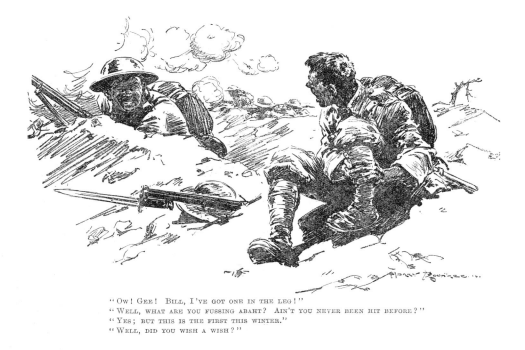

"Ow! Gee! Bill, I've got one in the leg!"
"Well, what are you fussing abaht? Ain't you never been hit before?"
"Yes; but this is the first this winter."
"Well, did you wish a wish?"

Figure 12.7   By 1916, romantic notions of warfare were gone. In the trenches, work was routinized in shifts, much as in factories. A 'blighty' – an injury that would allow a soldier-worker to be hospitalized back in Britain – was welcomed, as indicated in this illustration from *Punch*, 8 November 1916, p.328

at the highest levels of military authority. Detection was thus a vital aspect of the practice of military medicine. In Britain in the early nineteenth century, when there were nearly as many soldiers and sailors on disability pensions as in the armed forces, the detection of malingering became a state priority. Malingerers had to pit their wits against medical officers seriously intent on their unmasking. The same applied during the First World War and was as important a function of doctors at the recruiting stations as at the front (Figure 12.8).

It was not always easy to unmask malingerers, however, in part because a recruit might himself be uncertain about his real physical or mental state. This might be gleaned from the next reading, an extract from the memoirs of Private Edward Casey, a self-styled 'misfit soldier'.

Exercise

Read 'The soldier's view' (Source Book 2, Reading 12.6).

1   What does this account suggest about Casey's attitude to the army and to army doctors?

2   Do you think he is really malingering?

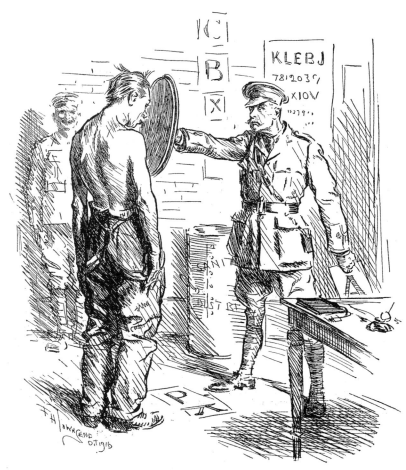

A BOLD BID FOR EXEMPTION.

Exasperated Medical Officer (picking up lid of sanitary dustbin—to compulsory recruit).
"CAN YOU SEE THAT?"
Compulsory Recruit. "YES."
Officer. "WHAT IS IT?"
Recruit. "TWO BOB OR 'ALF-A-CROWN.'"

Figure 12.8   This image suggests cowardly rather than clever malingering in the face of manly duty. But it also suggests the dredging of recruits from the ranks of the less physically fit. Reproduced from *Punch*, 11 October 1916, p.271

Discussion

1   Casey is clearly terrified by life under fire, and determined to get away from the front. At the same time, he is also afraid of the doctors, and concerned that they will somehow discover that he is not really suffering from shell shock: he spends a lot of time working out exactly how to present a convincing case. (And in the course of it, shows that soldiers were familiar with the causes, symptoms, progress and likely treatment of shell shock.)

2   Although Casey states that he feigned his symptoms, his account gives the impression that he was seemingly simultaneously suffering from some degree of shell shock – he mentions having a lump on his head and not being able to remember when he was injured. Given that his memoir was written long after the war, we also have to wonder whether Casey preferred to admit to repeated bouts of shell shock or to present a story in which he took his fate into his own hands by malingering.

It was often specifically in relation to malingering and the self-infliction of wounds that the politics of change in military medicine were debated. Florence Nightingale, for example, denied that malingering existed among British troops in the Crimea, in order to garner support for her 'soldier-victims' of a medically 'reactionary' War Office (quoted in Woodward, 1863, p.325). Her case for the reform of the army medical service would have been seriously compromised if a significant proportion of the sick troops had been labelled malingerers. Earlier in the century, one of the main arguments against dismantling the regimental system of the British army was that regimental surgeons were uniquely placed to detect malingerers. More centralized systems of military medical organization with high-ranking medical administrators at a distance were deemed ineffectual. Thus when this feature of modern military management was introduced, new methods of detecting malingerers had to be devised. At least in part, this was why the military gave encouragement to medical specialisms; the expectation was that the experts would be better able to detect troops feigning specific illnesses. Clearly, the worth of specialisms *to the military* was as much for their detective as for their corrective function.

The politico-economic context of medicine in war

To draw attention to malingering, or for that matter any aspect of military interest in the health and welfare of troops, is to highlight certain simple truths about war and medicine which tend to be obscured in medico-centric accounts. One of the most obvious is that military medicine, whether pursued in peace or in war, is both product and agent of its political and economic times. This is self-evident once you recall that the purpose of maintaining healthy troops is to win wars, the object of most conflicts being economic and ideological domination. Medicine in the armed forces is also subject to rigorous budget constraints, which of course are politically determined.

Although little research has been conducted into the political economy of military medicine, the signs of it are everywhere. The title alone of a famous work by a British inspector general of hospitals, Robert Jackson, *A Systematic View of the Formation, Discipline and Economy of Armies*, published in 1804, provides one such clue. From the contents of Jackson's book it is clear that he harboured no illusions about why it was necessary to prevent soldiers and sailors from acquiring disabling conditions and diseases. Like others with commissions in military and naval medicine before and after him, Jackson was acutely aware that the ultimate purpose of military hygiene was to enable imperialist expansion, the success of which depended on the prolonged good health of the troops. It was explicitly for this reason that in the eighteenth century the Royal Navy supported research that led to the use of lime juice against scurvy, and it was for this reason, too, that towards the end of the nineteenth century the colonial powers funded, via their military establishments, schools of tropical medicine and public health.

The practice of medicine and surgery in the armed forces also needs to be viewed in terms of immediate political and economic interests. Historian Colin Jones, in a scholarly overview of French military medicine from the time of Richelieu to Napoleon, has illustrated how economic expediency above all encouraged Napoleon's military surgeons to undertake the amputation of wounded limbs where in many cases limb-preserving 'conservative surgery' might have sufficed (Jones, 1989, pp.209–40). The long and expensive hospital convalescence required for the conservation of limbs was deemed militarily unnecessary in a mass army of expendable conscripts. (It is in this context, rather than in the narratives of medical genius, that Larrey's efforts at hip amputations need to be set.) In the different context of the First World War, where the value of conserving forces in the face of their wholesale slaughter was soon apparent, medical directives were modified accordingly. As a British army memorandum of 1917 put it:

> The primary objects of army hospitals are to get the disabled, physically and mentally, fit to fight again; or, if this is not possible within a reasonable time, to return him to civil life at his highest possible value in the labour market, so that he may cost the public purse the less. If this can be more rapidly and effectually obtained by a relatively high scale of equipment (e.g. orthopaedic surgery), or a larger personnel (e.g. the nursing service), it may be more economical to provide them.
>
> (Mitchell, 1917, p.1)

Like the supposedly purely 'medical' function of medicine in war, the purportedly 'humanitarian' performance is also open to political, economic and ideological scrutiny. The provision of welfare services for invalided ex-servicemen was often overtly politically motivated. Until the Second World War, the primary motive of nation-states in providing such services was to monitor and control the demobilized in order to prevent political revolt. To this end, the Hôtel des Invalides was established by Louis XIV in 1670, and the Chelsea Royal Hospital by Charles II in 1682 (Hudson, 2000; Jones, 1989). The medical profession, too, exploited the threat of revolutionary activity among the war-disabled: orthopaedic specialists warned of social upheaval from thousands of disabled soldiers in order to persuade the government to set up rehabilitation centres under their command. Such rhetoric carried force, for unlike more traditional war victims (widows and orphans) or the downtrodden veterans of earlier wars, those of the First World War had the vote, and were therefore able to exert real pressure on government. In Germany, they staged violent political revolt (Cohen, 2001; Whalen, 1984).

In other ways, too, medical practitioners were involved in the politics of war-disablement. Since they were invested with the power to decide whether or not an injury was war-related, there was a high degree of complicity with the state in the granting or refusing of disability pensions. In this connection, as with the detection of malingering, their role in wartime was comparable to their peacetime role in workmen's compensation claims (the civilian territory for medical adjudication of injuries, real or feigned). It is not coincidental that Sir John Collie, one of few British medico-legal experts on malingering before 1914, was appointed one of the medical directors at the Ministry of Pensions during the war.

12.4 Conclusion: war and medicine reconsidered

By this point, the limits of the war-as-good-for-medicine thesis should be clear. Whether seen narrowly in terms of advances in techniques and research, or more broadly in terms of specialization and professionalization, the thesis is equivocal at best. Although some features of medical knowledge and practice have obviously been expanded, altered or elaborated by war, others have remained unaffected. Still others have been temporarily interrupted, demoted in political importance, marginalized or halted altogether. Generalization is impossible. Quite apart from whether the perspective is that of patients or professionals, or whether the calculation is made in the short or the long term, the worth of war for any aspect of medicine and public health must be seen to vary according to the type of war as well as its time, place, duration and – not least – its political and economic outcome. In selected cases – perhaps for selected periods – it might be possible to claim that medicine reaps in peace what it sows in war; but equally, it can be argued that medicine only reaps in war what it sows in peace. To the institutions of military medicine, the audit may be different. To it alone (eventually) war came to preach valuable 'lessons', and for those with professional stakes in the expansion of military medicine, it scarcely mattered that a particular campaign may have been disastrous, medically as well as militarily. Indeed, the greater the medical shortcomings of any war, the greater its potentially educative role for future wars and hence for bolstering the interests of military medicine. The unhappy tales of woe in the Crimea, in Cuba (over typhoid and yellow fever during the Spanish–American War of 1898) and in the Transvaal were in this sense priceless. Such disasters at least provided powerful rationales for the reform of military medicine (although actual reform may have been another matter).

By now it will also be apparent to you that a part of the problem in trying to determine the relations between medicine and war lies in the question of 'effects' itself. 'Effects' assumes that there is a direct, mechanically causal interaction between war and medicine. War is perceived as a force in and of itself, and medicine merely as a recipient, passive or otherwise. It is this search for the direct consequences of war on medicine that separates both war and medicine from the societies, economies and cultures in which they are set.

While it is true that the conditions of war are in some respects peculiar and can occasion responses in medicine different from those in peacetime, it would be ludicrous to suppose that war is wholly an extraneous phenomenon which merely periodically interrupts the 'orderly progress' of society. Such a notion rests upon a polarity between war and society: between war, as a place of violence, and economic and political life as a place of non-violence. But recent studies of war and society refute the notion (Marwick, 1988; Smith, 1986). To assume that medicine in war can be treated as 'other', or merely reactive to war, is to deny that medicine is itself part and parcel of the society and economy in which its therapeutic and professional politics are pursued. Whatever else war and medicine may be, neither is autonomous.

Thus the interactions of war and medicine must vary according to the practical and ideological nature of the medicine and the society at the time a war occurs. To some extent, it also follows that the effects of any particular war on medicine must ultimately be elusive, for if war and medicine are themselves parts of wider socio-political phenomena, the impact of war on any aspect of medicine, public health or professionalization can never be precisely calculated. There is an additional reason why the relationship between war and medicine cannot easily be cast in narrowly causal terms for the near-century between the Crimean War and the Second World War. It is this: for this period, the boundaries between peace and war are not easily drawn, and the relations between civilian and military medicine are blurred. It is not simply that 'the distinction between army doctors and general practitioners [was] gradually disappearing', as one British clinician maintained in 1938 (Jules, 1938, p.17). More fundamental was the breakdown of the assumption 'that war is an abnormal situation, [and] that peace is – or ought to be – the normal lot of mankind' (Titmuss, 1963, p.77). Although western society was by no means in a state of constant war, it was increasingly 'militarized'; war and the preparations for it came to be regarded by many as normal and desirable social activities (Mann, 1988, p.124). Not only were military values and attitudes carried into the civilian sphere, but, more profoundly, society and economy were coming to be disciplined – rationalized, regulated and regimented – in accordance with industrial–military conceptions of efficiency. As the size and scale of industrial production and social 'disorder' grew, the more did military management appear as a model to cope with it. At a cultural level, as the late nineteenth century growth of the Boy Scout movement and the Salvation Army make clear, moral, mental and physical efficiency or robustness for nations and individuals alike was to be generated through the inculcation of military manliness.

The history of the 'militarization' of medicine has not begun to be written. Even for continental Europe, where military medicine was more prominent than in Britain and America, the relations of military to civilian medicine remain largely unstudied. There is space here only to note some of the more superficial signs and symbols of the process towards the end of the nineteenth century in Britain, where, precisely because of less obvious military traditions in medicine, the process of militarization was more striking. Indeed, one such sign was the observation and lament of this European difference by some British doctors. In a well-publicized lecture of 1903, for instance, specifically on the relations between the military and civilian medical services in Britain, a London physician dwelt enviously on the fact that:

> On the continent there is not that distinction between the military and civilian branches of the profession which exists here. Practically every civilian medical man has once been in the army and would merely revert to his former position in the eve of war, while in terms of peace both work side by side in the large state hospitals. In Russia a large part of the civilian practice is in the hands of the military medical officers and their

military hospitals would appear to play almost the same role that our large voluntary hospitals do in this country.

(Low, 1903, p.999)

Alongside statements such as this can be set the increased voluntary participation of practitioners in wars and in the reserve forces for war; their campaigns for the reform of the status, pay and conditions of service of doctors in the army and navy; the unprecedented outpouring of reminiscences by doctors who had served in military campaigns since Waterloo (of which the extract by Wrench is a good example); the cultivation of the image of medicine on the battlefield as the noblest expression of the 'gospel of humanity'; and, not least, the rewriting of civilian medicine (surgery in particular) in terms emphasizing its debts to military medicine.

Scarcely separable from these developments was the professionalization and increasing 'civilianization' of military medicine. By 1900, there were some fifty specialist military medical journals internationally, and military medical associations were well represented in bodies such as the British Medical Association and the international congresses of medicine and surgery. Reflecting and hastening these developments was the rise to prominence within the international medical establishment of postgraduate military medical academies, such as that of the Royal Army Medical Corps, removed from Netley to London in 1902. It was in these schools that many of the world's leading bacteriologists and (what we would now call) immunologists and parasitologists were based.

In view of these signs of the melding of military and civilian medicine in the late nineteenth century, especially around bacteriology, it is not surprising that military metaphors should have come to dominate medicine as a whole. Whereas before the late nineteenth century diseases were commonly spoken of environmentally, in terms of relations between 'seed and soil', that language declined with the rise of the science of germs in the context of militarized society. From that time to this, our illnesses have had to be *fought* (usually with the help of magic *bullets*). As we *battle* AIDS by seeking the means to restore *defence systems*, so we wage *war* on heart disease, and continue to run *campaigns* for research funding to fight such a dreaded *enemy* as cancer. (You can see an example of the use of such metaphors in Figure 9.1.) 'Biomilitarism', as one discourse analyst has labelled it, is now *the* language of modern biomedicine (Montgomery, 1991). Thus the very conception of our bodies and, by extension, the medical acts performed on them, remain within the militarized social relations of medicine that emerged during the late nineteenth century.

Clearly, then, the relations between medicine and war are not as simple and straightforward as is sometimes assumed. To see them as if in a world apart from the rest of the history of society, economy, culture *and* medicine is untenable. Nor can we regard them as merely causally interactive, largely self-contained and mutually beneficial. Rather, as war comes to be seen (at least for much of the period focused on here) not as a phenomenon outside society and culture but as the epitome or apotheosis of the wider socio-economically informed process of militarization, so medicine must be seen as part of that process. Pursued in these terms, the history of medicine and war might reveal more than most historians have yet dared to imagine about the construction of disease entities, the structuring of both medical and military institutions, and the daily practice of medicine as we have come to know it.

References

Abel-Smith, B. (1964) *The Hospitals, 1800–1948: A Study of Social Administration in England and Wales*, London: Heinemann.

Abrams, P. (1963) 'The failure of social reform: 1918–1920', *Past and Present*, vol.24, pp.42–64.

Allbutt, Sir T.C. (1921) 'Medicine in the twentieth century' in Sir T.C. Allbutt, *Greek Medicine in Rome with Other Historical Essays*, London: Macmillan, pp.541–61.

Bayly, H.W. (1934) *Triple Challenge: A Doctor's Memoirs of the Years 1914 to 1929*, London: Hutchinson.

Bennett, J.D.C. (1990) 'Medical advances consequent to the Great War, 1914–1918', *Journal of the Royal Society of Medicine*, vol.83, pp.738–42.

Berridge, V. (1990) 'Health and medicine' in F.L.M. Thompson (ed.) *The Cambridge Social History of Britain 1750–1950*, vol.3 *Social Agencies and Institutions*, Cambridge: Cambridge University Press, pp.171–242.

Bourke, J. (1996) *Dismembering the Male: Men's Bodies, Britain and the Great War*, London: Reaktion.

Carson, J. (1993) 'Army alpha, army brass, and the search for army intelligence', *Isis*, vol.84, pp.278–309.

Clarke, R.G. (1937) 'The evolution of a casualty clearing station on the western front', *Bristol Medico-Chirurgical Journal*, vol.54, pp.1–20.

Cohen, D. (2001) *The War Came Home: Disabled Veterans in Britain and Germany, 1914–1939*, Berkeley: University of California Press.

Cooter, R. (ed.) (1991) *In the Name of the Child: Health and Welfare, 1880–1940*, London: Routledge.

Cooter, R. (1993) *Surgery and Society in Peace and War: Orthopaedics and the Organization of Modern Medicine, 1880–1948*, London: Macmillan.

Cooter, R. (2003) 'Of war and epidemics: unnatural couplings, problematic conceptions', *Social History of Medicine*, vol.16, pp.283–302.

Cope, Z. (1961) 'The medical balance sheet of war' in Z. Cope, *Some Famous General Practitioners and other Medical Historical Essays*, London: Pitman, pp.169–83.

Davis, A.F. (1967) 'Welfare, reform and World War I', *American Quarterly*, vol.19, pp.516–33.

Deutsch, A. (1946) 'Some wartime influences on health and welfare institutions in the United States', *Journal of the History of Medicine and Allied Science*, vol.1, pp.318–29.

Dumas, S. and Vedel-Petersen, K.O. (1923) *Losses of Life Caused by War*, ed. by H. Westergaard, Oxford: Clarendon.

Duncan, L.C. (1914) 'The comparative mortality of disease and battle casualties in the historic wars of the world', *Journal of the Military Service Institution of the United States*, vol.54, pp.141–77.

Dwork, D. (1987) *War is Good for Babies and Other Young Children: A History of the Infant and Child Welfare Movement in England, 1898–1918*, London: Tavistock.

Firth, C.H. (1902) *Cromwell's Army*, London: Methuen.

Garrison, F. [1922] (1970) *Notes on the History of Military Medicine*, Hildesheim and New York: Georg Olms.

Garrison, F. (1929) *Introduction to the History of Medicine*, 4th edn, Philadelphia: W.B. Saunders.

Hardy, A. (2000) '"Straight back to barbarism": anti-typhoid inoculation and the Great War', *Bulletin of the History of Medicine*, vol.74, pp.265–90.

Hardy, A. (2001) *Health and Medicine in Britain since 1860*, Houndmills: Palgrave.

Hudson, G.L. (2000) 'Disabled veterans and the state in early modern England' in D.A. Gerber (ed.) *Disabled Veterans in History*, Ann Arbor: University of Michigan Press, pp.117–44.

Ireland, M.W. (1921) 'The achievement of the army medical department in the world war in the light of general medical progress', *Journal of the American Medical Association*, vol.76, pp.763–9.

Johnson, P.B. (1968) *A Land Fit for Heroes: The Planning of British Reconstruction, 1916–1919*, Chicago: University of Chicago Press.

Jones, C. (1989) *The Charitable Imperative: Hospitals and Nursing in Ancien Régime and Revolutionary France*, London: Routledge.

Jules, H. (ed.) (1938) *The Doctor's View of War*, London: Allen & Unwin.

Keegan, J. (1976) *The Face of Battle*, London: Jonathan Cape.

Lane, J. (2001) *A Social History of Medicine: Health, Healing and Disease in England, 1750–1950*, London: Routledge.

Lawrence, G. (1992) 'The ambiguous artifact: surgical instruments and the surgical past' in C. Lawrence (ed.) *Medical Theory, Surgical Practice*, London: Routledge, pp.295–314.

Leese, P. (2002) *Shell Shock: Traumatic Neurosis and the British Soldiers of the First World War*, Houndmills: Palgrave.

Leneman, L. (1994) *In the Service of Life: The Story of Elsie Inglis and the Scottish Women's Hospitals*, Edinburgh: Mercat.

Lerner, P. (2000) 'Psychiatry and casualties of war in Germany, 1914–18', *Journal of Contemporary History*, vol.35, pp.13–28.

Lerner, P. (2003) *Hysterical Men: War, Psychiatry, and the Politics of Trauma in Germany, 1890–1930*, Ithaca: Cornell University Press.

Low, V.W. (1903) 'The relationship of the military medical service to the civil profession', *Lancet*, vol.2, pp.997–1001.

MacCormac, W. (1871) *Notes and Recollections of an Ambulance Surgeon, Being an Account of Work Done Under the Red Cross during the Campaign of 1870*, London: J. & A. Churchill.

Mann, M. (1988) *States, War and Capitalism: Studies in Political Sociology*, Oxford: Blackwell.

Marwick, A. (ed.) (1988) *Total War and Social Change*, London: Macmillan.

Mitchell, P. (1917) *Memoranda on Army General Hospital Administration*, London: Bailliere, Tindall & Cox.

Mitchell, T. and Smith, G. (1931) *Casualties and Medical Statistics of the Great War*, London: HMSO.

Montgomery, S.L. (1991) 'Codes and combat in biomedical discourse', *Science as Culture*, vol.12, pp.341–90.

More, E. (1989) '"A certain restless ambition": women physicians and World War I', *American Quarterly*, vol.41, pp.636–60.

Moulin, D. de (1988) *A History of Surgery: With Emphasis on the Netherlands*, Dordrecht, Boston and Lancaster: Martinus Nijhoff.

Murard, L. and Zylbermann, P. (1996) *L'Hygiène dans la republique: la santé publique en France, ou l'utopie contrariée, 1870–1918*, Paris: Fayard.

Prinzing, F. (1916) *Epidemics Resulting from Wars*, ed. by H. Westergaard, Oxford: Clarendon.

Prüll, C. and Sinn, M. (2002) 'Problems of consent to surgical procedures and autopsies in twentieth century Germany' in A. Maehle and J. Geyer-Kordesch (eds) *Historical and Philosophical Perspectives on Biomedical Ethics: From Paternalism to Autonomy?*, Aldershot: Ashgate, pp.73–93.

Ryle, J.A. (1939) 'Active service medical societies', *British Medical Journal*, vol.2, p.1202.

Sargent, P. and Holmes, G. (1915) 'The treatment of the cranial injuries of warfare', *British Medical Journal*, vol.1, pp.537–8.

Schmiedebach, H.-P., (1997) 'The mentally ill patient caught between the state's demands and the professional interests of psychiatrists' in M. Berg and G. Cocks (eds) *Medicine and Modernity: Public Health and Medical Care in*

Nineteenth- and Twentieth-Century Germany, Cambridge: Cambridge University Press, pp.99–119.

Searle, G.R. (1971) *The Quest for National Efficiency: A Study in British Politics and Social Thought, 1899–1914*, Oxford: Blackwell.

Shephard, B. (2000) *A War of Nerves: Soldiers and Psychiatrists, 1914–1994*, London: Jonathan Cape.

Smith, F.B. (1988) *The Retreat of Tuberculosis, 1850–1950*, London: Croom Helm.

Smith, H. (ed.) (1986) *War and Social Change: British Society in The Second World War*, Manchester: Manchester University Press.

Stevens, R. (1971) *American Medicine and the Public Interest*, New Haven: Yale University Press.

Summers, A. (1988) *Angels and Citizens: British Women as Military Nurses, 1854–1914*, London: Routledge.

Titmuss, R. (1963) 'War and social policy' in R. Titmuss, *Essays on 'The Welfare State'*, 2nd edn, London: Allen & Unwin, pp.75–87.

Watson, F. (1950) *Dawson of Penn*, London: Chatto & Windus.

Weindling, P. (1999) 'A virulent strain: German bacteriology as scientific racism, 1890–1920' in Waltraud Ernst and Bernard Harris (eds) *Race, Science and Medicine, 1700–1960*, London: Routledge, pp.218–34.

Weiner, D. (1993) *The Citizen-Patient in Revolutionary and Imperial Paris*, Baltimore: Johns Hopkins University Press.

Whalen, R.W. (1984) *Bitter Wounds: German Victims of the Great War, 1914–1939*, Ithaca: Cornell University Press.

Winter, J.M. (1985) *The Great War and the British People*, London: Macmillan.

Woodward, J.J. (1863) *Outlines of the Chief Camp Diseases of the United States Armies as Observed during the Present War: A Practical Contribution to Military Medicine*, Philadelphia: J.B. Lippincott.

Source Book readings

E.M. Wrench, 'The lessons of the Crimean War', *British Medical Journal*, 1899, vol.2, pp.205–8 (Reading 12.1).

M. Seacole, *Wonderful Adventures of Mrs Seacole in Many Lands*, Oxford: Oxford University Press, [1857] 1988, pp.124–6, 143–4, 166 (Reading 12.2).

J. Winter, *The Great War and the British People*, London: Macmillan, 1985, pp.117, 120–1, 123–4, 134–5, 138–40 (Reading 12.3).

Report of the War Office Committee of Enquiry into 'Shell-Shock', London: HMSO, 1922, Cmd 1734, pp.17, 55–7 (Reading 12.4).

L. Bryder 'The First World War: healthy or hungry?', *History Workshop Journal*, 1987, vol.24, pp.142–8, 150 (Reading 12.5).

'The Misfit Soldier': Edward Casey's War Story, 1914–18, ed. by J. Bourke, Cork: Cork University Press, 1999, pp.52–4 (Reading 12.6).

Access to Health Care, 1880–1930

Deborah Brunton

Objectives

When you have completed this chapter you should be able to:

- describe the wide range of methods of promoting health, preventing disease and providing care that were available to patients of different social groups and classes;

- be aware of the inequalities of services – in terms of both quality of care and access to different services – open to different social groups and classes;

- assess the significance of the roles of central and local governments, the private sector and voluntary associations in providing medical services;

- understand the concept of 'medicalization' and assess the degree of power doctors had over people's lives in the early twentieth century.

13.1 Introduction

The late nineteenth and early twentieth centuries have often been described as a period of progress, when the poorer classes gained access to a whole range of medical services previously reserved for the wealthy. In the past, this opening up of care was largely attributed to the state. Across Europe, central and local governments created health insurance schemes and new welfare services to provide the poor with access to care, from general practitioners (GPs) to outpatient and hospital care, and treatment for specific complaints such as tuberculosis and venereal disease. This movement culminated in the 1940s, when it was the boast of the British government that the National Health Service provided care for all 'from the cradle to the grave'. However, more recent studies by historians of medicine have shown that improved access to health services was also provided through charities. Old voluntary organizations, such as hospitals and dispensaries, expanded their work and strove for greater efficiency, employing professional administrators. New charities were founded, providing novel services, including help for mothers and babies. Improved access to health care also came about through private insurance schemes to provide GP and inpatient care to the working classes.

While historians of medicine agree that this period saw greater provision of medical services, especially for the poorer classes, some researchers have questioned whether improved access to care was an unalloyed good. They have argued that not everyone benefited equally from improved services. Improvements in access to care were unequally distributed. New medical services were often limited to the very poorest, or to particular groups, such as working men or women and children, and levels of provision varied between countries and regions. Provision of care did not guarantee a high standard of service: detailed research by some historians has shown that the poorer classes often received a lower quality of care than their wealthier counterparts. Others have argued that there were drawbacks to more accessible medical services. They have described the early twentieth century as a period of 'medicalization'. As patients gained greater access to medical professionals – doctors, nurses and health educators – they became passive consumers of medical services. At the same time, the medical profession no longer simply dealt with the sick, but increasingly took a role in monitoring the lifestyle and behaviour of healthy people. As a result, people became increasingly dependent on medical practitioners to guide their lives.

In this chapter, I explore these issues through a study of the health-care services available in Britain at the end of the nineteenth and in the first decades of the twentieth centuries, using a wide range of sources. Where material is available, I make comparisons with the care available elsewhere in Europe. I cover all aspects of health care – from disease prevention, through care in the home, general practitioner services and finally care in institutions. I explore the access to medical services among different social groups and assess how much control practitioners had over their patients' lives by 1930. This requires you to look again at many of the medical services described earlier in this book – but this time from the patient's viewpoint.

13.2   Patterns of disease

Before looking at how people dealt with ill health, you need to know what sort of medical conditions were prevalent. In Chapter 7, you discovered that between the nineteenth and twentieth centuries, all over Europe, the prevailing pattern of mortality changed. Infectious diseases, which had killed huge numbers of people, were gradually brought under control. As life expectancy increased, degenerative diseases, associated with old age, began to cause more deaths. However, although people were living longer, they actually spent more time off work because of illness. James Riley's studies of the records of friendly societies, which offered health insurance (these are discussed in more detail later), have shown that workers were no longer dying from infectious diseases. Instead, they survived illness, but spent a long time recovering their health and strength (Riley, 1989, pp.159–92).

The friendly society records show that the complaints that caused workers to take time off were not the same as those that dominate mortality statistics (Table 13.1).

Table 13.1 **Comparison of mortality with sickness recorded by friendly societies in England and Wales**

Leading causes of death in England and Wales among men, in 1908		Leading causes of sickness in three friendly societies, 1896–1919	
Cause	% of total	Cause	% of total
Heart disease	14	Accidents	16
Tuberculosis	14	Poorly identified	13
Old age	8	Influenza and catarrh	13
Cancer	8	Bronchitis	9
Bronchitis	7	Rheumatism	4
Pneumonia	7	Lumbago[1]	4
Cerebral haemorrhage	5	Gastritis[2]	2
Accidents	5	Carbuncle[3]	2
Bright's disease[4]	3	Tonsillitis	1
Influenza	3	Skin ulcers	1
Apoplexy	2		

[1] Lower back pain, caused by muscular inflammation or arthritis
[2] Inflammation of the stomach lining, causing pain and discomfort after eating
[3] A local infection, similar to, but larger than, a boil
[4] Now recognized as a number of kidney diseases, all associated with the presence of albumin in the urine
(Adapted from Riley, 1997, pp.191–2, Tables 7.1 and 7.2)

If we ignore accidents and 'poorly identified' complaints, the most common ailments among the working-class men insured by the friendly societies were respiratory infections – influenza, colds and bronchitis – followed by joint and muscle problems, such as rheumatism and lumbago. Few workmen reported sick with degenerative diseases. Nor did they take time off for tuberculosis (TB), one of the major killers at this time. TB was a chronic, but not disabling, disease, and men were able to work until they developed advanced symptoms.

Friendly societies insured a select group – fairly young, fit, working men – so their records are not representative of the whole population. General practitioners saw a larger cross-section of society. Records from their practice suggest that they treated a fairly similar range of complaints to those recorded by the friendly societies – respiratory infections, rheumatism and digestive complaints, such as dyspepsia and diarrhoea. GPs did not spend much time treating degenerative diseases since they could do little for such conditions. Their case records show how patterns of disease varied by class, area and season. Middle- and upper-class patients consulted doctors about obesity, gout and nervous complaints – conditions that were rarely reported by working-class patients. The poor suffered from rickets (a consequence of a poor diet), dysentery and diarrhoea (reflecting the difficulty of keeping food clean and fresh) and infectious diseases. GPs working in industrial areas had to deal with the results of accidents and occupational diseases: miners, for example, who worked in a damp and dusty environment, suffered from high levels of bronchitis, pneumonia and pleurisy. Everywhere, the incidence of respiratory diseases increased in the winter months, while digestive complaints were more frequent in the summer (Digby, 1999, pp.192–3, 208–14).

Men were more likely than women or children to visit a GP (for reasons I discuss later), but not because women and children were any healthier. Children continued to suffer from a range of infectious diseases – tonsillitis, scarlet fever, chickenpox, whooping cough, measles and mumps. A survey of the health of working-class women in the 1930s found that they suffered from headaches, constipation, anaemia, rheumatism, gynaecological problems (often associated with childbirth), bad teeth, and 'bad legs', resulting from varicose veins, ulcers and phlebitis (inflammation of the veins) (Spring Rice, [1939] 1981, p.37).

Fears about TB, VD and degeneration are discussed in more detail in Chapter 9.

While people suffered from a wide range of complaints, two diseases prompted particular public concern – tuberculosis and venereal disease (VD). Both were seen as causes of national degeneration, causing high levels of disease which weakened the population and led in turn to the birth of feeble children (Figure 13.1).

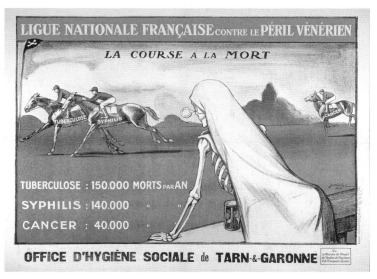

Figure 13.1 This poster, issued in 1926 by the National French League against the Danger of Venereal Disease, neatly encapsulates the perceived risks associated with three diseases in the 1920s. Death watches a three-horse race, in which Tuberculosis (150,000 deaths per year) narrowly beats Syphilis (140,000 deaths per year), while Cancer causes only 40,000 deaths. These mortality statistics do not correspond to those recorded by the Registrar-General for England and Wales; in 1910, deaths from tuberculosis were thirty-two times greater than those attributed to syphilis. However, the Registrar-General's report acknowledged that there was a serious under-reporting of syphilis deaths by doctors, who did not wish to stigmatize their patients, and so recorded syphilis deaths under other disease categories. Wellcome Library, London

There was also a widespread belief among the public and medical practitioners that the pace of modern life – in which information flashed through the air by telegraph, and people travelled by train and steamship at previously unimaginable speeds – caused ill health. The modern lifestyle was associated with physical disorders, including dyspepsia, diabetes and liver complaints. It was also blamed by some practitioners for an apparent epidemic of nervous diseases, such as hysteria and neurasthenia. Symptoms of anxiety, depression, insomnia, pain, involuntary movements and nervous tics were believed to result from the strain of modern life on the nervous system. In Russia, neurasthenia was associated with a cultivated 'western' lifestyle (Goering, 2003).

13.3 Preserving health

Surrounded by the ever-present threat of ill health, not surprisingly, people expended a good deal of time and energy on trying to stay well. The late nineteenth century saw a new emphasis on promoting health, which was defined as 'a state of complete physical, mental, and social well-being and not merely the absence of disease or infirmity' (quoted in Riley, 1997, p.199). Health was not simply a desirable end in itself. The pursuit of health was portrayed as a moral duty: parents had a responsibility to protect both the health of their children and their own health, so that they could support their families. Health also became a political concern: the future strength of the nation was seen to rest on the good health of children – the future generations of soldiers and workers. At the beginning of the twentieth century, popular beliefs about the best means of preserving health were little different from those prescribed two thousand years earlier in classical Greece – good diet, fresh air, exercise and cleanliness. Such a lifestyle would keep the body in the best possible condition to fight off germs and diseases.

While all classes regarded good health as desirable, access to various means of preserving or promoting it varied according to economic circumstances. For the upper and middle classes, with substantial amounts of disposable income, a wide range of options were available. They could access information about how to protect their health through books and articles in magazines. Many of these books were written (or at least claimed to be written) by doctors and other health-care professionals. An article about pregnancy in the opening number of *Woman* magazine in 1932, for example, was allegedly written by 'Mumsie, the wife of a famous children's doctor' – a persona neatly combining medical authority and the status of an ordinary wife and mother (Beddoe, 1989, pp.14–15). The 1920s saw a boom in baby-care books, aimed at middle-class mothers, which not only gave practical advice on feeding, bathing and clothing, but also set out the stages of physical and psychological development, thus unwittingly creating the first generation of mothers worried that their babies walked and talked 'late' (Unwin and Sharland, 1992).

Generally, the wealthier classes enjoyed the sort of varied diet thought to promote good health. They could afford meat, fish, fresh fruit and vegetables (Burnett, 1979, pp.213–39). However, some wealthy individuals worried that they ate too much, and dieting to obtain a slim figure was a well-established activity by the 1920s. Others were concerned that their diet was too rich, and in the pursuit of health adopted simple, more 'natural' diets. They stopped consuming alcohol, tea, coffee and meat, and ate fruit, vegetables and cereals (the word 'muesli' was adopted into the English language at this time). The popularity of 'health foods' (such as 'Hovis' wholemeal bread) and vegetarianism grew from the mid-nineteenth century to become a mass movement in Germany and surrounding states by 1900, although it was much less popular in Britain. The quest for a healthy diet was closely linked with other movements – such as unorthodox medicine and feminism, whose supporters argued that overly elaborate diets tied women to the kitchen (Meyer-Renschhausen and Wirz, 1999). Even ordinary foodstuffs were marketed for their health-giving properties (Figure 13.2).

Exercise and fresh air, two more building blocks for good health, would appear to be open to all. However, only the upper and middle classes had the cash and the leisure time to participate in the craze for healthy exercise which began in the late

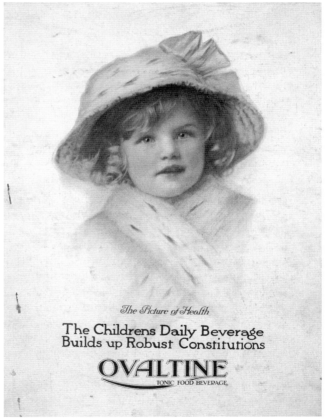

The Picture of Health

The Childrens Daily Beverage
Builds up Robust Constitutions

OVALTINE
TONIC FOOD BEVERAGE

Figure 13.2 In this advertisement, the image, caption and description of Ovaltine, a proprietary brand of malted milk drink, clearly link food with health. The appeal here is to a mother's desire to build up her children's health and strength; the message would have been a poignant one at a time before immunization, when many children died from infectious diseases. Other advertisements stressed the benefits for adults, promising that a cup of Ovaltine at bedtime would ward off 'night starvation'. Wellcome Library, London

nineteenth century. They could afford to buy bicycles, tennis rackets and golf clubs. They could also, following the German example, go rambling and hiking in the countryside, and pay to attend gymnastic exercise classes. Exercise was clearly gendered. Men and boys took part in team games (such as rugby, football and cricket), athletics and German gymnastics, which made use of apparatus such as vaulting-horses and parallel bars. Such activities were thought to develop a competitive spirit and build strong muscles, desirable qualities in the next generation of workers and soldiers. Women, too, were encouraged to exercise – not to build muscles, which were regarded as undesirable in the female sex, but to cultivate health. For women, exercise was thought to prevent curvature of the spine, chlorosis (a mysterious complaint, whose main symptoms were tiredness and a pale complexion) and hysteria, and a strong, fit body was thought to guarantee easy births and healthy offspring. Cycling, tennis, golf, team games requiring skill rather than strength (such as hockey) and Swedish gymnastics, which involved stretching the body with the aim of developing flexibility and coordination, were seen as beneficial forms of female exercise (Fletcher, 1984, pp.1–55; Stewart, 2001, pp.151–72).

Good hygiene – a clean home and a clean body – would also appear to have been available to all classes, but again, it was easier for the wealthier classes to achieve these goals. Newer houses, with bathrooms and laundries, modern plumbing and sanitary facilities, and servants to do the hard work, ensured that the middle and upper classes could enjoy regular baths (hot and cold), clean clothes and clean homes.

Exercise and good personal hygiene were not just a means of protecting health but were also pursued for aesthetic reasons. Women, for example, took exercise to promote grace and suppleness, and bathing was presented as a way for them to pamper themselves with scented soaps and oils, not just to get clean (Stewart, 2001, pp.65–72). The *Ladies Diary and Housekeeper* for 1917 provided beauty hints, allegedly written by 'an eminent MD', who suggested that 'a cheerful disposition' would prevent wrinkles and gave a recipe for a cream to soothe the blistered hands of overenthusiastic sportswomen. A revolution in women's clothing came about through a similar mixture of aesthetics and concerns about health. By the 1900s, tightly laced corsets were seen as a hazard to health, squashing women's internal organs (thus threatening the health of future babies) and preventing them from inhaling health-giving fresh air. Very long skirts also prevented women from taking exercise. Despite objections from some men, who found women wearing culottes or bloomers 'manly' and rather disgusting, women increasingly wore lighter clothing with shorter skirts and flexible stays and brassieres. By the 1920s, short tennis dresses were even considered to be chic (Stewart, 2001, pp.72–4, 169). At this time, men's clothing also became lighter (Figure 13.3).

However, for a large proportion of the population, altering diet, clothing or behaviour in the pursuit of better health was well nigh impossible. The working classes, who made up the vast majority of the population, survived on tight budgets. In 1913, the typical workers' wage of £1 per week just covered the essentials of food and rent, and left limited opportunities to follow a healthier

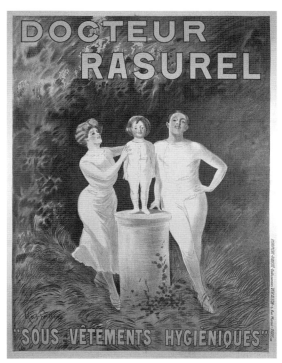

Figure 13.3   Advertisement for Dr Rasurel's hygienic underclothing, 1906. Note the associations between the clothes being advertised and health. The reader is assured that the clothes are 'hygienic'; they carry the name of a doctor, and the family pose surrounded by green plants, presumably in the open air. Rural settings were always seen as being more healthy than the urban environment. Wellcome Library, London

lifestyle (Pember Reeves, 1913). The staples of the working-class diet were white bread, margarine and tea. These cheap foods filled up hungry stomachs, but did not provide a balanced diet (Burnett, 1979, pp.182–212). In 1901, one-quarter of the population were not getting enough to eat: as late as the 1930s, research showed that half the British population were eating a diet deficient in some vitamins and minerals (Burnett, 1979, pp.245, 301–19). Just as members of the poorer classes found it difficult to afford a good diet, they also lacked the money, time, equipment and transport, never mind the energy after a long day at work, to take exercise. Personal hygiene too was difficult to achieve. Many working-class women struggled to keep their homes clean, but the poor condition of their houses, the lack of a bathroom and often hot water, and shared laundry facilities meant that the poor were inevitably dirtier than the middle classes. Doctors and midwives going into poor homes sometimes complained of the smell of their patients.

By the beginning of the twentieth century, for the first time governments and charities stepped in to try to improve the diet, exercise and hygiene of the poorest sections of society. While organizations all over Europe shared the goal of guaranteeing the physical health of the nation, the level of provision varied between different countries, reflecting national political agendas.

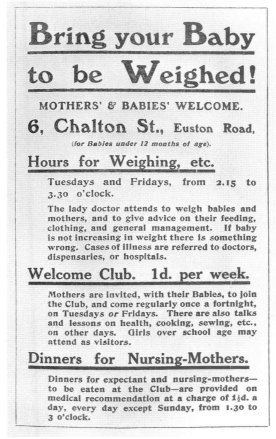

Figure 13.4   Leaflet advertising the new Mother's and Babies' Welcome in St Pancras, London, 1907. A charity, founded in 1907, the St Pancras Welcome offered a comprehensive range of services to mothers and babies. These were not free, but available for a small fee. Wellcome Library, London

As you read in Chapter 9, the health of mothers and infants was one target for action. France was among the first to introduce infant welfare schemes, as low birth rates, high infant mortality and defeat in the Franco-Prussian War led politicians to fear for the future strength of the nation. Diarrhoea among bottle-fed babies was singled out as a preventable cause of high infant mortality. From the 1890s, charities and local authorities set up infant welfare clinics called *gouttes de lait*, which encouraged mothers to breastfeed, gave out free milk to those that could not, and provided free regular medical examinations to check on babies' development. Charities also provided free meals to pregnant women and the mothers of small children. To improve the health of older children, municipal authorities set up school canteens to provide free and subsidized meals. These schemes proved very popular: in Paris in 1901, over 1,400 babies were brought to clinics: in some towns, up to one-third of all mothers and infants attended. Government bodies in Britain looked to France as a model of good practice, but did not simply copy French child welfare programmes, fearing that to provide food would usurp the role of the family breadwinner and overstep the proper limits of action. Hence, the few 'milk banks' set up in Britain around 1900 offered subsidized rather than free milk. Instead, charities focused their efforts on education. Lectures and demonstrations on 'mothercraft' were offered at welfare centres (Figure 13.4). In Britain, efforts to provide free school meals for older children were hindered by the same reluctance to interfere in family life. Even after they were given powers to provide school meals in 1906, many local authorities were reluctant to do so and, by 1912, only around one-third of local authorities provided school meals (Dwork, 1987, pp.93–166, 167–84).

Historians are divided over the impact of such policies. Some have argued that the authorities in Britain chose to provide education, rather than food, as a cheap but ineffective solution to the problem of child poverty. They have portrayed education in 'mothercraft' as patronizing and often impractical. Other researchers, such as Deborah Dwork, are more sympathetic, arguing that, given the government's reluctance to interfere in the family, education was a practical and effective way of helping mothers, and one which the mothers themselves appear to have found useful (Figure 13.5).

Governments also provided working-class children with access to physical exercise (PE) through school. Again, wider politics dictated the level of provision. By the 1930s, schoolchildren in Germany, Czechoslovakia, Russia and Italy were taught games, drill and gymnastic exercises. These facilities were much admired by British government ministers (although they did not approve of the regimes that funded them), who attempted to establish PE as a regular part of the school curriculum. Exercise was presented as a cheap form of preventive medicine, which would help to prevent 'flat-feet, curvature of the spine, adenoids, deafness, "mental deficiency" and respiratory problems' (quoted in Welshman, 1996, p.34). However, in Britain, local authorities were again slow to act, and provision of PE was patchy in the state school system. Hampered by a lack of trained instructors, and the fact that many children could not afford appropriate clothing and shoes, the periods of exercise were shorter and less frequent than those provided in private schools.

As you read in Chapter 7, education in hygiene was provided by both charities and local government. In Salford, before the First World War:

> The Ladies' Health Society worked bravely among us ... Together with the 'Sanitary Society', they visited the 'lowest classes' and found 'much that is saddening: but there are bright spots – clean homes, pretty little sitting-room kitchens ... clean hearths, chests of highly polished mahogany drawers, a steady husband, a tidy wife and children' ... The Society also sold ten hundredweights of carbolic soap and distributed six hundred-weights of carbolic powder [disinfectant] ... The corporation lent out its whitewash brushes, distributed free, bags of lime and bottles of a preventive medicine popularly known as 'diarrhoea mixture', and urged hygiene on all the populace.
>
> (Roberts, 1971, pp.57–8)

A is Advice, which is given you free ;
B is for Babies, one, two and three.
C is the Centre in Molesey we've made ;
D our good Doctor who lends us his aid.
E stands for Economy, taught to us there,
F is the Future for which we prepare.
G is for Glaxo, fine babies it builds ;
H is for Hygiene, which saves Doctor's bills.
I is for Ideal,—and Infants too,
J is the Joy they bring to you.
K stands for Kiddies, the big and the small.
L is the Love we have for them all.
M stands for Mothers, who all come to see ;
N, our Nurse Barnes, on every Friday.

O is for Ovaltine, a splendid food ;
P stands for Powders, which sometimes do good.
Q are the Questions we all like to ask,
      To answer them all Nurse has quite a task.
R stands for Rules, which must be obeyed ;
S stands for Scales on which we are weighed.
T is for Tea, at 1d. a cup,
U stands for Us, who all drink it up.
V is for Virol, it will make you grow strong, and
W, your Weight will go up before long.
X is our 'Xcellent audience here ;
Y is for Year—come again please, next year.
Z is the Zeal, which is shown by each helper
At the E. & W. Molesey Infant Welfare Centre.

Figure 13.5   Infant Welfare Centre ABC, East and West Molesey Infant Welfare Centre, c.1930. Documents such as this have prompted historians to view the education provided by Infant Welfare Centres as patronizing. Here, mothers are taught in the same way as infants, by learning an 'ABC'. Alternatively, the 'ABC' can be seen as a light-hearted celebration of the work of the centre, presented in a simple and appealing manner. Wellcome Library, London

Children were taught basic hygiene – about the need to bath weekly, to wash their hands and faces daily, and to scrub their fingernails – as part of the school curriculum. Girls (but not boys) were taught about healthy clothing – garments should be loose, warm and frequently washed.

These campaigns are described in more depth in Chapter 9.

However, the poor were not the only targets of health education. Campaigns against tuberculosis and venereal disease were aimed at all classes. Advice was dispensed through exhibitions, lectures, classes, posters, radio talks and films. Tuberculosis, the public was told, was best combated by a generally healthy lifestyle – fresh air, exercise and hygiene. The 1939 film *Stand Up and Breathe*, made by the National Association for the Prevention of Tuberculosis (NAPT), promoted all sorts of outdoor recreation as a means of guaranteeing health. Venereal disease could be avoided by restricting sexual activity. Campaigns sought to inform the public of the dire effects of VD – some exhibitions included graphic wax models of syphilitic lesions – in the hope that people would refrain from sex outside marriage, or, if they became infected, that they would come forward for treatment. In this educational material, 'loose' women were often portrayed as the source of infection, trapping vulnerable men (Figure 13.6). Innocent wives were the ultimate victims of VD. Infected by philandering husbands, they had sick or stillborn children (Davidson and Hall, 2001).

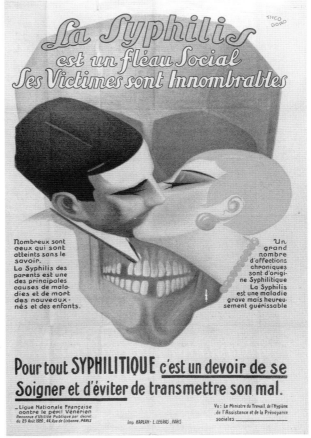

Figure 13.6   Poster warning of the dangers of syphilis, c.1930. The text reads: 'Syphilis is a social scourge. Its victims are innumerable. Many suffer from it without knowing. Syphilis among parents is one of the main causes of sickness and death among newborn children and infants. A great number of chronic infections originate in syphilis. Syphilis is a serious disease, but fortunately curable. For those infected it is a duty to obtain treatment and to avoid transmitting the disease.' Notice the image of a glamorous woman, with fashionable haircut, makeup and jewellery, set against the less detailed image of the man. Women who had sex outside marriage – often pejoratively called 'amateur prostitutes' or 'problem girls' – were frequently blamed for infecting men with syphilis. Wellcome Library, London

13.4   Domestic care

Despite their best efforts, everyone fell ill at some point in their lives. Although historians of medicine write a great deal about how the sick were cared for by doctors and in hospitals, in the past (as nowadays) minor complaints were diagnosed and treated at home, almost entirely without the help of medical professionals, using special diets and home-made or bought-in remedies. As with preserving health, poor families had relatively few resources for treatment. They might seek advice from neighbours or friends, or perhaps a health visitor. Those prevalent joint and respiratory ailments described earlier might respond to simple forms of treatment. Linseed or onion poultices were used to treat boils or painful joints, and hot footbaths were given as a remedy for colds. These would have been within the resources of all but the very poorest. In rural areas, ancient magical remedies, such as using snails to treat warts, persisted well into the twentieth century. Poor families might also be able to produce some simple foods aimed at helping a sick member feel better – for example, gruel, soup or egg dishes.

Better-off members of society were able to adopt more elaborate forms of domestic treatment. Medical practitioners had an indirect input into their home care through advice given in books on nursing and even diaries. The *Ladies Diary and Housekeeper* (1917) contained useful notes for emergencies in alphabetical order, from 'Abdomen' to 'Wounds', including what to do in cases of strangulation and how to tell if someone was dead. In cases of hysteria, the *Ladies Diary* recommended not sympathizing with the patient, but throwing cold water in her [*sic*] face, then administering an anti-spasmodic draught. (Perhaps life in the Edwardian home was not as quiet as we think!) Middle-class households had more resources with which to prepare home-made remedies. For example, a well-stocked larder was a prerequisite for making the cough mixture consisting of melted butter, black treacle and lemon, which was recommended in *Everywoman a Nurse* (1927). The middle and upper classes could also afford to treat illnesses using special diets. Nursing manuals published between the 1890s and the 1920s provided recipes for dishes to tempt the invalid's appetite and aid recovery, including beef tea (a broth made by boiling meat in water), rice pudding and egg dishes. Brandy was given as a stimulant to the very sick. Tonic wines, fortified with quinine or iron, and red wine (perhaps because of its colour) were reputed to strengthen the blood. By the end of the century, families could purchase patent invalid foods. Cod liver oil, now given as a source of vitamin D, was recommended as a rich food which helped patients to gain weight.

All classes purchased medicines to deal with illness within the family. These medicines were self-prescribed, and were often seen as a cheap alternative to paying for a doctor's services. Despite practitioners' bitter complaints that such medicines could do little good, and might even be harmful, the market in over-the-counter medicines boomed. In the mid-nineteenth century, the British population spent about £500,000 per year on patent medicines – by 1914, this sum had increased ten-fold (Digby, 1999, p.228). Drugs and medicines were readily available – they were sold by retail chemists (Boots the Chemist thrived in this period, building up a chain of shops), grocers, corner shops and even by mail order, and were heavily advertised in newspapers and periodicals. Over-the-counter remedies ranged from the innocuous to the extremely potent. Thomas Beecham (after whom Beecham's Powders are named) began his career selling a preparation based on aloes, ginger and soap. At the same time, chemists sold morphine preparations, and new chemical drugs such as sulphonal (a sleeping drug). As well as medicines based on orthodox medicine, homeopathic and herbal remedies were also freely available.

Medicines were marketed to reach all classes. Hoechst, one of the largest German pharmaceutical firms, was not above selling exactly the same pain-relieving drug under four different names and at four different prices. The following reading is an extract from Robert Roberts's book *The Classic Slum*, which gives a picture of the trade in patent remedies in a corner shop in the 1900s.

Exercise

Read 'Self-medication' (Source Book 2, Reading 13.1). Who buys these proprietary medicines and what conditions do they hope to treat with them? What is the author's view of the effectiveness of these remedies? How does it compare with that of the purchasers?

Discussion

Roberts's account describes a flourishing trade in patent medicines. Everyone seems to buy remedies – even the very poor, who can buy a few pills for a halfpenny – and to take them frequently. Medicines were taken routinely, to counter constipation and as tonics to strengthen the body, as well as to treat illnesses. The remedies claimed to treat a huge range of complaints, often associated with a particular organ and rather vague symptoms (such as 'premature decay'). However, Roberts suggests that constipation related to the starchy diet is the most common reason for buying them.

Roberts is clearly sceptical of the effects of many of these remedies and he claims that some were clearly detrimental, such as the tooth whitener. Some are all too effective – like the 'knock-out drops' given to babies – but are given for the wrong reasons. Despite Roberts's scepticism, the purchasers clearly have great faith in these nostrums, since they keep returning to buy more. They also make careful judgements between them – though Roberts claims that the efficacy of a medicine was less of a selling point than its colour, texture and packaging. In his comments about 'Therapion', and the fact that many of these patent medicines included some sort of laxative, Roberts hints at a reason for the popularity of these patent medicines – they made the purchaser feel better.

13.5 Calling in help

When people did seek help for their ailments, most sought some form of outpatient care. For the upper and middle classes, during much of the nineteenth century, this meant calling in a general practitioner. The poorest could apply for help at the outpatient department of a charitable hospital or dispensary. Another source of help was to apply for assistance from local government – in some countries the local authorities employed doctors to care for the poor. In Britain, medical help was available through the Poor Law – the body responsible for all aspects of welfare. There was what historians call a 'mixed economy of care' – patients could either pay for the services of practitioners, or apply for free care from charities or local government agencies. The end of the nineteenth and beginning of the twentieth centuries saw a huge expansion in the availability of outpatient services – both through these existing outlets and through new facilities. The result was a patchwork of services, where the same care was available from numerous outlets, leading administrators to worry about inefficiencies and the over-provision of medical services.

General practitioners

General practitioners were the backbone of medical services. They dealt with almost every sort of complaint, from the serious to the trivial. Although it is often assumed that previous generations were prepared to put up with discomfort, in 1876, an anonymous correspondent to a friendly society magazine complained that 'one of the most distinctive traits of this generation is its almost fidgety care about its health' (quoted in Riley, 1997, p.199). Working men went to the doctor with minor injuries, colds and headaches. One Yorkshire doctor recorded treating a patient for indigestion, toothache, hoarseness and hair loss (Riley, 1997, pp.199–200). At the other end of the scale, GPs delivered babies in patients' homes, even applying anaesthetics and using forceps to speed the delivery. In rural areas, they performed major surgery. Harry Pearson Taylor, a GP on the Shetland Isles, recalled amputating a boy's arm after it had been crushed in a threshing machine. With the minister of the local church, he

> improvised an operation table, and got the little man on it. I disinfected the area as well as I could under the circumstances, and got all I wanted ready. I chloroformed the boy, and the Minister kept him under while I disarticulated the elbow joint. The Minister, who ... knew quite a lot about medicine and surgery, had put a tourniquet on the upper arm. The weather remained so bad for several days that I was storm stayed in the island, which gave me an opportunity to attend to the patient myself. Of course there were no nurses in those far back days, and had I been able to get back to Yell [his home island], the Minister would have had to undertake the duties of a nurse.

(Taylor, 1948, p.76)

Despite the primitive conditions of his treatment, the child made a full recovery. However, the bulk of a general practitioner's work was more mundane. GPs prescribed medicines for a range of illnesses, treated injuries and local infections, lanced boils and syringed ears.

Middle- and upper-class patients paid directly for care from general practitioners, but they did not all pay the same fees. GPs charged according to the patient's income. In 1917, the *Ladies Diary and Housekeeper* provided a table of charges, based on the rental value of homes, suggesting that GPs would charge from 2s 6d to 10s 6d for a visit, and from 1 to 5 guineas for a midwifery case. By the early twentieth century, some medical practitioners built successful practices among the upper working classes, by lowering their fees to as little as 1s or even 6d – a price that put their services within reach of many working-class patients (Digby, 1999, pp.100–3).

In the late nineteenth century, working-class men began to obtain access to general practitioners through insurance schemes. In Britain, these schemes were run by friendly societies or sick clubs (Figure 13.7), in France, they were called *sociétés de secours mutuels* (mutual aid societies) and in Germany, *Krankenkassen* (literally a 'sick box'). All worked on the same principle: for a small weekly payment, workers were entitled to financial help when ill, and had access to treatment from the society's doctor. A substantial portion of the male working population had

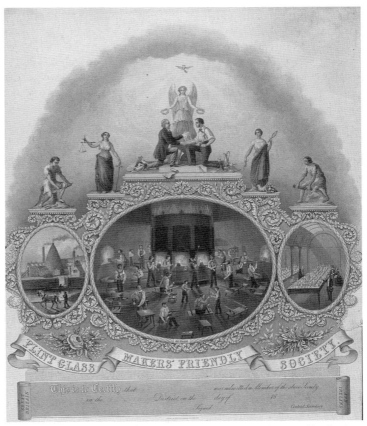

Figure 13.7   Membership certificate of Flint Glass Makers' Friendly Society, nineteenth century. This elaborate certificate exemplifies the virtues aspired to by members of the Flint Glass Makers' Friendly Society. The main vignettes show scenes of glass processing – the common occupation of members. The female allegorical figures represent industry (with her spindle) and justice (with the scales and sword). Wellcome Library, London

some form of insurance cover. In Britain, friendly society membership peaked in 1900, when around half of the entire adult male population was insured. In France in 1902, over two million people belonged to some form of insurance scheme (Mitchell, 1991, p.181). However, working women and the families of workers were often excluded from many of these schemes, and thus were less likely to go to a GP. In the twentieth century, state health insurance schemes gradually replaced the direct provision of medical care to the poor. As you read in Chapter 9, health insurance was set up in Germany in 1883, and in Britain in 1911 under the National Health Insurance Act. These schemes, which initially covered only the poorest workers, operated in the same way as private insurance, except that the workers' contributions were augmented by contributions from his employer and the state.

The combination of low fees and private and state health insurance produced a huge expansion in the number of patients who consulted a general practitioner. In Britain, the number of GPs doubled between 1860 and 1914, while the number of patients attending each practitioner remained roughly constant (Hardy, 2001, p.17). However, not everyone was equally well provided with care. Even in the twentieth century, patients in remote Scottish islands faced a journey of several hours to consult a doctor. The situation was much worse in the eastern regions of Russia, where in 1913 the ratio of licensed practitioners to population was less than 1 in 10,000 (Hyde, 1974, p.18).

While more people gained access to GP services in the first decades of the century, not everyone received the same quality of treatment. Patients who paid a higher fee received a better quality of care. General practitioners would call on wealthier patients in their homes, discuss the case, and offer advice as well as therapy (Figure 13.8). Better-off patients were more likely to receive a thorough physical examination, using diagnostic instruments. They were also more likely to have specimens sent for laboratory tests, and to receive new treatments, such as vaccine therapy or insulin for diabetes (described in Chapter 4). They also benefited from referral to specialists for further diagnosis or treatment (Digby, 1999, p.200).

Well-off patients could afford to employ several practitioners if they were unhappy with the treatment offered by their original doctor. However, this was a mixed blessing, if the doctors disagreed. For example, when Sir Leslie Stephen fell ill in 1902, he was initially attended by the family practitioner, Dr Seton. The family then called in Sir Frederick Treves, a distinguished surgeon, to give another opinion. Seton thought Sir Leslie was improving, Treves thought that he was seriously ill and required an operation. The family accepted Seton's view, and he remained in charge of the case until the autumn of 1903, when another surgeon, Hugh Rigby, was called in. He brought in a GP (Dr Wilson) to visit every day. The efforts of all these medical men had little effect – Sir Leslie died in February 1904 (Trombley, 1981, pp.77–80).

Patients paying the lowest fees or receiving care through an insurance scheme received a much more basic consultation. In the next reading, Anne Digby examines state-funded care provided through the National Health Insurance Act of 1911.

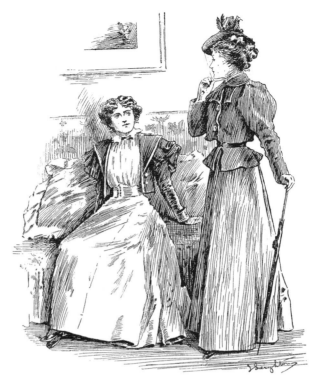

Figure 13.8   In this cartoon, the two well-dressed ladies share the following exchange: "'Isn't it tiresome! I've just got a lovely new bicycle, and now my doctor absolutely forbids me to cycle! What would you advise me to do?" "Change your doctor."' The cartoon neatly captures the new craze for bicycling among women at the end of the nineteenth century – a fashionable pursuit, as well as a means of getting healthy exercise. It also reveals something of the upper-class attitude towards doctors – they are there to serve, and can be dismissed if the patient disagrees with the practitioner's opinion. From *Punch*, 29 January 1898, p.45

Exercise

Read 'Services under the National Health Insurance Act' (Source Book 2, Reading 13.2). In her view, did the National Health Insurance scheme provide good-quality care to all? Were both patients and doctors satisfied with the quality of the service?

Discussion

Digby makes clear that 'panel' patients received a lower-quality service in virtually every aspect of care than did private patients – including the surgery accommodation, the range of medicines prescribed, the length of consultation and the quality of the dressings. However, patients seemed happy with the service – relatively few of them changed their doctor or complained about the care they received. Digby suggests, however, that this may have been because they had low expectations of a service that they saw as similar to that provided by earlier sick clubs. Despite the long hours and heavy workload, doctors also seemed reasonably happy working under the National Health Insurance scheme, which provided them with a guaranteed income. However, she also notes instances of doctors not accepting that panel patients should receive poor care: for example, some were accused of 'over-prescribing' (i.e. not conforming to the expected standard of prescribing) and others complained about the use of poorer-quality bandages for their panel patients.

Digby's account may give the impression that patients were powerless in the face of a form of rationing of care, imposed by government and the medical profession. In fact, they exerted control over how they used the National Health Insurance system. Some commentators complained that patients abused the system by going to see their doctor for no good reason (Figure 13.9). Although doctors might appear to be 'fobbing off' their patients with stock medicines, in fact practitioners complained that patients expected to leave the surgery with a bottle of medicine (most drugs were dispensed in liquid rather than tablet form in this period). They

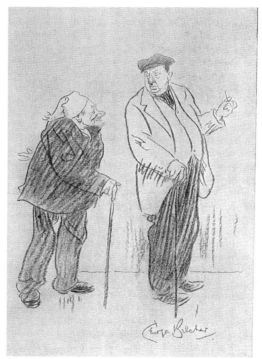

Figure 13.9   While contemporary commentators (as well as historians) expressed concern about the poor standards of care provided by panel doctors under the National Health Insurance scheme, patients were criticized for overusing the service. The caption to this cartoon, entitled *A Cheap Diversion*, reads: "'Let's go to the music-hall?" "Naw." "Let's go to the sinnemer, then?" "Naw." "Well, come on, let's go and see my panel doctor?" "Right-o.'" From *Punch*, 1913, p.46. Wellcome Library, London

were therefore forced to act in response to patient demand. Some of these frequently prescribed medicines had little pretensions to do any good. Elsewhere in her book, Digby reports that one doctor handed out coloured aspirins. In another practice, one of the stock medicines 'was labelled "Mist. ADT" or "Mist. Any Damn Thing" ['Mist.' is an abbreviation of the Latin word for 'mixture'] which was given to "somebody you thought there was nothing wrong with, and you could do nothing for"' (Digby, 1999, p.198). More alarmingly, another practitioner

> prescribed a mixture ... called Mist. Explo. It was a clear yellow liquid made from a few bright yellow crystals dissolved in water. The crystals were apt to ignite if left to dry in the sunlight, hence the name Mist Explosive. I don't remember the exact chemistry of this wonder drug but it was a derivative of picric acid and quite harmless when well diluted and used as a bitter tonic.
>
> (Porter, 1999, p.196)

Such medicines seem little different to patent medicines, which doctors so frequently condemned.

Irregular and unorthodox practitioners

In the twentieth century, unlicensed practitioners continued to be an important source of medical advice. Faced with illness, people of all classes consulted relatives, neighbours with a reputation for curing or the local retail chemist – who had no medical training but a wide knowledge of therapies. Substantial numbers of patients from all classes chose to consult unorthodox practitioners who offered 'natural' forms of healing. Herbal medicine remained popular among working-class patients, and flourished in the industrial north and midlands of England. There were perhaps 2,000 herbalists practising before the First World War, and many more working part-time (Brown, 1985). By contrast, homeopathy declined in popularity in Britain and over much of Europe (with the exception of Germany and Holland). In 1874, there were around 300 practitioners in Britain; by 1909, there were 196 (Nicholls, 1988, p.182). The decline of homeopathy did not herald any general slide in the popularity of unorthodox medicine. The early twentieth century saw the rise of Christian Science – a sect founded in 1879, whose followers rejected orthodox medical treatment in favour of mental and spiritual healing – and of osteopathy – a system of treatment devised in 1874, which was based on manipulating the joints.

Clinics and outpatient services

In addition to acquiring greater access to general practitioners in the late nineteenth and early twentieth centuries, poor patients also received more medical help from the outpatient departments of charitable hospitals and dispensaries. As you read in Chapter 2, hospital outpatient departments were an increasingly popular source of care: between 1860 and 1900, the number of patients attending the outpatient department of the London Hospital increased from 25,000 to 220,000. By 1910, there were 1.75 million attendances each year at outpatient and casualty departments across London, and provincial hospitals experienced similar levels of demand. Consequently, huge queues regularly built up, and patients had to wait for up to six hours to see a doctor. In an effort to reduce demand, some hospitals introduced a small charge for repeat consultations unless patients could prove they were unable to pay. Treatment was similar to that in a GP's surgery – a rapid examination and a routine prescription, although some patients were referred to specialist departments or admitted to the hospital as inpatients.

Charitable dispensaries, funded by wealthy donors, were an important source of care for working-class patients in the nineteenth century right across Europe – they were founded even in Russia, where there was no strong tradition of medical charity. At the end of the nineteenth century, the charitable institutions inspired the creation of provident dispensaries, which operated as a form of health insurance. In return for a small weekly subscription (one Northampton dispensary charged 1d for adults and 2d for families), members received basic medical treatment at the dispensary's premises. The work of these dispensaries has received little attention from historians. The York Dispensary is the subject of one of the few detailed studies, and, if it is typical, then dispensaries were lively institutions, responsive to a wide range of medical needs within the community. Founded in 1788, the York Dispensary quickly became an important source of medical care: in the 1880s, around 5,000 patients – roughly 10 per cent of the city's population – called there each year. Attendance at the dispensary peaked in 1903–4, when 9,000 patients used it, but fell after the introduction of National Health Insurance. However, the numbers of women, children and the elderly – all uninsured under NHI – increased after 1913. As well as providing consultations with a general practitioner, the dispensary had a dental service, and an inpatient and outpatient maternity service. It also played a role in dealing with outbreaks of epidemic disease (Webb, 1988).

Around this time, other specialized dispensaries and clinics, dealing with specific diseases or particular groups of the population, opened their doors. Tuberculosis dispensaries were established by charities and local government as part of the campaign to control the disease. By 1938, there were 482 TB dispensaries in Britain, dealing with over 100,000 cases per year. In them, patients received physical examinations to check the condition of their lungs. They were given advice on diet and lifestyle to help combat the infection, and on how to avoid spreading the disease. Treatment was limited to cough mixtures and cod liver oil, which was supposed to strengthen the body and help increase weight. VD clinics providing free and confidential treatment to everyone were opened as a means of controlling the spread of infection. However, they were not attractive places – many clinics were poorly funded and rather forbidding. Clinics provided as part of the School Medical Service were more popular. Children in poorer families had little access to medical care, which their parents were unable to afford – unless a child was very ill, the parents were unlikely to call on the services of a GP. Not surprisingly, when local authorities were given powers to institute medical inspections of schoolchildren in 1906, they found many untreated complaints. '[I]nspection showed whole classes of children infested with head vermin; many had body lice. The worst would sit isolated in a small sanitary cordon of humiliation. They would later be kept at home, their heads shaven, reeking of some rubbed-in disinfectant' (Roberts, 1971, p.58). The First World War gave a new impetus to the School Medical Service: faced with the massive death toll on the battlefields, one commentator explained, 'it behoves us to see that the rising generation is reared amid healthy surroundings and sent forth into the world under the best possible conditions' (quoted in Webster, 1983, p.73). Local authorities began to open clinics to treat common minor complaints. By 1920, there were 288 clinics in England and Wales, dealing with head lice, ringworm and orthopaedic conditions, providing dental inspections, free spectacles and (through local hospitals) the removal of tonsils and adenoids (enlarged lymphatic tissue between the nose and the throat, which can interfere with breathing) (Hirst, 1989, pp.327–42; Webster, 1983, pp.71–6).

Nurses, district nurses and midwives

While access to GPs and outpatient services was growing, access to nursing care was expanding in some sectors and declining in others. The numbers of trained professional nurses who were employed in wealthy households to care for seriously ill family members fell in the first decades of the twentieth century. These nurses stayed in the patient's home, carrying out the doctor's instructions, monitoring the patient's condition and providing general care – making beds, bathing the patient, giving medicines and keeping the sickroom in good order. The role of the private nurse was not an easy one: she had an ambiguous social position – above domestic servants but below family members. The ideal private nurse, according to one textbook, should possess 'average intelligence' but 'more than the average amount of tact' (Wightman, 1912, p.10). Private nursing slowly died out after 1918, at the same time as did the live-in domestic servant. By this time, few households had enough room to accommodate a live-in nurse, and patients wealthy enough to afford a private nurse could get the same services in a nursing home (discussed below).

At the same time, poor patients were enjoying increasing provision of nursing care. The late nineteenth century saw the creation of new charities to provide the sick poor with nursing care in the home. Some of these organizations were secular, but a substantial proportion were religious, with care provided by orders of nursing sisters. These nurses paid short visits to their patients, caring for the sick, giving advice and sometimes helping with housework. From these fragmented charities, a coordinated district nursing service developed in Britain, which remained part of the voluntary sector until the 1950s. The backbone of the service was the Queen Victoria Jubilee Institute for Nursing the Poor in their Own Homes founded in 1889. In 1896, it had 539 nurses across the country: by 1914, there were over 2,000 Queen's Nurses. Existing nursing charities became affiliated to the institute, which provided six-month training courses for 'village nurses' who worked in rural areas (Dingwall *et al.*, 1988, pp.173–97).

In response to public demand, district nurses increasingly took on midwifery work, especially in rural areas. The demand for their services was in part driven by the increasing regulation of midwifery, and a reduction in the number of women working as midwives. From the early twentieth century, midwives attended the majority of births. Most were paid directly by their clients, and, as with other medical services, the better-off were able to afford practitioners who were better trained. Respectable working-class women would save up to employ a trained midwife to deliver their babies. The poorest women employed untrained midwives, often called handywomen, who charged lower fees and stayed on after the birth to help look after the household (Llewelyn Davies, [1915] 1978). However, in the early twentieth century, these untrained midwives were gradually pushed out of practice by the registration of midwives and new regulations on training (Dingwall *et al.*, 1988, pp.145–72; Loudon, 1992, pp.172–92, 206–33).

13.6   Hospital care

In most aspects of medical care, the rich generally enjoyed better access to medical services and better-quality services than the poor. The only exception to this rule was hospital care. As you read in Chapter 2, in the nineteenth century the 'deserving' poor – whose respectability was guaranteed by the need for them to have a letter of admission from a subscriber or employer – could receive medical and surgical treatment in charitable hospitals. The very poor could obtain care through Poor Law hospitals, which in 1926 were transferred into the hands of local authorities. As the voluntary hospitals became associated with high-quality care, some commentators complained that the poor received far better hospital care than the rich. If a poor person needed to undergo an operation, he or she might be treated in the latest, most modern facilities in a teaching hospital. A rich client would have to go through the same procedure in his home, in a room rigorously scrubbed but lacking specialized equipment.

In the late nineteenth century, hospital facilities were gradually opened up to all classes. The upper and middle classes could receive treatment in private wards or in beds on general wards. These were not cheap: when Guy's Hospital accepted paying patients in 1884, they were charged 1 guinea per week for a ward bed and 3 guineas for a bed in a private cubicle. By 1902, private hospitals could charge as much as 4 guineas (Abel-Smith, 1964, pp.149, 194). Alternatively, wealthy patients could pay for care in private nursing homes, which began to appear in the 1890s. By 1921, there were 26,000 nursing-home beds in England and Wales. Convalescent hospitals also offered a comfortable environment in which to recover from illness – Thomas Cook, the holiday firm, even had a facility in Egypt (Abel-Smith, 1964, pp.133, 339).

Those patients who were unable to afford private care, but not so poor as to qualify for charity gained access to hospitals either by directly paying a contribution towards the cost of their care or through some form of insurance. The British Provident Association offered a 1-guinea policy which paid for up to three weeks in hospital. More often, workers paid into a 'Saturday fund' – these were schemes where, in return for a small, regular contribution, patients were ensured access to hospital facilities (Abel-Smith, 1964, pp.327–8, 338–9).

While hospitals were increasingly open to all classes, there were still serious geographical inequalities. Far more beds were available in London than in any other city, and there were more facilities in urban than in rural areas. From the 1860s, small cottage hospitals helped to fill this gap, providing care to all classes in rural areas. From the outset, cottage hospitals were funded partly by patients' contributions and partly by donations. They proved popular, and numbers grew rapidly: the first cottage hospital was founded in 1859, and by 1880 there were 180 such facilities. Most were small institutions – many had around twenty beds – staffed by local general practitioners. Although cottage hospitals could not boast the high standard of facilities of the voluntary hospitals, many had operating theatres where GPs or consultant surgeons performed quite complex surgery.

Not all hospitals offered equally good levels of care. The next reading gives a patient's view of being treated in two voluntary hospitals and a Poor Law hospital.

Exercise

Read 'Care in hospital' (Source Book 2, Reading 13.3). What differences does Bella Aronovitch note between the voluntary hospitals and the Poor Law hospital? How does she describe the attitude of staff towards her, and what does she think of them?

Discussion

Aronovitch notes several differences between the voluntary and Poor Law hospitals. Larger wards, fewer staff, the numbers of geriatric patients and the uniforms mark out the Poor Law hospital. However, there are many similarities. She describes all the hospitals as being highly ordered institutions, organized to suit the staff, not the patients – for example in the rules on visiting times. None of the staff make any efforts to ensure that patients are kept amused, and as a result the whole environment is very depressing.

According to Aronovitch, all the hospital staff maintain a rather supercilious attitude towards her. No one is willing to discuss her treatment, or the likely outcome of her case. Indeed, some even joke about her condition in her presence. The consultants have the most superior attitude. Perhaps the consultant in the first hospital, who shakes hands with his private patients, would have spent more time talking to them. A woman doctor she finds easy to talk to – but she clearly still joins in the professional 'conspiracy of silence'. Curiously, Aronovitch seems to accept the doctors' view that 'this is the way things are' and does not question their competence or complain about the ineffectiveness of the care she receives.

13.7 Conclusion: the medicalization of society?

All the evidence you have looked at so far suggests that historians are right to see a 'medicalization' of society in the sense that when ill, people were more likely to consult a qualified medical practitioner in 1930 than they had been in 1880. The extension of medical services – combined with the increase in chronic complaints – meant that working-class patients in particular had much greater contact with general practitioners, health visitors and nurses. However, it is also clear that there were continuing variations in the level of health-care provision. Not all social groups enjoyed the same access to medical services. Working men were the chief beneficiaries of insurance schemes, infants and children had their own clinics, but women remained poorly served. Poorer sections of society did not enjoy the same quality of services as the wealthier classes.

Did the greater availability of treatment bring greater power to medical practitioners? Did patients become powerless consumers of medical advice?

Before reading the rest of this conclusion, pause and review the material given in this chapter, and try to identify any evidence of doctors' power over their patients. Is there any evidence of patients exerting control when dealing with illness?

The material presented here suggests that patients did regard medical practitioners as authorities and respect their advice and instructions. People were eager to consult practitioners and were prepared to wait for a consultation and advice. Despite the complications of her case, Bella Aronovitch did not question the competence of her doctors. However, patients were by no means passive or dependent on doctors. They took responsibility for their own health and illness, dealing with bouts of minor illness within the home and buying tonics and pills in the face of doctors' disapproval. Even when seeking medical help, patients exercised considerable choice over where to obtain help; if their finances permitted, they could call on several doctors, or choose to go to unorthodox practitioners. They forced doctors to fulfil their demands for medicines – even if the medicines themselves were of limited therapeutic value. Patients were not in thrall to the medical profession – while recognizing and respecting the specialist knowledge of practitioners, they maintained forms of control over their health and their use of medical services.

There is also good evidence which suggests that the public took control over their own health by choosing not to seek medical help, or by rejecting offers of help and treatment (Figure 13.10).

The Women's Health Enquiry survey of working-class women of 1933 showed that a large proportion of working-class women suffered from chronic illnesses which went untreated (Spring Rice, 1981, pp.28–43). The next reading is an extract from this survey, published in 1939.

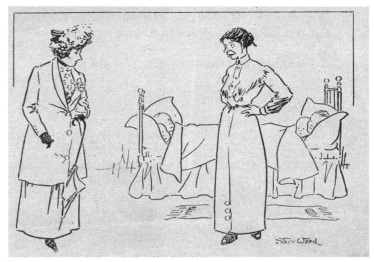

Figure 13.10   Not all visits from well-meaning charity workers were welcome. Lady-visitors who dispensed advice on child care were often portrayed as being nosy and interfering, and dispensing useless advice. In this cartoon, from the *London Mail*, 1915, the mother says to the district visitor: 'Lumme miss! There ain't no danger of infection. Them children wot's got the measles is at the 'ead of the bed, and them wot ain't is at the foot.' The working woman's comical response is presumably prompted by the visitor's advice to isolate the children suffering from measles – which was quite impossible in the small homes of the working classes. The cartoonist conveys the stereotyped character of the two women by their clothes. The middle-class visitor's fussy outfit of hat, gloves and umbrella contrasts with the plain and practical clothing worn by the mother. Wellcome Library, London

Read 'The health of working-class women' (Source Book 2, Reading 13.5). What reasons does the author give for the women not receiving treatment? In the light of this source, do we need to revise our idea that state intervention ensured health care for all sections of society?

The author suggests that while cost was the greatest barrier to health care, the women had many reasons for not seeking treatment: a 'disinclination to fuss' over themselves, greater concern with the health of their families, exhaustion, ignorance and prejudice. The women surveyed had a fear of any sort of operation – from minor dental work to major surgery.

The results of the Women's Health Enquiry survey showed that many women were not well served by government health care services – relatively few went to panel doctors or used clinics. The reading suggests that while ensuring that the population could afford medical advice and therapy was an important step towards ensuring health care for all, it was not the whole story. In order for the women in this survey to seek medical help, they also needed support in getting to the hospital or clinic and in looking after the home while they underwent treatment. Women also had to be cured of their fear of surgery.

Patients also rejected offers of care for venereal disease and tuberculosis. VD sufferers were reluctant to undergo the long and painful therapies used to treat syphilis and gonorrhoea, and often did not complete the courses of treatment. People infected with TB also refused opportunities for treatment, for fear of being stigmatized. There was a widespread fear of people with TB. Long after doctors realized that tuberculosis was infectious, many people continued to believe that the disease was hereditary, and would be passed on from parent to child. Patients were often unwilling to come forward for treatment or to follow the advice given, for fear of being identified as a 'lunger'. One patient wrote: 'It is depressing to find how frightened people are becoming of us. I am being turned out of my rooms, and this will make my fourth move in this particular town' (Bryder, 1988, p.223). People infected with TB were dismissed from their jobs, and even those who recovered from the disease found it very difficult to find employment.

Inpatient care in specialist sanatoria, with its emphasis on fresh air at all times and a rich diet (described in Chapter 9), was also unpopular. In the following reading, Linda Bryder describes patients' attitudes towards the strict sanatorium regime.

Exercise

Read 'Resistance to care – sanatorium treatment' (Source Book 2, Reading 13.4). Are the patients happy to accept the prescribed regime? How successful are the sanatoria staff in imposing strict discipline on their patients?

Discussion

Despite the gravity of their illness, the patients in TB sanatoria are not passive. They complain about the food, the spartan conditions and about having to sleep in the open air in bad weather (and not without good reason, it would seem!). They also fight against the rules and attempt to maintain normal patterns of life, by mixing with patients of the opposite sex and drinking. Ultimately, they reject the whole sanatorium experience by simply leaving – and Bryder's figures suggest that a very large proportion of patients did not go through the prescribed course of treatment.

Staff in the sanatoria are clearly keen to enforce the rules – they fight against complaints by trying to discredit the patient's judgement (although Bryder notes that the introduction of heating may have been a response to patients' discomfort). Their main sanction is to send patients home for breaking the rules. This may explain why staff are so dismissive of patients who discharge themselves – they are not only rejecting the care offered, but also subverting the main sanction used to enforce discipline.

Even patients in private sanatoria rebelled against the discipline. In 1909, Alice Clark, a young woman from a wealthy family with a history of TB, went to Nordrach-sur-Mendip, the oddly named English sanatorium modelled on a German institution. The regime there was particularly strict: patients had to conform to a rigid timetable, take their own temperatures four times a day and eat a prescribed diet. Alice Clark

> found Nordrach-sur-Mendip a ... cruel experience, for she was by now very sick and weak, complaining how bedroom windows were kept wide open at night even in subzero temperatures or during snowstorms, how she was required to empty her own chamber pot while in a high fever, and how she was forbidden to employ a nurse to attend to her. Separation from family and friends proved especially troubling to her. Within a few weeks she was writing that she felt she had been making better progress at home.
>
> (Holton, 1999, p.87)

Despite being allowed a sympathetic nurse (a fellow campaigner for votes for women), Clark left the sanatorium, and subsequently recovered.

Even when ill, then, patients maintained a degree of independence over whether to seek help, and whether to follow medical advice. They showed a similar response to education by health professionals, aimed at teaching them how to maintain a healthy lifestyle. This was not a new phenomenon. In the eighteenth century, physicians had written popular books on how to preserve health. However, the early twentieth century saw a huge expansion in the way this information was disseminated – through new media such as film and radio – and in the target audience. How well people absorbed these messages about healthy living is very hard to gauge. Books, exhibitions and health films were certainly very popular, attracting large audiences. A survey by the Women's Co-operative Movement found that working-class women wanted more sources of information, advice and support during pregnancy and when bringing up small children (Llewelyn Davies, 1978). Another survey of working-class women in the 1930s found that about half of the respondents had learned some skills though a welfare centre or clinic. A smaller number claimed to have received some education through a health visitor or district nurse. However, even if people were willing to listen to advice, this does not mean that they put it into practice. Some did – a few women practised the breathing exercises they learned in school into adult life (Spring Rice, 1981, pp.82–90).

One aspect of life which is often seen as having been 'medicalized' in the twentieth century is that of childbirth. Historians argue that until the nineteenth century, pregnancy and birth were dealt with within families, with minimal input from medical practitioners. By the late twentieth century, pregnancy was labelled as a form of illness by some practitioners, births took place in hospital and pregnant women, new mothers and their babies were subjected to constant supervision by medical personnel. What about the early twentieth century? Had birth come under the control of the medical profession by 1930?

The answer has to be that it had not. Although obstetrics and gynaecology emerged as specialist areas of medicine around this time, doctors and nurses did little to monitor the health of pregnant women – in part because there was little they could do to help women in the event of complications. Even after local authorities in England and Wales established antenatal clinics, many women attended only once or twice. The medical profession did exert some control over birth, as a consequence of a concern about persistently high levels of maternal mortality. Not surprisingly, practitioners chose to focus on clinical problems associated with birth, such as sepsis and haemorrhage, rather than on social factors, such as poor diet and long working hours, which were also associated with death in childbirth. Their chosen solution to these problems was to encourage women to give birth in hospital, in sterile conditions and with medical staff on hand. The proportion of births taking place in hospitals began to rise at this time – from 15 per cent in 1927 to 24 per cent in 1933. This shift towards hospital birth was not entirely due to pressure from medical practitioners. Women welcomed the prospect of giving birth in hospital under anaesthesia – which midwives working in the home were not permitted to offer – and grasped the opportunity to take a few days' rest away from domestic responsibilities after the birth. The three-quarters of all babies that were born at home were also brought under a degree of medical supervision. In the twentieth century, midwives were required to be registered and to have gone through a set training programme. They were required to call in a GP if there were complications, and were told to use aseptic techniques (although these were very difficult to achieve in poor households) (Lewis, 1980, pp.117–61; Loudon, 1992, pp.234–53).

Even in 1930, doctors had at best limited influence over pregnancy and childbirth. Their input would have varied between classes. A middle-class women, able to afford regular visits from a general practitioner, and to pay for childbirth in a hospital or nursing-home, would have been under regular, if not constant, medical supervision. A poor mother would have had little contact with medical services during pregnancy and would have called in a midwife to attend at the birth (Llewelyn Davies, 1978). Overall, then, early twentieth-century medical practitioners had greater influence over the sick and the healthy than had their nineteenth-century counterparts, but this influence was not all-pervasive, and nor did it go unchallenged.

References

Abel-Smith, B. (1964) *The Hospitals 1800–1948*, London: Heinemann.

Beddoe, D. (1989) *Back to Home and Duty: Women between the Wars 1918–1939*, London: Pandora.

Brown, P.S. (1985) 'The vicissitudes of herbalism in late nineteenth and early twentieth-century Britain', *Medical History*, vol.29, pp.71–92.

Bryder, L. (1988) *Below the Magic Mountain: A Social History of Tuberculosis in Twentieth-Century Britain*, Oxford: Clarendon Press.

Burnett, J. (1979) *Plenty and Want: A Social History of Diet in England from 1815 to the Present Day*, London: Scolar Press.

Davidson, R. and Hall, L.A. (eds) (2001) *Sex, Sin and Suffering: Venereal Disease and European Society since 1870*, London: Routledge.

Digby, A. (1999) *The Evolution of British General Practice 1850–1948*, Oxford: Oxford University Press.

Dingwall, R., Rafferty, A.M and Webster, C. (1988) *An Introduction to the Social History of Nursing*, London: Routledge.

Dwork, D. (1987) *War is Good for Babies and Other Young Children: A History of the Infant and Child Welfare Movement in England, 1898–1918*, London: Tavistock.

Fletcher, S. (1984) *Women First: The Female Tradition in English Physical Education, 1880–1980*, London: Athlone Press.

Goering, L. (2003) '"Russian nervousness": neurasthenia and national identity in nineteenth-century Russia', *Medical History*, vol.47, pp.23–46.

Hardy, A. (2001) *Health and Medicine in Britain since 1860*, Basingstoke: Palgrave.

Hirst, J.D. (1989) 'The growth of treatment through the School Medical Service', *Medical History*, vol.33, pp.318–42.

Holton, S.S. (1999) 'To live "through one's own powers": British medicine and "invalidism" in the life of Alice Clark (1874–1934)', *Journal of Women's History*, vol.11, pp.75–96.

Hyde, G. (1974) *The Soviet Health Service: A Historical and Comparative Study*, London: Lawrence and Wishart.

Lewis, J. (1980) *The Politics of Motherhood: Child and Maternal Welfare in England, 1900–1939*, London: Croom Helm.

Llewelyn Davies, M. [1915] (1978) *Maternity: Letters from Working-Women*, London: Virago.

Loudon, I. (1992) *Death in Childbirth: An International Study of Maternal Care and Maternal Mortality, 1800–1950*, Oxford: Clarendon Press.

Meyer-Renschhausen, E. and Wirz, A. (1999) 'Dietetics, health reform and social order: vegetarianism as a moral philosophy. The example of Maximilian Bircher-Benner', *Medical History*, vol.43, pp.323–41.

Mitchell, A. (1991) 'The function and malfunction of mutual aid societies in nineteenth century France' in J. Barry and C. Jones (eds) *Medicine and Charity before the Welfare State*, London: Routledge.

Nicholls, P.A. (1988) *Homeopathy and the Medical Profession*, London: Croom Helm.

Pember Reeves, M. (1913) *Round About a Pound a Week*, London: G. Bell.

Porter, R. (1999) *The Greatest Benefit to Mankind: A Medical History of Humanity from Antiquity to the Present*, London: Fontana.

Riley, J.C. (1989) *Sickness, Recovery, and Death: A History and Forecast of Ill Health*, Basingstoke: Macmillan.

Riley, J.C. (1997) *Sick, Not Dead: The Health of British Workingmen during the Mortality Decline*, Baltimore and London: Johns Hopkins University Press.

Roberts, R. (1971) *The Classic Slum: Salford Life in the First Quarter of the Century*, Manchester: Manchester University Press.

Spring Rice, M. [1939] (1981) *Working-Class Wives: Their Health and Conditions*, London: Virago.

Stewart, M.L. (2001) *For Health and Beauty: Physical Culture for Frenchwomen, 1880s–1930s*, Baltimore and London: Johns Hopkins University Press.

Taylor, H.P. (1948) *A Shetland Parish Doctor*, Lerwick: T. & J. Manson.

Trombley, S. (1981) *All That Summer She Was Mad: Virginia Woolf and her Doctors*, London: Junction Books.

Unwin, C. and Sharland, E. (1992) 'From bodies to minds in childcare literature: advice to parents in inter-war Britain' in R. Cooter (ed.) *In the Name of the Child: Health and Welfare, 1880–1940*, London: Routledge, pp.174–99.

Webb, K.A. (1988) *'One of the most useful charities in the city': York Dispensary 1788–1988*, York: University of York.

Webster, C. (1983) 'The health of the school child during the Depression' in N. Parry and D. McNair (eds) *The Fitness of the Nation – Physical and Health Education in the Nineteenth and Twentieth Centuries: Proceedings of the 1982 Annual Conference of the History of Education Society of Great Britain*, Leicester: History of Education Society of Great Britain, pp.70–85.

Welshman, J. (1996) 'Physical education and the School Medical Service in England and Wales, 1907–1939', *Social History of Medicine*, vol.9, pp.31–48.

Wightman, C.F. (1912) *Home Nursing Manual: With Chapters on Personal Hygiene and Care of Infants*, London: George Gill.

Source Book readings

R. Roberts, *The Classic Slum: Salford Life in the First Quarter of the Century*, Manchester: Manchester University Press, 1971, pp.97–9 (Reading 13.1).

A. Digby, *The Evolution of British General Practice, 1850–1948*, Oxford: Oxford University Press, 1999, pp.318–22 (Reading 13.2).

B. Aronovitch, *Give It Time: An Experience of Hospital 1928–32*, London: André Deutsch, 1974, pp.38–43, 50–2, 55–6, 60, 62–7, 71–2, 74 (Reading 13.3).

L. Bryder, *Below the Magic Mountain: A Social History of Tuberculosis in Twentieth-Century Britain*, Oxford: Clarendon Press, 1988, pp.205–11 (Reading 13.4).

M. Spring Rice, *Working-Class Wives: Their Health and Conditions*, London: Virago, 1981, 1st edn 1939, pp.39–43 (Reading 13.5).

Glossary

aetiology   cause of disease.

alienist   term used originally in France (*aliéniste*) and commonly in the nineteenth century, derived from the French word *aliéné*, meaning lunatic. Now routinely used by historians of psychiatry in preference to more modern and anachronistic terms such as psychiatrist.

allopathy   the dominant system of western or scientific medicine, also referred to as 'regular' medicine to distinguish it from alternative systems of medical thought such as **homeopathy** or **herbalism**.

anaesthesia   loss of consciousness or sensation in part of the body as a result of the application of chemicals (called anaesthetics) which temporarily depress the function of nerves.

antisepsis   prevention of infection by means of killing micro-organisms with the use of chemicals or heat.

artificial selection   as practised in animal husbandry: the choice of which individuals to mate or prevent from mating in order to achieve desired characteristics in breed.

asepsis   techniques to prevent infection by excluding all micro-organisms. Any contact between **bacteria** and wounds are prevented by sterilizing all instruments and dressings that come into contact with the wound, and requiring that practitioners wear gowns and masks, thus creating a sterile environment around the patient.

asylumdom   a term coined by D.J. Mellett in his book *The Prerogative of Asylumdom* (New York: Garland, 1982) to denote the institutional, bureaucratic and legislative machinery, as well as the care ethos, associated with asylum-based responses to lunacy in Britain.

auscultation   the practice of listening to sounds within the body either by directly placing the ear to the surface of the body (immediate auscultation) or using a device, such as a stethoscope, to magnify the sounds (mediate auscultation).

autopsy   the examination and dissection of a body to determine the cause of death and identify changes caused by disease.

bacteria   living, single-celled organisms, some of which cause disease.

bacteriology   the study of the **bacteria** that cause disease, and the development of **vaccines** and **sera** used to prevent and treat them.

bilharzia   (or schistosomiasis) water-borne parasitic infection caused by the worms of the species *schistosoma*, in which snails are intermediate hosts.

biochemistry   the study of the chemical processes that take place in living organisms.

boarding-out lodging the insane outside asylums, normally within more domestic and often rural settings, more familiar to them than asylums, generally with guardians or relatives in single dwellings and cottages. A system that had its origins in family and parochial care, but that was systematized and overseen by central authorities in most countries from around the mid-nineteenth century. Also embracing the accommodation of the insane in lunatic colonies and cottages within, or close by, the asylum.

caste Hindu hereditary social group, similar to a social class; there was little social interaction between different castes.

cholera serious infectious disease, spread by water. It swept across Europe repeatedly in the nineteenth century, causing mass panic. Victims suffered severe vomiting and diarrhoea, and could die in a matter of hours.

clinico-pathology a medical methodology that combines detailed observation of the patient's symptoms during life with scrutiny of organic lesions revealed by **autopsy**.

East India Company the commercial enterprise that effectively ruled India until the **Indian Mutiny** in 1857.

enclavist policies that promoted the health of colonial administrators and soldiers, who lived in camps (or enclaves), at the expense of native peoples.

endemic disease that is present within a population at all times.

endocrinology the study of **hormones**.

epidemic disease that periodically appears in populations, sometimes causing large numbers of deaths.

eugenics term coined in 1883 by Francis Galton to refer to the science of heredity and breeding, it became a branch of human genetics concerned with improvement of national populations and/or races, through measures termed **positive eugenics** and **negative eugenics**. Since 1933, it has been commonly associated with Nazi racial policies.

hard inheritance transmission to offspring of only those characteristics with which their parents were born; an idea associated with Francis Galton and August Weismann.

herbalism complete therapeutic system based on the use of plant remedies, devised by Samuel Thomson in 1822.

histology the study of the microscopic structure of animals and plant tissues, and their function and formation.

historiography the process of writing history or the body of literature produced by historians. It is often used in discussions of how the understanding of events has changed over time. New interpretations can arise through the study of new sources, the application of a new approach to material or a reconsideration of well-known sources.

homeopathy a system of treatment using infinitesimal doses of drugs, designed to produce the symptoms of disease and thus stimulate the body's healing responses.

hormone chemical produced by a gland which acts as a messenger to stimulate or inhibit the function of another organ, and thus regulate physiological activity within the body.

hospitalism an infectious disease, or possibly diseases, of unknown cause associated with hospitals in the early nineteenth century, which caused wounds to become severely infected.

hydropathy also known as hydrotherapy; unorthodox system of medical treatment devised by Vincent Priessnitz in which patients took cold baths and showers, were wrapped in wet sheets and drank copious amounts of water. This was supposed to expel 'poisons' which caused all disease.

hypnotism also known as mesmerism or animal magnestism; a form of medical treatment originally developed by Anton Mesmer (1734–1815). Mesmer believed that all living beings had a subtle magnetic fluid that flowed through their bodies, and that this flow could become blocked, resulting in disease. To remove such blockages and alter the flow of fluids or energies, he used magnets or metal bars attached to buckets of 'magnetized' water, or channelled the magnetic influence from his body to that of another person which induced in them a hypnotic trance.

Indian Medical Service founded in the late eighteenth century to provide medical support to the **East India Company**. After 1858, its main role was to support the Indian Army.

Indian Mutiny also known as the Indian Uprising; revolt against the policies of the **East India Company** in 1857, which was suppressed after a year of fighting and led to the British government assuming direct control of the country through the government of India.

indigenes people, plants and animals native to a particular place.

irregular healers all those who offered some sort of medical treatment, despite having no formal training.

lazaret refuge or hospital for the isolation of the sick, especially for lepers.

leishmaniasis **protozoan** parasitic disease spread by sandflies that affects either the skin or the spleen and liver.

materia medica study of the actions and uses of drugs and medicines. Physicians learned this, not to make up their own drugs, but to be able to prescribe and to ensure that the apothecaries made up their prescriptions properly.

medical cosmology a phrase coined by N.D. Jewson to describe his all-encompassing view of medicine, covering theory, practice, practitioners and patients, and the relationships between them.

medical police wide range of policies adopted in the late eighteeth and early nineteenth centuries to protect the health of the people. These included the provision of hospitals, street cleaning, control of medical practice and regulations on marriage.

mercantilism also known as cameralism; political doctrine that related the strength of nations to the size of their populations. A large population was seen as a means to a healthy economy (with many workers and consumers) and a strong state (as a large population would supply many recruits to the armed services). Mercantilist doctrines were used to legitimate the provision of basic health care and disease control measures in northern Europe in the eighteenth century.

metabolism the physical and chemical changes necessary for life: the uptake of food, its digestion and the excretion of waste products. All cells have an individual metabolism and large organisms have a 'total metabolism'.

miasma 'bad air' arising from decomposing organic matter; miasmas were believed to cause diseases such as cholera and typhus.

morbidity rate the number of people in a population who have a particular disease or are sick, usually measured as cases per thousand.

mortality rate the number of people dying in a population, usually measured as deaths per thousand.

natural selection as taught by Charles Darwin, preservation by means of a struggle for existence of characteristics that adapt organisms to survive in their environments and thus leave more offspring.

negative eugenics measures to reduce the fertility of undesirable social groups, including birth control, segregation, sterilization and euthanasia.

organic analogy especially in Germany, doctrine that the body-politic is like the human body, an organism greater than the sum of its parts, which may become diseased and degenerate, and whose health depends on the quality and proper functioning of its components.

pathogen any virus, micro-organism or substance that causes disease.

pathogenic the changes caused by disease.

pathology the study of disease, especially of the physical changes to the anatomy of the body as a result of disease.

pauper the formal status of being a pauper involved losing certain rights, such as the right to vote (although poor people were in any case unlikely to qualify for the franchise). The term 'pauperization' is also used to describe the process by which the poor became dependent on welfare and unable to survive without it.

pharmacology the study of drugs, including their chemical structure and their effect on the body.

physiology the study of the functioning of the body during life.

policlinic   medical clinic, usually independent of a hospital, that offers a variety of treatments to outpatients.

Poor Law hospital   hospital funded by local rates as part of a welfare system in England and Wales (and, under separate laws, in Scotland).

positive eugenics   measures to increase the fertility of desirable social groups, including child benefits, education grants and tax incentives.

primary care   treatment by general practitioners, in the twentieth century this was usually freely accessible to all persons through the state or health insurance.

protozoa   single-cell organisms.

puériculture   especially in France, ensemble of **positive eugenic** methods for producing healthy children through the cultivation of personal hygiene and domestic environments; associated with **soft inheritance**.

racial hygiene   improvement of the biological qualities and health of a population by means of **positive** and **negative eugenics**; associated with **hard inheritance**.

Rassenhygiene   especially in Germany, study of 'the conditions of preserving and developing a race' (Alfred Ploetz, 1896); from the First World War, extreme nationalist programme to purify the superior Aryan race of degenerate and Semitic elements, notably through mass extermination; associated with **hard inheritance**.

reductionist   the view that there is no fundamental difference between the processes that occur in living bodies and those that are found in the inorganic world.

relapsing fever   infectious disease, characterized by recurrent fever and carried by lice and ticks.

sanatorium   plural sanatoria; hospital dedicated to the cure of invalids, convalescents and the chronically sick, but associated particularly with tuberculosis.

seasoning   acclimatization to a new environment.

secondary care   more specialized treatment, often in some type of hospital.

separate spheres   the idea that men and women had separate roles in life – women in the private realm of the home, raising children, and men in the public world of work.

serum   plural sera; preparation made from the blood of infected animals that contains immunoglobulins, and attacks invading micro-organisms.

Social Darwinism   the application of Darwinian evolutionary biological concepts – especially 'the survival of the fittest' – to races and societies, often in a crude and distorted form. Popularized in Britain by the philosopher Herbert Spencer (1820–1903) in the 1850s as a means of achieving 'social progress'.

social medicine   also called social hygiene; a wide range of policies aimed at improving health through better diet, hygiene, health education and the provision of new medical services. These policies were popular in Europe in the early twentieth century.

soft inheritance   transmission to offspring of characteristics acquired by their parents during their lifetimes; associated with Jean-Baptiste Lamarck.

subscription   a regular (usually annual) charitable donation to a hospital, dispensary or asylum that gave a donor the right to recommend patients for care at the institution.

trench fever   epidemic disease, characterized by recurrent fever, carried by lice, and common among soldiers in the First World War.

unorthodox practitioners   practitioners of unorthodox medical systems such as **herbalism**, **homeopathy** or **hydropathy**. These included people who were entirely self-taught, *and* practitioners who had received a formal medical training, but chose to offer unorthodox forms of therapy.

vaccination   technique of infecting a person with cowpox – a mild disease – in order to induce immunity to smallpox. Although the original **vaccine** was produced from cows, infants were later vaccinated using the fluid which appeared in the vaccination lesion of a previously vaccinated child.

vaccine   preparation of weakened or killed **bacteria** that provokes an immune response and thus protects against future attacks of disease.

VAD   Voluntary Aid Detachment nurse; volunteer nurse who served during the First World War. VADs had limited training.

voluntary hospital   hospital maintained by charitable donations, or **subscriptions**, rather than by government support.

wise-women   women known in their community for their expertise in attending births, nursing the sick and laying out the dead.

Index

Ackerknecht, Erwin 3, 190, 194, 204
    'An early account of public health
        history' 181–2
Africa 223–36
    health of Europeans in 223–6
    mental illness in 235–6
    missionary medicine in 232–4
    and tropical medicine 226–31,
      233
        sleeping sickness 227, 230–1
    western and indigenous medicine
      234
AIDS 92, 358
air pollution 199
alienists 315
    low status of 321–2
    as 'moral entrepreneurs' 316–17,
      319–21
    and the redefinition of madness
      311–14
Allbutt, Sir Thomas Clifford 341
allopathic medicine 28, 135
alternative medicine 28, 120
    irregular and unorthodox healers
      xviii, 119, 135–8
Amalgamating Savages, Maoris as 215,
  216, 217
American Civil War 335, 349
amputations 61
    and anaesthesia 76, 79
    and antisepsis 80, 82
    and general practitioners in rural
      areas 378
    speed in performing 75
    in wartime 333, 344, 355
anaemia, diagnosis of 111
anaesthesia xiii, 47, 74, 75–80, 84, 85,
  86
    and childbirth 378, 392
    chloroform 76
    ether 75–6
        and mesmeric anaesthesia
          137–8
    and experimental procedures
      79–80
    and power relations in medical
      practice 76, 78–9
    satirical cartoons on 76–8
    side-effects of 56, 76
anatomy 100
    pathological anatomy 3, 10–11,
      15–16, 68–71
        and resective surgery 70–1

animal experimentation 27, 102
antenatal clinics 392
anthrax 102, 112
anthropogenetics 280
antibiotics, and tropical diseases 228
antisepsis xiii, 47, 80–4, 85, 86
apothecaries 119, 121, 122
    in hospitals 34
    and physicians 63
Arnold, David 221
    'Health, race and nation' 222–3
Aronovitch, Bella, 'Care in hospital'
  387, 388
Aryan language, and Nazi eugenics
  286
aseptic techniques 47
asylumdom 298, 325
asylums in Britain xii, xiii, xv, xvi,
  298–326
    and the community 315–16
    domestication of 314–16, 327
    eighteenth-century 299–300
    English Metropolitan
      Commissioners in Lunacy 301
    Essex County Lunatic Asylum,
      Brentwood 315
    and eugenics 271
    and the 'great confinement' 300
    Hanwell Asylum 316
    industrialization, urbanization
      and the growth of 305–9, 326
    Lancaster County Asylum 309–10
    Lincoln Asylum 316
    medical factors in the growth of
      311–24
    and moral therapy/management
      306, 313, 314, 316–21, 327
    nineteenth-century increase in
      numbers 298, 302, 327
        contemporary views on
          302–3
    and nineteenth-century lunacy
      legislation 300–1, 302, 313
    panopticon structures 317, 318
    pauper lunatics in 303, 324–5
    public attitudes to 316
    size of 298
    social control and the family
      309–11, 326
    use of 'shock' treatment in 319–21
    West Riding Lunatic Asylum 312
    York Retreat 305, 306, 314, 316,
      317
    see also mental illness; Scottish
      asylums
Auenbrugger, Leopold 13

auscultation 14, 17
Australia, colonial medicine in 212,
  214
Austria, public health practices 259
Austria-Hungary
    birth rates 241
    and the First World War 336
    sanitary reform 245
autopsies
    in the First World War 351
    and hospital medicine 3, 4, 19, 28,
      92
        Paris hospitals 12, 17
    and laboratory medicine 24, 25,
      105

babies *see* maternal and child welfare
bacteriology 26, 27, 102, 104, 115
    and diagnosis 110
    and the First World War 349
    mobile bacteriological laboratory
      97
    and public health practices 239,
      241–7
    and surgery 83
    and typhus 257–9
    and vaccine therapy 112–14
Baldwin, Peter 194, 195
Banting, Fred 114
barbers/barber-surgeons 61, 64, 65–7
Barger, George 98
Bartlett, Peter 325
Bayle, Gaspard-Laurent 13
Bayliss, William 101
bedside medicine 1, 2, 3, 18, 20–1, 28–9
Beecham, Thomas 377
Behring, Emil 114, 244
Belgian Congo, epidemic of sleeping
  sickness 230–1
Belgium
    boarding-out of lunatics 325–6
    and the First World War 336
    licensing of medical practitioners
      122
    medical education 121, 122, 128
    medical journals 127
    medical societies 128, 130
    social medicine in 254
Bell, Benjamin 75
Bennett, John Hughes 24–6
Bergmann, Ernst von 83
    painting of (1890) 87
Berlin
    Institute for Infectious
      Diseases 93